SEPARATE BEDS

A History of Indian Hospitals in Canada, 1920s–1980s

Separate Beds is the shocking story of Canada's system of segregated health care. Operated by the same bureaucracy that was expanding health care opportunities for most Canadians, the "Indian Hospitals" were underfunded, understaffed, overcrowded, and rife with coercion and medical experimentation. Established to keep the Aboriginal tuberculosis population isolated, they became a means of ensuring that other Canadians need not share access to modern hospitals with Aboriginal patients.

Tracing the history of the system from its fragmentary origins to its gradual collapse, Maureen K. Lux describes the arbitrary and contradictory policies that governed the "Indian Hospitals," the experiences of patients and staff, and the vital grass-roots activism that pressed the federal government to acknowledge its treaty obligations.

A disturbing look at the dark side of the liberal welfare state, *Separate Beds* reveals a history of racism and negligence in health care for Canada's First Nations that should never be forgotten.

MAUREEN K. LUX is an associate professor in the Department of History at Brock University.

Separate Beds

A History of Indian Hospitals in Canada, 1920s–1980s

MAUREEN K. LUX

UNIVERSITY OF TORONTO PRESS
Toronto Buffalo London

Toronto Buffalo London
www.utppublishing.com
Printed in the U.S.A.

ISBN 978-1-4426-4557-8 (cloth)
ISBN 978-1-4426-1386-7 (paper)

♾ Printed on acid-free, 100% post-consumer recycled paper

Library and Archives Canada Cataloguing in Publication

Lux, Maureen K. (Maureen Katherine), 1956–, author
Separate beds : a history of Indian hospitals in Canada, 1920s–1980s
Maureen K. Lux.

Includes bibliographical references and index.
ISBN 978-1-4426-4557-8 (bound). – ISBN 978-1-4426-1386-7 (paperback)

1. Native peoples – Hospitals – Canada – History – 20th century. 2. Native peoples – Hospital care – Canada – History – 20th century. 3. Native peoples – Health and hygiene – Canada – History – 20th century. 4. Discrimination in medical care – Canada – History – 20th century. 5. Medical policy – Canada – History – 20th century. I. Title.

RA450.4.I53L89 2016 362.1089'97071 C2015-907180-1

This book has been published with the help of a grant from the Federation for the Humanities and Social Sciences, through the Awards to Scholarly Publications Program, using funds provided by the Social Sciences and Humanities Research Council of Canada.

University of Toronto Press acknowledges the financial assistance to its publishing program of the Canada Council for the Arts and the Ontario Arts Council, an agency of the Government of Ontario.

Canada Council for the Arts Conseil des Arts du Canada

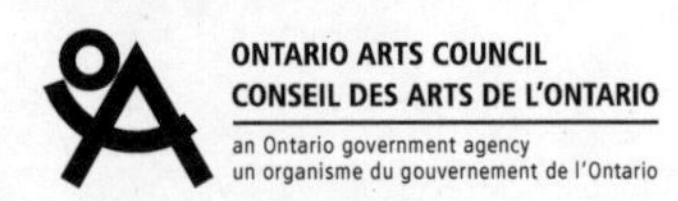

Funded by the Government of Canada Financé par le gouvernement du Canada

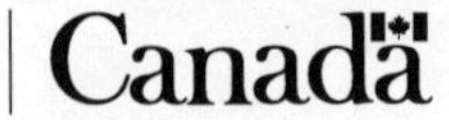

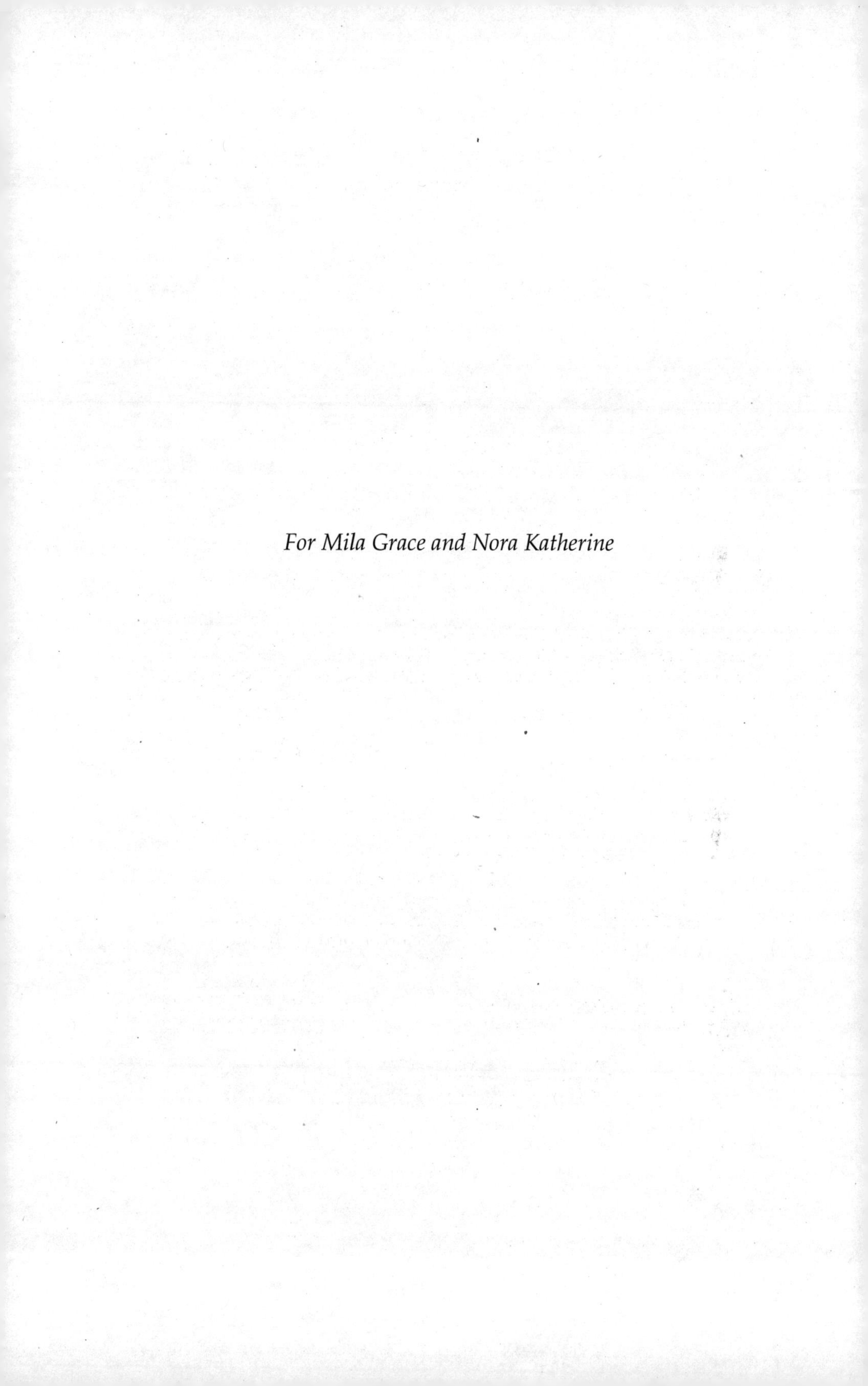

For Mila Grace and Nora Katherine

Contents

Illustrations

Acknowledgments

As I write, Canada's historic Truth and Reconciliation Commission is presenting its final report documenting the dark history and the damaging legacy of residential schools. *Honouring the Truth, Reconciling for the Future* demands that all Canadians not only acknowledge that our privilege came at a terrible cost, but that we might also listen and learn how to build a respectful future. I hope that in a small measure this work heeds the Commission's call that we learn from the past to build that future.

Many people aided my research, though all errors and omissions are mine. At the Stó:lō Research and Resource Management Centre, Tia Halsted took the time to walk me through the history and the grounds of the former Coqualeetza Indian Hospital. Janice Kennedy at the Battlefords Tribal Council Indian Health Services provided invaluable insight into the past, present, and future importance of community-directed health services. Gail Boehme took time from her Director's role to explain how the All Nations Healing Hospital came to replace the Fort Qu'Appelle Indian Hospital. Carol Greyeyes introduced me to Matthew Joseph, who spent a day teaching me the "people's history" of Fort Qu'Appelle. Kathy Kinew at the Assembly of Manitoba Chiefs helped ease access to archival records. I would also like to thank Siksika Chief Fred Rabbit Carrier and Councillor Kendall Panther Bone for their guidance and advice. These busy people patiently fielded my requests for help; without their encouragement and support this research would not have been possible. Thank you all. Most importantly, they also introduced me to their communities' most valued Elders.

I had the honour to meet and learn from Elders Agnes Cyr at Fort Qu'Appelle and Hazel McArthur at Stoughton, who experienced the hospitals in different ways. They are both gone now. Frank Malloway Sr invited me into his home and shared his history at Sardis, BC. Over lunch and tea in Winnipeg, Grace Anderson taught me about work in an Indian hospital; her daughter Renata Meconse took the time to chauffeur me around. At Siksika, Dave Melting Tallow graciously shared his most painful experiences with a stranger. I hope that I have told their stories with the honour and respect with which they were given. Finally, I would like to thank Linda and Roy Little Chief. Roy never let me forget why this history needs to be told.

I could not have asked for a more supportive and collegial group of scholars than Brock's history department, especially Renée Lafferty-Salhany, Carmela Patrias, John Sainsbury, Danny Samson, Dave Schimmelpenninck, and Liz Vlossak. History of medicine colleagues Erika Dyck, Geoff Hudson, and Peter Twohig have helped more than they know. I had the benefit of able and cheerful research assistants Charity Blaine, Austin Brooks, Steven Lee, and Leslie Wiebe. I would particularly like to thank Alma Favel-King, who lived the struggle over the North Battleford Indian Hospital. I also thank Julie Grahame of the Yousuf Karsh estate for permission to reproduce Mr Karsh's compelling portraits.

A Canadian Institutes of Health Research/Associated Medical Services operating grant supported my research. Some of the material in Chapter One appeared as "Care for the 'Racially Careless': Indian Hospitals in the Canadian West, 1920–1950s," *Canadian Historical Review* 91, no. 3 (2010); sections of Chapter Five appeared as "We Demand 'Unconditional Surrender': Making and Unmaking the Blackfoot Hospital, 1890s to 1950s," *Social History of Medicine* 25, no. 3 (2011).

Finally, I thank my family for the constant love and support that sustains me; the babies carry the hope for our brighter future so it is to them that I dedicate this book.

St Catharines
December 2015

SEPARATE BEDS

A History of Indian Hospitals in Canada, 1920s–1980s

Introduction

On a cool August morning in 1946, war hero and Canadian governor general, Field Marshall Viscount Alexander of Tunis, with a wave of his hand, officially declared Edmonton's sprawling Charles Camsell Indian Hospital open. Among the guests were the hospital's namesake, Charles Camsell (recently retired deputy minister of mines and resources), Indian Affairs bureaucrats, Catholic clergy from the Edmonton Residential School, medical staff, and "several Indians." The local press reported that Lady Alexander alone toured the wards (while her husband waited outside), where "many dark heads" had "prettied up" to greet the viscountess.[1] On the children's ward eight-year-old patient Doreen Callihoo from nearby Villeneuve, Alberta, presented her with a bouquet of roses.[2] High drama intended to demonstrate the gift of modern medicine, the opening ceremony also alerted Canadians to the arrival of a progressive and benevolent state actively guarding the national health. The Indian Health Service (IHS), once the poor stepchild of Indian Affairs, came under the expert management of the newly created department of National Health and Welfare. The Edmonton institution, not the first "Indian hospital" to be opened (though the largest, with up to 500 beds), was part of an aggressive postwar expansion that by 1960 included twenty-two institutions with more than 2,200 beds for the treatment of Aboriginal people (First Nations and Inuit).[3]

Much in that opening ceremony informs this study of Indian hospitals in Canada. It signalled the state's changing relationship with Aboriginal people in the latter half of the twentieth century. The rise of expert and objective medical authority supplanted often-meddlesome Christian missionaries, and redefined what was commonly referred to as the "Indian problem," or the anxieties Canadians experienced by

Aboriginal people's continued legal and cultural differences. The long-standing policy of assimilation, or "integration to citizenship" as it came to be known, would be pursued by other means. Moreover, with both growing population and presence in towns and cities, Aboriginal people came under greater scrutiny for their perceived threats to the nation's hygiene and morality. Indian hospitals not only promised to contain disease, but also assured concerned Canadians that theirs was a humanitarian government that extended the benefits of modern health care and a "fair deal" to the long neglected. At a time when Canada was consciously defining and investing in the "national health" that would culminate in Medicare, racially segregated institutions reassured citizens that their access to modern hospitals need not be shared with Aboriginal patients. Doreen Callihoo represented the people's gratitude – docile, infantile, and muted – effectively obscuring other meanings of Indian hospitals.

Indian hospitals represented a very different promise to the "several Indians" and "many dark heads" at the opening ceremony. The impact of the colonizing practices of the state and settler society – repressive legislation and economic dispossession – had plunged First Nations communities into hunger and disease.[4] Neglect and parsimony characterized the government's response, though rudimentary care, particularly vaccination, attempted to limit the spread of disease from reserve to town. Epidemic disease often prompted intense medical attention that, together with the police, confined and quarantined, only to leave when the immediate threat abated. Though never consulted, many First Nations leaders who had long sought relief from the burdens of illness and the socio-economic conditions of its rise, welcomed Indian hospitals, particularly those established near reserves. While communities recognized and attempted to ameliorate the underfunded hospitals' many shortcomings – the coercion, the overcrowding, and the high-handed, paternalistic management – the qualifier "Indian" came to define them as community institutions. First Nations hospital employees who performed the poorly paid domestic chores, also provided comfort and advocated for children and elders in their own language. Their presence as cultural brokers and interpreters for patients blunted the hospitals' colonizing impulses, reminding us to look beyond acts of resistance as the sole manifestation of subordinate power.[5]

Scholars of colonial medicine have drawn attention to the inadequacies of a simple binary of colonizer and colonized to explain a complex relationship. Certainly in Canada the rhetoric situated Western medicine as evidence of the colonizer's superiority, most often in order to disparage or repress competing systems of indigenous healing. As historian Waltraud Ernst argues, our understanding of the other social dimensions of medicine are lost in an approach that "conceives of medicine as determined mainly by the agenda of colonialism." The putatively colonized may well use Western medicine and its institutions in ways and for reasons never intended by the colonizer. Ernst continues: "There is more to medicine within a colonial setting than the discourse of colonialism."[6] Many communities saw nothing necessarily incompatible in incorporating Western biomedicine into their indigenous healing practices. Indeed, medical plurality is the norm in much of the world. With its single biomedical system that points to organized medicine's influence – and its insecurities – in marking out its ground to the exclusion of all others, Canada is an anomaly. Nevertheless, indigenous healers and midwives survived the formal and informal efforts to suppress their work in the nineteenth and twentieth centuries, though much was lost.

As systems of knowledge (including scientific biomedicine), all medical traditions emerge from rational cultural understandings of the place of humans in the environment. Consequently, there are many Aboriginal healing complexes that reflect the diversity of indigenous cultures in Canada. At the risk of oversimplification, one can say they share a world view that positions humans as but one part of the Great Circle of Life that includes the spirits of both the animate and the inanimate; there are few distinctions between the natural and supernatural, between medicine and spirituality. Healers, those best able to communicate with the spirit world, view illness as a loss of balance between mind, body, and spirit. Their cures vary from herbal treatments for commonplace ailments to community-wide spiritual rites of healing and regeneration such as the Sun Dance and the Potlatch. The Midewiwin that originated among the Anishinaabe (Ojibwa) in the early nineteenth century in western Ontario and subsequently spread west and south to neighbouring groups, is a hierarchical medicine society that teaches healing and the maintenance of spiritual and social harmony.[7] Midwives, too, continued their practice; for example, in the early years of settlement on the prairies they often shared their skill and expert knowledge of botanicals with struggling settler families.[8]

Under the changing circumstances of colonialism Christian missionaries worked with Indian Affairs officials and police to undermine healers and ban their practices. Furthermore, restrictions on people's movement off reserve limited access to healing medicine, while intensive cultivation and agricultural settlement destroyed medicinal plants. Moreover, indigenous healers acknowledged that some of the sicknesses brought by newcomers might best be treated by settler medicine. At the three on-reserve hospitals established in the 1920s – southern Alberta's Blood and Blackfoot Hospitals, and the Six Nations' Lady Willingdon Hospital (the latter two institutions originally owned by the First Nations) – communities developed a medical pluralism or syncretism that assimilated biomedicine into their healing practices. However, for others such as the Inuit, who were relocated to southern institutions for years at a time, the emotional and cultural impact on patients and families was especially devastating. Clearly, the meanings of Indian hospitals differed widely among Aboriginal peoples, but the proximity of elders and community created some social and cultural space to integrate Indian hospitals into indigenous notions of good health. Indeed, by the 1990s, as communities regained some limited autonomy in health care, Aboriginal medicine would emerge from the secrecy imposed by state assimilationist policies that sought to undermine cultures and the languages that bore it.

First Nations communities also interpreted the IHS hospitals as the state's concrete, if belated, recognition of its legal and treaty responsibility for health care.[9] Signatories to the eleven so-called Numbered Treaties in the west and north understood medicines and health care to be included in the treaties' terms. Medicine and medical care were discussed during many of the treaty negotiations, although the promises invariably failed to appear in the written text. The sole exception was Treaty Six (1876), whose text promised a "medicine chest." Vaccinations and other medical care at annual meetings where treaty annuities were paid confirmed the clear link of health care to the treaty relationship. The federal government certainly anticipated this interpretation of Indian hospitals. In his 1946 announcement of an expanded IHS, the minister of national health acknowledged the existence of the "medicine chest clause" in Treaty Six. But he promptly denied it in his next sentence. His explanation at the time, which remained policy, was that IHS was motivated by "humanitarian reasons and as very necessary protection to the rest of the population of Canada."[10] The understanding of Indian hospitals as fulfilling a treaty right, held by many treaty people (and a wide swath of the Canadian public), would be most vigorously contested in the 1960s as IHS attempted to offload its responsibilities to provinces. That understanding remains contested. By rejecting a treaty right to health care, the state claimed instead to be pursuing a humanitarian policy (leaving it free to make frequent changes) that also characterized Aboriginal people as the objects of charity. Moreover, the minister's statement alerted Canadians to the dangers to their health and welfare that lurked in Aboriginal communities.

Indian hospitals reflected the changing role of health care in an emerging welfare state, but they were also firmly rooted in persistent, century-long government policies that, regardless of political stripe, sought to protect, civilize, and assimilate Aboriginal people.[11] Such a remarkably consistent policy stemmed from the notion that Aboriginal people could not be considered true individuals in the classical liberal model that was hegemonic in Canada by the twentieth century.[12] The liberal view of the individual as one whose body and mind were theirs alone stood in sharp contrast to Aboriginal world views that saw human beings as but one part of the larger circle of life. Theirs was a universe where individual wellness required community support and collective rites for its restoration and where the value of goods was realized in their redistribution. The Aboriginal legal status as wards of the state presumed the absence of rational citizenship and the inability to acquire it without fundamental social, cultural, and political change. As theorist Uday S. Mehta argues, at liberalism's core rests the "thicker set of social credentials that constitute the real bases" of citizenship.[13] The social credentials – race, ethnicity, gender, and class – defined the individual and marked those to be excluded, above all Aboriginal people.[14] Critical race scholar David Goldenberg draws attention to the "liberal paradox" where states, as they commit themselves to the principles of liberty and equality, construct a "multiplication of racial identities and the sets of exclusions they prompt and rationalize, enable and sustain."[15] Indeed, as Adele Perry notes, in Canada the liberal order and the nation that defined it "would find its own unique ways of rendering some people outsiders and, in the process, making itself."[16] Canada's liberalism, simultaneously "a utopian project of individual liberation *and* one of colonialism and subordination," cultivated its core of normal healthy white citizenship by marginalizing and excluding Aboriginal bodies.[17] This "liberal order" of governance attempted to subordinate and contain Aboriginal conceptions of the world and society; beginning in the 1880s schooling would accomplish this goal.

Historian Ian McKay calls residential schools "Christian/liberal manufactories of individuals, pre-eminent laboratories of liberalism" where Aboriginal children were "forced to be free, in the very particular liberal sense of 'free,' even at the cost of their lives."[18] Christian churches owned and managed the schools while government subsidized missionary zeal on a per diem basis rather than face the unpredictable and ongoing costs of managing the institutions. But subsidies based on student enrolment to cover all institutional costs – food, clothing, wages, and building maintenance – prompted churches to maximize revenues by enrolling more students and feeding them less. Children spent less time in the classroom and more time toiling in the laundry, the kitchen, the fields, and the barns to maintain the institutions. This approach was rationalized as a practical education and useful training for life on the reserve. Early deaths at the schools or shortly after discharge were all too frequent. Far removed from reserves and the influence of concerned parents, residential schools significantly damaged the health of their charges, who often brought disease back to the reserve.[19] As early as 1907 Dr Peter Bryce, the chief medical officer for the Department of Indian Affairs (DIA), reported on the appalling condition of children in residential schools and found an "intimate relationship between the health of the pupils while in the schools and that of their early death subsequent to discharge."[20] Bryce's report was widely distributed and caused considerable public criticism of the DIA, though little change. Two years later Bryce advocated that a number of schools be converted into sanatoria in recognition of the extent of illness in the schools.[21] Some limited measures were undertaken in subsequent years to guard schoolchildren's health, such as isolation rooms for infectious disease and increased per capita grants to the institutions. Nevertheless, as historian Brian Titley notes, the DIA was often more concerned with controlling its image than with improving the children's health.[22] The surviving "ex-pupils" and their families were effectively isolated on reserves. The contradictions inherent in the project to assimilate through isolation would be recalibrated in the formation of the welfare state, with similarly damaging results.

Foucault's famous "carceral archipelago" made scholars aware of the continuities among institutions of isolation where experts attend to those requiring reform or cure.[23] This "collusion of knowledge and power" created institutions that "consolidated administrative authority, bureaucratic regulation" and colonial control.[24] In the broader colonial project of racial exclusion and segregation, Western medicine, far from benign and apolitical, occupies what David Arnold calls a central place in the "ideological as well as the technological processes" of colonial rule.[25] With the rise of the welfare state, where governing agencies assumed increasing responsibility for aspects of life previously the remit of families or charities, isolation was, as Carolyn Strange and Alison Bashford argue, not a departure from liberal governance "but central to its internal logic." Public funds flowed into projects that, under the guidance of experts in human sciences and medicine, sought to normalize the behaviour of those who could not be trusted with the freedoms that healthy citizens enjoyed.[26] In what Robert Menzies and Ted Palys call the "gravitational forces" exerted by the state, medicine, and society to confine and isolate Aboriginal people, the Indian hospitals have much in common with the asylum, the school, the reserve, and the penitentiary.[27]

The meanings of Indian hospitals are also found in an increasingly shrill medical and bureaucratic discourse about the threat of rampant "Indian tuberculosis."[28] By the 1930s, reserves, the prime sites of segregation and colonization, seemed no longer adequate to contain disease. As historian Mary-Ellen Kelm notes, North American medical literature that pathologized the "discursive Indian" shifted its focus in the 1930s. From the deleterious impact of settlement and civilization (and the inadequate response of Aboriginal bodies) that led to notions of the "dying race," medical discourse increasingly concentrated on the threat that Aboriginal contagion posed to society.[29] Dr David Stewart, superintendent of Manitoba's Ninette sanatorium, advised that reserves were not "disease-tight compartments." Tuberculosis, he warned, "leaked" into ordinary communities through berries and handicrafts peddled by Aboriginal people. More alarming, the "racial carelessness and ignorance" of First Nations "soaked with tuberculosis" were spreading as Aboriginal populations were actually growing and "mingling with the general population," despite grave predictions of their imminent demise.[30] What historian Warwick Anderson calls the image of "disease-dealers" emerged to occupy physicians and bureaucrats alike.[31] Despite steadily declining tuberculosis rates in Canada generally, the healthy and clean were now vulnerable to the threat of "Indian" tuberculosis, which only fuelled the rhetoric. Though the disease's retreat began in the 1890s, well before any medical interventions, sanatorium directors like Stewart, represented by the Canadian Tuberculosis Association (CTA), naturally took full credit.[32] As medical experts whose social and political authority rose as tuberculosis rates fell, the CTA (which also included provincial health bureaucrats) urged the federal government to take responsibility for its wards. In a bold use of state power, by 1945 the CTA effectively designed the system of federally owned and operated Indian hospitals. Initially rationalized as tuberculosis sanatoria,

Indian hospitals in fact admitted patients suffering from all conditions based on race, not disease. The institutions not only isolated the alarming public peril of tuberculosis but also ensured that the CTA's member institutions would continue to be reserved for white patients. To paraphrase Foucault, an ascendant bureaucracy with its focus on Indian hospitals represented an effort not to isolate less, but to isolate better.[33]

Race, Class, and the Sanatorium Cure

Sanatoria – enduring institutions that adapted to the changing understandings of the disease, from "consumption" to tuberculosis – were established in Canada in the late nineteenth and early twentieth centuries. Fashioned after European spas with chalet-style architecture in bucolic settings far removed from the city's dank air and crowds, they offered "open air" treatment, bed rest, and nourishing food. Prominent citizens and volunteer groups ("anti-tuberculosis leagues") established most provincial sanatoria before the First World War, but the institutions soon came to rely on public funds. As the most popular, indeed the only, approach to the disease, sanatorium treatment required extended stays that focused on improvement and regulation of the self, where the "soul of the citizen" came under scrutiny.[34] A physician and former patient at the first Canadian sanatorium, in Muskoka in central Ontario at the turn of the century, G.D. Stanley recalled (fifty-three years later) that the "cure" consisted of fresh air, six daily feedings of milk and raw eggs, and, for him, exercise. Patients were expected to help each other: "The intimate association of one man with the others around him in entertaining one another, in extending help to one another … all combined to create a fellowship that was indispensable … and one of the outstanding treasures of my life."[35] His recollections evoke the picture of young, homosocial health and vitality, not disease. Stanley no doubt suffered from "incipient consumption" at a time when it was possible to feel "a little bit consumptive."[36] As treatment at Muskoka made clear, however, only the white upper classes suffered from the disease that could be cured at such institutions. By the 1920s, interventions that artificially collapsed the diseased lung, to induce it to "rest," augmented but did not supplant the focus on improving citizens. The director of Saskatchewan's Fort Qu'Appelle Sanatorium explained that the cure was not medicine or surgery but "an idea: a way of life … the development of faithful endeavour, helpfulness, earnestness, good humour, kindliness and forbearance."[37]

As wards of the state deemed insufficiently advanced to benefit from training in rational citizenship, Aboriginal people were not generally accepted for treatment in provincial sanatoria. Neither Tranquille Sanatorium in Kamloops, British Columbia, nor Ninette Sanatorium in Manitoba admitted Aboriginal patients, and the Central Alberta Sanatorium only accepted them "when space was available."[38] Saskatchewan, with three public sanatoria by 1930 and more than 700 beds, made segregated space for them in the northern Prince Albert Sanatorium, while in the south the Saskatoon and Fort Qu'Appelle sanatoria reserved their beds for "taxpayers," though for a time the latter maintained a forty-bed "Indian wing" in order to repay debts to the federal government. Deserving patients, those judged by Indian agents as worthy of care and advanced enough to benefit from treatment, might be admitted, but only on the authority of the director of Indian Affairs in Ottawa. Social, not necessarily medical, criteria determined who might receive care: young residential school students whose families demonstrated progress along the path to assimilation.

Historians continue to debate the role of sanatorium treatment in the decline of tuberculosis.[39] Most agree that isolation of the ill may have protected the larger community from infection. However, sanatorium directors preferred to admit those whose disease was not too far advanced, those who stood a chance of recovery, leaving the most ill, or what were called the "hopeless cases," in the community. Historian F.B. Smith argues that the emphasis on sanatorium treatment, likely the least efficient use of public funds, served to enhance the medical reputation of sanatorium directors.[40]

A resilient institution that successfully incorporated changing understandings of tuberculosis, from open-air treatment to chest surgery to chemotherapy, the sanatorium has been studied as a site of exclusion and isolation. Confinement created healthy, self-governing citizens who, as Alison Bashford argues, were "released back into the community, as part of this new cultivation of the hygienic self."[41] The disciplinary function of the sanatorium emerged more clearly as tuberculosis became associated with the working classes and the poor. Reflecting nostalgically on his days as medical superintendent of Manitoba's Ninette Sanatorium, Dr A.L. Paine believed the pre–drug therapy regime created patients with "moral strength, courage and perseverance in fighting their disease." Through their struggle, patients became "more mature, better adjusted and educated, and with a higher potential for giving and receiving than ever before."[42] But as one expert admitted, "one can marvel at how many recovered, though, in the final analysis, failures outweighed successes."[43] Armed with these attributes of safe and healthy citizenship, the cured – or at least the improved – citizen could leave the institution as a self-governing individual knowing they no longer posed a risk to their families or community.

Antimicrobials developed in the late 1940s made tuberculosis much more manageable, but institutional treatment remained necessary for those who could not be trusted to follow the long course of chemotherapy. As Dr Wherrett, executive secretary of the CTA advised in a Department of Labour radio series *Canada at Work*, the sanatorium experience not only restored health, but also improved workers. "Rest is still the basic core of treatment," he advised, "but its effects are fortified and augmented by new drugs and daring surgery." Wherrett recommended state support for the rational (male) citizen to relieve anxieties about his dependents while taking the cure; mortgage payments and life insurance premiums should be paid by the province to "preserve these props to family security."[44] Confinement in the sanatorium preserved classed and gendered notions of the healthy family and society: "It's a smart secretary too who sees that she doesn't lose her shorthand or let her typing slip. Should she happen to be weak on spelling she can use the months in hospital to become a better speller – a joy to any boss." While science provided "miraculous tools" to fight tuberculosis "from us it has a right to expect the knowledge and understanding which will hasten mankind's victory over tuberculosis."[45] The medical discourse of improvement through confinement is obvious, and clearly directed at those who either through ignorance or social standing had not yet acquired the ability to be rational, healthy citizens. As antimicrobial treatment made the sanatorium cure increasingly obsolete, sanatorium directors and the IHS again collaborated, filling their wards with Aboriginal, particularly Inuit, patients.

In Indian hospitals the treatment for tuberculosis was not aimed at the soul as much as at the chest. The expansion of IHS institutions coincided with the increased use of what Wherrett termed "daring surgery." Aboriginal people – seen as incapable of healthy citizenship, that is, unable to return to their presumed inadequate reserve homes without infecting others, or "reactivating" their tuberculosis – spent long years in hospital. Surgeons removed ribs, collapsed lungs, and, emboldened by effective antibiotics, surgically removed the last foci of infection in Aboriginal bodies. Indian hospitals, particularly Charles Camsell Indian Hospital with its close association with the University of Alberta medical school, provided "interesting clinical material" for teaching and research. As Jordan Goodman, Anthony McElligott, and Lara Marks argue, the concept of "usefulness" brings together medical experimentation, knowledge, and the state where otherwise "use*less* bodies were rendered use*ful* by being made use*able*."[46] Eight-year-old Doreen Callihoo, after presenting roses to Lady Alexander in 1946, would spend eleven of the next twelve years in the Charles Camsell Indian Hospital. She recalled that as a child she received streptomycin injections and twice-weekly painful pneumothorax treatments (air injected into the chest to collapse the lung). As an adolescent, she had two separate thoracoplasties (removal of several ribs at a time to collapse the lung), disfiguring procedures performed under local anaesthetic. She left the hospital after a year of antimicrobial medications, but returned the following year to undergo a pneumonectomy (the surgical removal of her lung) because of bronchiectasis, a chronic lung infection. But she survived. In her recollections for an in-house history twenty-three years later, she thanked the staff for the care she received because, as she put it, after spending her entire childhood in the institution "they were my family."[47]

Isolation and Integration

Indian hospitals need also to be viewed in the context of politics and the practice of postwar Canada's articulation of modern hospitals and the national health. North American hospital history emphasizes the expansion and transformation of the hospital in the late nineteenth and early twentieth centuries from almshouse to medical marketplace. In Canada, before 1890, hospitals, financed by charity and government, housed the sick poor while their social betters convalesced in the comforts of home. By the 1920s hospitals began to attract patients who demanded, and would pay for, the benefits that medicine seemed to promise: relatively safe and effective surgery, professional nursing, and technological innovations such as X-rays.[48] The modernizing hospital, where the poor were kept separate from the paying patient, actively shaped class inequality within and beyond its walls.[49] But even the "patient of moderate means" found access to hospital care increasingly difficult, leading to demands for the state to take a greater role in protecting and enhancing the national health. One of the first acts of the new Department of National Health and Welfare, created in 1945 as the flagship of the welfare state, was to take control of IHS and its expanding number of hospitals. A separate arm of the bureaucracy also invested public funds into National Health Grants that for nearly two decades beginning in 1948 provided matching funds for provincial projects of hospital construction, medical training, and disease control.[50] By 1953 Canada had added forty-six thousand new hospital beds.[51] The same bureaucracy managed Indian hospitals on the presumption and promise that they would operate at half the costs of provincial hospitals; in several communities the Indian and local hospitals were literally side by side. This ensured that IHS hospitals would never draw qualified staff or other resources away from community hospitals, with dire consequences for Aboriginal patients. Indian hospitals reflected and constructed racial inequality by making it seem natural that modernizing hospitals would be white hospitals.

Finally, the meanings of Indian hospitals are found in rapidly shifting federal policies in the 1960s that sought ultimately to sever the legal and treaty relationship. With national hospital insurance in 1957, IHS planned to close its hospitals and divert its funds to community hospital expansion to accommodate First Nations patients. Local organization and grass-roots activism, particularly (but not exclusively) in Treaty Six communities in central Saskatchewan and Alberta, coalesced to protect Indian hospitals as the only concrete acknowledgment of the Crown's treaty promise of health care represented by the "medicine chest." More threatening, national health insurance in 1968 would absorb First Nations into provincial programs and ultimately dissolve the links between the economic and political roots of ill health on reserves and the state's responsibility for health care. Using the same liberal (and Liberal) language of equality and "non-discrimination," it was an ominous foreshadowing of the infamous White Paper the following year that proposed to dismantle completely the treaty, customary, and legal relationship with Aboriginal people. While the White Paper's proposals were withdrawn within the year in the face of concerted and organized opposition, health and health care policy continued as contested terrain. Indian hospitals emerged as sites of resistance where communities sought a measure of self-determination to address the poverty, overcrowded housing, contaminated water, and inadequate infrastructure that gave rise to much illness.

Constructing Disparity

This thematic study examines the rationales for segregation in Indian hospitals and the particular focus on tuberculosis; staffing and hospital operations; coercion and the hospital experience; IHS efforts to shift responsibility for health care to the provinces; and community resistance and the articulation of the treaty right to health care. But such a singular historical focus on Indian hospitals risks repeating and reinscribing the state's vertical approach to health care, which sought to treat ill health without acknowledging or mitigating its economic, environmental, and political circumstances. Bad water and crowded houses are as important to this story as hospital beds and bureaucrats; the links between them form the backdrop to this study. The colonization of lands and resources, and the socio-economic inequities that create and maintain ill health, continued through the twentieth century, particularly as governments encouraged industrial resource development. Lest the connections between ill health and material realities become obscured in the telling, a brief and unsettling sketch of one community's experience with dispossession and its consequences at mid-century illustrates this study's broader themes.

Fort Alexander, 132 kilometres northeast of Winnipeg, was a trading and provisioning post on the Winnipeg River in the eighteenth and nineteenth centuries. Signatories to Treaty One in 1871, the Anishinaabe of the Sagkeeng First Nation made their homes nearby on reserved lands that straddled the river's mouth where it spilled into Lake Winnipeg. In 1927 the Manitoba Paper Company built a pulp mill and the company town of Pine Falls, complete with a hospital, eight kilometres upriver from the Fort Alexander community. Indian Affairs contracted with the local physician to provide health care for Anishinaabe residents, but when townspeople objected to their presence in the hospital, the government built an adjacent annex that in 1937 became the Fort Alexander Indian Hospital. During the Second World War local Anishinaabe men found work at the mill, although at war's end most lost their jobs to non-Aboriginal workers; some found work cutting pulpwood in the bush.

The Fort Alexander community, which relied on the Winnipeg River for its water supply, also suffered the environmental impact of the upstream mill and town. Pine Falls pumped its raw sewage into the river, and the pulp mill discharged twenty thousand gallons of toxic sulphur, lime, and sulphur dioxide into the river four or five times per day. Most of the sulphur dioxide occurred as a gas, which was stored until the prevailing winds blew away from the town of Pine Falls. It was then discharged into the air, though whether the toxic gas blanketed the reserve was "not considered too important."[52] Those who could afford it purchased water at the "unheard of price" of $0.60 to $0.75 per 45-gallon drum; even so, tests confirmed this "town water" was dangerously contaminated as well.[53] Between 1949 and 1958, in a population of less than 1,300, 462 infants were admitted to the Fort Alexander Indian Hospital with gastro-enteritis, and 19 died. In July 1958 alone, 33 infants were admitted and one died.[54] The IHS field nurse reckoned that mothers were negligent for bottle-feeding instead of breastfeeding their infants, although she did allow that many were forced to do so in order to work.[55] Accordingly, she advised that children should be taken from their parents as soon as possible and enrolled in the Fort Alexander Residential School. [56] But the school's water supply, also contaminated by raw sewage, was suspected as the cause of an infectious hepatitis outbreak in 1954.[57] Tuberculosis was also a problem that sent thirteen residents, escorted by RCMP, to sanatoria for treatment in 1957; however, a report to IHS suggested that gastro-enteritis caused by the polluted water supply "certainly outranks tuberculosis as a killer."[58]

Those made destitute by economic circumstances could apply to Indian Affairs for monthly rations, and the hospital's medical superintendent could recommend rations for the ill or incapacitated. For a family of two adults and four children (children received half an adult ration), calculated on a diminishing scale, adults received 950 calories per day, and children 805 calories per day (which included 330 calories in the one-pint milk ration for children under twelve).[59] A decade earlier Indian Affairs had conducted nutrition experiments at other Manitoba First Nations communities; they made clear the links between disease and an average diet that provided only 1,470 calories per day. Historian Ian Mosby compared those studies to a postwar University of Minnesota experiment that induced starvation in thirty-six adult volunteers with a diet of 1,570 calories.[60] As an IHS report noted, at Fort Alexander "the people who are in need because the man of the house is ill will get sufficient food for the family if the Medical Superintendent of the Fort Alexander Hospital is so inclined and not as a basic right."[61]

The thirty-bed Pine Falls Hospital with two resident doctors served the town's 3,200 residents. In the five years from 1955 to 1959 the occupancy never exceeded 43 per cent. The adjacent Fort Alexander Indian Hospital that served 2,800 residents of the Clandeboye Indian agency, with a rated capacity of thirteen beds had twenty beds and five bassinets. In 1959 the occupancy averaged 128 per cent. A provincial Hospital Survey Board, after inspecting the Indian hospital in early 1960, was "impressed with its inadequacy." Not only was the facility "obsolete" and constantly overcrowded, there were no fire exits, and inadequate isolation facilities. The Survey Board recommended its closure and an addition to the Pine Falls Hospital to accommodate the increased patient load; it urged that the addition not be segregated for the use of "Indian" patients, though "it might be necessary to provide a few separate beds."[62] The stark Fort Alexander experience, not atypical for communities in the path of resource development, highlights the synergies between environmental degradation, racial inequality, and the creation of health disparities.[63] It serves to remind us that ultimately Indian hospitals isolated and treated the consequences of colonization, and operated to maintain if not widen health disparities.

This history of Indian hospitals from the 1920s to 1970s is situated at the intersection of race, medicine, and public policy in the wider context of twentieth-century Canadian health care. This does not presume to be a comprehensive history of all the hospitals, but a thematic approach to the commonalities in the institutions operated by the bureaucracy initially known as IHS.[64] Although it was a national bureaucracy, the IHS established no hospitals east of the Ottawa River, reflecting both the Aboriginal population's distribution, and the political and medical anxieties in the west.[65] There has been little sustained scholarly attention to the history of the Indian Health Service or its hospitals. Progressive accounts, written by those most closely involved with the IHS and the Canadian Tuberculosis Association, focus on the bureaucracy's humanitarianism and particularly their role in the "conquest" of tuberculosis.[66] More recently, scholars have examined gender and colonialism in the IHS nursing service.[67] T. Kue Young's critical examination of the Sioux Lookout Indian Hospital in the context of cultural and socio-political dimensions of health and health care among northern Ontario's Cree and Anishinaabe, argues that without political and economic autonomy, medical and technological interventions have a limited impact on health status.[68]

This book builds on the compelling narratives of the subjective experience of Inuit in southern hospitals, and on oral histories of life in Indian hospitals that give voice to individual experience as embodied resistance.[69] It contextualizes these threads of experience in the larger fabric of twentieth-century health policy. To do so is not to create victims, but to acknowledge the often perilous world constructed at the intersection of race, medicine, and the imperatives of the nation's health. Indian hospitals, created and operated in the interests of Euro-Canadians as a modern reiteration of an older practice of quarantine, worked to maintain difference. By resisting the state's attempts in the 1960s to shed its legal and treaty commitments, First Nations were also pointing to the damaging futility of treating those made ill by poverty and deprivation, only to return them to the same conditions. When communities argued that they might best know their own health needs, and pursued a measure of autonomy to improve health, they were met with a bureaucratic and political resolve, striking in its intensity, to undermine and frustrate those efforts. To view Indian hospitals, like "Aboriginal history" generally, as ancillary to grander themes, obscures the links between marginalization, poverty, and disease. It is a "powerful fiction," then as now, to treat as distinct and unrelated two enduring twentieth-century narratives: the progressive march towards improved health care for Canadians and the seemingly intractable ill health in Aboriginal communities.[70] How it became normal and natural to see those narratives as separate is the subject of this history of "separate beds."

Chapter One

Making Indian Hospitals

Indian hospitals emerged from deep anxieties about Aboriginal people and their perceived threat to the public's health. Initially begun in concert with mission schools to keep ill children within the Christian embrace, with uneven support from the state, mission hospitals provided limited care to a "dying race." Literally and figuratively, through disease, isolation on reserves, and particularly the assimilationist policies in schools, "Indians" were expected to disappear as Canada embraced modernity in the twentieth century. That they did not, and indeed increased their presence in towns and cities, created considerable concern. By the 1930s, medical discourse shifted from civilization's supposed deleterious influence on Aboriginal people to the threat Aboriginal illness posed to the nation's health. With an increasingly strident rhetoric of the threat of "Indian tuberculosis," sanatorium directors working with provincial physician bureaucrats, pushed the federal state to protect society by creating Indian hospitals. Formalizing an already well-entrenched system of racially segregated care, Indian hospitals also made it seemingly natural that the sanatorium and the modernizing hospital would be reserved for white patients.

In the 1920s the Department of Indian Affairs (DIA) took control of some mission hospitals and nursing stations, providing limited physician and nursing services while continuing to subsidize missionary efforts. Though sporadic and piecemeal, increasing DIA involvement in health care was motivated by the foremost need to economize while isolating illness on reserves to protect the health of white communities, foreshadowing the more significant post–Second World War expansion of Indian hospitals. The department relied on mission and community hospitals, providing funds for construction and maintenance.

Unwilling to interfere with missionary control of hospital care unless forced by to do so by public criticism, the department confined its meagre medical efforts to isolating epidemic disease on reserves and hiring five travelling public health nurses to cover all the western reserves and schools. Dr Peter Bryce, appointed chief medical officer in 1904 to control medical costs, by 1907 began advocating for increased spending to stem the appalling death and disease rates of children in the department's schools.[1] Bryce's recommendations, calling for non-denominational schools and increased government financial commitment, were not well received. The DIA's Duncan Campbell Scott, rising from copy clerk in 1880 to chief accountant in 1893 to superintendent of education by 1909, found Bryce's recommendations "scientific … [but] quite inapplicable to the system under which these schools are conducted."[2] After 1913, when Scott became deputy superintendent general (deputy minister) of Indian Affairs, Bryce's services were no longer required and he was pensioned in 1921.[3] That the DIA operated without a chief medical officer for fourteen years until 1927, and that the newly created Department of Health in 1919 did not include responsibility for Indian health, indicate a distinct lack of interest in health matters. Yet, at the same time, Canadians of the middling classes, increasingly health conscious, insisted on purchasing medical care in modernizing hospitals.

The transformation of the hospital from repositories of the sick poor to institutions that attracted paying patients actively shaped class and racial inequality within and beyond its walls.[4] Segregated wards and hospitals for racialized minorities were the norm in the Canadian west, mirroring the racial segregation in society.[5] For example, Chinese and Japanese patients in the early twentieth century suffered in Vancouver General Hospital's basement "Ward H" alongside "dirty indigent cases," those with particularly loathsome terminal illnesses.[6] Chinese tuberculosis patients in the 1940s were relegated to Vancouver's St Joseph's Oriental Hospital. Patients complained about the constant traffic noise from the railway lines on one side of the hospital, and the stench from the cannery on the other; there was little nursing care; patients were expected to clean the toilets; the food was unpalatable; and the Catholic missionaries actively proselytized dying patients. Many in the Chinese community avoided X-ray clinics for fear of being confined at St Joseph's. As community advocates noted, "Some have declared emphatically that they would rather die than go to St Joseph's Hospital." Public health nurse J.B. Peters urged: "When the Chinese were given the same type of facilities for treatment as occidental races they would cooperate in the same way."[7] Patients and their supporters who resisted such hospital care were deemed "racially indifferent" to health care and a danger to the community, further recommending their incarceration and segregation.

Community hospitals throughout the west and north also maintained "Indian wards" and segregated annexes; even hospitals that relied for their financial survival on DIA funds maintained strict racial separation. The Bella Coola Hospital on British Columbia's west coast received funds from the department for construction and equipment, but its "Indian ward" consisted of one bed and a chair, with neither chimney nor fire; Bella Coola was not an exception in British Columbia.[8] Like the Indian annex next to the Pine Falls Hospital, the St Boniface Sanatorium, owned by the Grey Nuns at St Vital Manitoba, maintained a separate Indian building.[9] Segregation likewise defined territorial hospitals in the post–Second World War period, when the privately owned hospital at Mayo, Yukon, simply refused to admit Aboriginal patients until the government built an Indian ward. In a tuberculosis survey in 1947 Whitehorse residents refused to share hospital gowns with "diseased Indians."[10] From its opening in 1948 the Yellowknife hospital confined Aboriginal patients to its ten-bed Indian wing with a separate entrance and waiting room.[11] As late as 1965 the Royal Commission on Health Services (Hall Commission) was told "there has been a tendency to place Indians in wards which are not as attractive or desirable as those used for white patients. Too often they have been treated in white institutions as indigent patients rather than as Canadian citizens."[12] The Indian annexes, Indian wings, and basement wards, demanded by community prejudice and inadequately funded by the state, actively shaped inequality and constructed an image of Aboriginal people as less worthy of care.

Government fiscal policy also worked to maintain the colour line in community and voluntary hospitals, especially its practice of paying somewhat less than the "indigent rate," or the rate paid by municipalities for the care of the poor. Defending the practice, federal bureaucrats argued that hospitals padded each bill to cover delinquent accounts, but since the department paid its bills eventually, hospitals should discount the rates charged for government patients. Not surprisingly, hospital administrators disagreed. In Alberta in the late 1940s the issue became particularly acrimonious when the manager of the Calgary Hospitals Board asked why the government expected Alberta communities to subsidize Aboriginal care: "Each Indian patient admitted and paid for by the government on the basis of $3.00 flat rate per day prohibits, during the period of his or her hospitalization, the admission of some civilian patient who likely would pay the full rates charged." Accordingly, he recommended that the "Calgary Hospitals Board adopts a policy of refusing to admit Indian patients."[13] The 846-bed Calgary General Hospital had treated only about eight Aboriginal patients in the previous six months.[14] To press the point the Indian Health Service (IHS) threatened that since the city's Calgary Stampede profited by Aboriginal participation, it would pay no accounts "incurred by Indians due to injury when competing in stampede activities."[15] Smaller community hospitals in Alberta also benefited in their efforts to attract and maintain paying patients. By 1950 Alberta hospitals had practically "ceased to accept a sick Indian except in the most emergent circumstances, and for the shortest possible time." Moreover, the hospitals "are overcrowded by patients from their own municipalities and for whose care they can depend on full rates."[16] State policy clearly aided hospitals' efforts to devote bed space to the right patient, the paying patient. As Lindsay Granshaw argues in reference to British hospitals, the active intervention of the state in providing hospital accommodation for the least advantaged in society removed them from the voluntary hospitals, thus reducing the stigma attached to the latter.[17]

The DIA only reluctantly moved from Indian wings to Indian hospitals. Beginning in the 1920s it came under increasing public scrutiny and criticism from provincial and national tuberculosis associations that charged the department was ignoring the threat posed by reserve populations, undermining their efforts to "clean up" provincial populations.[18] But unless Aboriginal communities funded their own hospital care, either directly or by paying for care in local community hospitals, if they could be admitted, the DIA only grudgingly invested in health care ("hospital" would be an exaggeration in many cases) in order to answer public criticisms. The conditions at Anglican boarding school on the Sarcee (Tsuu T'ina) reserve near Calgary, the subject of repeated medical inspections early in the century, had continued to deteriorate by 1920. Inspector Dr Corbett drew attention to one particular child in what had become grotesquely familiar reports:

> She lies curled up in a bed that is filthy in a room that is untidy, dirty and dilapidated in the northwest corner of the building with no provision of balcony, sunshine or air. Both sides of her neck and chest are swollen and

five foul ulcers are discovered when we lift the bandages. This gives her pain and her tears from her fear of being touched intensifies the picture of her misery.[19]

The "dirty and dilapidated" room was the school's infirmary. The following year inspectors found dirty floors and windows, and bed linens "stained with blood and puss [*sic*] marks old and recent."[20] Finally, the long-neglected school was fitted out with new sleeping porches and deemed a "hospital" with Dr F.T. Murray in the dual role of physician and Indian agent. Meanwhile the whole reserve became a "hospital area," with movement off reserve restricted while Calgarians were warned of the nearby threat of contagion.[21] Elder Helen Megunis, who attended the school in the 1920s, recalled: "We have lived an isolated life, after I became a young girl in my teens we were still isolated, there was no TVs, phone, electricity, plumbing, newspapers. It was strange, visiting Calgary during the stampede was our only contact with alien people of Calgary [*sic*]."[22] While it seems clear that infection crossed reserve boundaries, the direction of that spread was never questioned. The continued isolation of the reserve that literally adjoined the burgeoning city of Calgary was made possible through the formal and informal restrictions on the people's movements, always enforced by the Royal Canadian Mounted Police. The justification for isolation had certainly shifted from ostensible efforts to protect the Aboriginal people from unscrupulous whites to efforts to contain disease on the reserve and thereby safeguard the public's health.

By 1932, with only a "practical nurse" and cook in attendance, it was judged "scarcely a hospital."[23] The reserve's poverty limited treatment to little more than custodial care. Even X-rays were impossible since the reserve remained without electricity until 1937, although the adjacent city of Calgary enjoyed its benefits since at least the 1890s.[24] But the conversion of the mission school to "hospital" was more than merely discursive; it indicated an increasing concern to monitor the racial boundaries of reserve and disease. It also marked a shift towards secularization (accelerated in the postwar period) that removed the sometimes interfering missionaries, who often acted as mediators and advocates for Aboriginal communities.[25] Creating the dual role of Indian agent/physician, while economical, also afforded closer state regulation and medical surveillance. The fate of the Tsuu T'ina seemed sealed when government anthropologist Diamond Jenness arrived to conduct "rescue anthropology" that documented the last gasp of a dying race.[26]

Despite predictions of their imminent demise, the Tsuu T'ina by the early 1950s improved their economic circumstances by developing the reserve's oil and gas resources, and given their experience with the reserve boarding school, they were anxious to access medical care. But IHS continued to pay somewhat less for care than Calgary hospitals charged, leaving the Tsuu T'ina to subsidize hospital costs if they wanted treatment. Meanwhile reserve living conditions, especially housing, deteriorated, and as the supervisor of Indian Agencies noted, there was little logic in using their funds to pay hospital bills when they required so many necessities "before we can conclude that the people are not experiencing a substandard existence."[27] Despite devoting precious funds to pay for their care, Tsuu T'ina patients found themselves in the indigent ward. The modernizing hospital with patients anxious to purchase its services saw no need to take up valuable beds and offend middle-class sensibilities by admitting Aboriginal patients. Moreover, the state's minimal commitment to Aboriginal health care actively cultivated an image of the people as a burden on the community.

The largest (and wealthiest) reserves in the country – the Siksika (Blackfoot) east of Calgary and the Six Nations reserve in Ontario – at the suggestion and insistence of the DIA, built reserve hospitals in the 1920s.[28] At the Siksika reserve, the Anglicans' Queen Victoria Jubilee Hospital, built in 1897 in conjunction with Old Sun's mission school, became increasingly irrelevant by 1912 when the school was moved closer to the only source of electrical power on the reserve at the village of Gleichen. In 1923 the Siksika band council agreed to contribute to the construction and maintenance of a new hospital using the funds from the surrender of nearly half their reserve. Pushed by poverty and the promise of a better standard of living, in 1910 the Siksika had surrendered for sale 50,586 hectares of their reserve; by 1920 their trust fund from land sales amounted to nearly $1 million. As DIA inspector J.A. Markle reported, the Siksika agreed to the surrender on the condition that $400,000 would be for their immediate use, while the interest on the remainder was to be expended for the benefit of the next generations. It seems unlikely that the Siksika agreed (if they were aware) that all DIA operations on the reserve as well as goods and services promised in the treaty were henceforth to be paid from the band's funds. As Markle put it, "[the band] will soon have a sufficient income of their own to meet all their wants and ... they will be no longer any expense on the government outside of what was guaranteed to them by the treaty, i.e. a cash annual annuity of $5 per head."[29] In January 1924 the sixteen-bed

Blackfoot Indian Hospital opened with two general wards, two semi-private wards, an operating room, dispensary, and living quarters for the matron and her four staff. At the Siksika council's insistence the hospital was to remain non-denominational and local Aboriginal healers were not to be disturbed in their medical work.[30] At Six Nations in 1927, at the suggestion of the DIA, the two-storey, twenty-bed Lady Willingdon Hospital opened at Ohsweken, for which the band council paid half the costs while also contributing to physician salaries. The DIA assumed complete control of the institution, limiting local Six Nations participation, despite their investment. Reserve women offered to form a hospital auxiliary to provide knit goods and incidentals, but the physician's influential wife rejected the proposal.[31] Both the Blackfoot and the Six Nations' Lady Willingdon hospitals would eventually come under complete government control by the 1950s.

Citing increased public criticism of the government in 1923, the Indian agent at Battleford in central Saskatchewan suggested an Indian hospital: "Many that should have gone to hospital have been attended at their homes on account of expense and several have died in filth and misery because there was no possible place to care for them and local hospitals would not take them having no accomadition [*sic*] for this class of patient which you cannot blame them after seeing some of these cases as we do in the course of our duties."[32] The next year the department considered building an Indian wing at the local Notre Dame Hospital where the Sisters of Providence would charge the government $2.50 per day for care. But hospital superintendent Sister Justinian demanded a separate Indian building with its entrance at the rear of the property instead of an Indian wing.[33] In the meantime Anglican bishop George Lloyd objected to the DIA "handing all our Anglican Indians in the Battleford area over to the tender mercies of a Roman Catholic institution at the time of sickness ... You must know as well as I do the unfair leverage this gives to the Roman Catholics."[34] Fearing that funding an Indian wing at the Catholic hospital might necessitate an Anglican institution as well, Indian Affairs' D.C. Scott let the matter rest. There would be no hospital care for Aboriginal people in the Battleford area until 1947.

Aboriginal communities also actively advocated for better care. Elders recall that a delegation from Pasqua reserve in southern Saskatchewan travelled to Ottawa in 1928 (covertly circumventing the travel and fund-raising restrictions of the Indian Act) to protest their exclusion from community hospitals. A 1923 petition from the British Columbia

Indian Anti-Tuberculosis League likewise demanded improved care.[35] Indian commissioner in the west, William Graham, also agitated for hospital care in the 1920s, arguing that a departmental hospital in the Regina area with fifty to sixty beds with minimal staff could be maintained for less than half the per diem cost they were currently paying to local institutions. How those savings might be accomplished was left to the imagination. In any event, Graham was sure that most costs could be paid from band funds; indeed, from 1922 to 1924 Aboriginal communities paid for half their hospital costs. If Aboriginal people could find hospitals that would admit them, and they funded their own care, D.C. Scott saw little reason to entertain the notion of an Indian hospital. In reply to Graham's plea that he was faced every week with people "actually suffering and some of them dying for want of care," Scott replied that the "present system is adequate."[36]

Provincial bureaucrats and sanatorium directors who made up the Canadian Tuberculosis Association (CTA) held no such illusions. Anxious to know the extent of disease on reserves, they joined with the DIA to undertake medical surveillance of a number of British Columbia communities in 1926. For two years the survey X-rayed, examined, and gave advice to Aboriginal communities, with no offer of treatment. Researchers found a clear link between tubercular bone and gland infection in residential schoolchildren and the raw milk used in the schools. They concluded that the infection could not have come from home since few reserve families used cow's milk.[37] The DIA prevented that report from becoming public, and its 1928 *Annual Report* noted only that tuberculosis was about "five times more common among Indians" than among the general population (this statistic would vary widely depending on the circumstances), and that the Aboriginal people were too ignorant to make use of food supplies that would produce "robust health."[38] This desire to create a detailed "colonizing archive" while refusing treatment caused considerable outrage in communities.[39] A decade later physician bureaucrats found that surveys on reserves with no chance of treatment "only irritate the tuberculosis and public health authorities and the Indians."[40] Nevertheless, it seems clear that D.C. Scott was allowed to suppress the report linking schools with bone and gland infection in children if he agreed to appoint a chief medical officer, a position vacant for fourteen years since Dr Peter Bryce's ouster.[41]

Dr E.L. Stone, a colonel in the Canadian Army Medical Corps during the Great War and, since 1922, physician and Indian agent at Norway

House in northern Manitoba, took up the work of chief medical officer in 1927.[42] Stone's appointment, like Bryce's before him, was prompted by the need to manage the work and the costs of physicians contracted by the DIA to provide part-time medical care, particularly the quarrels between the physicians and the DIA's accountant who discounted their fees.[43] Departmental physicians, under strict supervision by the Indian agent lest they provide too many services, could do little more than recommend hospital care for their patients; ultimately bureaucrats and bookkeepers determined who was admitted to hospital and for how long, with a keen eye to the bottom line.[44] While Aboriginal patients were relegated to indigent wards or Indian wings and subjected to community prejudice, the DIA accepted the situation since its financial commitment was predictable and easily controlled.

In 1932 the top bureaucratic position in the Department of Indian Affairs (deputy superintendent) passed from the accountant D.C. Scott, to the physician Dr Harold McGill. Four years later the department itself was dismantled and made a branch of the Department of Mines and Resources with a severely reduced budget. Immediately, Indian agents were instructed to remove patients from hospital; there would be no funds for tuberculosis surveys or treatment in hospital or sanatoria; expenditures for drugs were reduced by 50 per cent; and "quarantine … [was] to be rigidly enforced, with guards if necessary."[45] The expedient of ignoring the ill or confining them to reserve schools or mission hospitals rather than admitting them to local hospitals was dictated by the department's uppermost concern for economy in all things. But there were other considerations that influenced the form and place of medical treatment for Aboriginal people in the Canadian west.

In May 1937 sixteen-year-old "Mary" (not her real name) was discharged from Onion Lake's St Barnabas Residential School in Saskatchewan with tuberculosis after suffering haemorrhages for more than a year. Overcrowded residential schools had earned an appalling reputation for breeding disease among underfed students; when children like Mary became too ill they were sent back to their parents, with disastrous consequences for their home communities. Mary's father demanded she receive sanatorium treatment at the Prince Albert Sanatorium, but Indian Affairs' Dr Norquay refused. Mary's older sister, who had also contracted tuberculosis at the school and was treated at the sanatorium, had subsequently become pregnant though she was unmarried. According to the physician, the sanatorium cure – bed rest and the development of the attributes of healthy citizenship – had clearly failed, and it was her father's fault. Mary was therefore refused treatment, though the doctor did approve a $5 ration voucher. But when Norquay discovered that Mary's father spent it all on fresh fruit "which would necessitate the rest of the family participating if the fruit was not allowed to spoil," he warned that "this sort of foolishness would result in the withdrawal of such favours."[46] To appeal to the doctor's superiors, Mary's father engaged a lawyer who argued, "The child was well when she went to the school and contracted the disease there ... They [parents] know that there is care for sick white children and believe the same care should be afforded to Indian children." Publicly funded provincial sanatoria provided free tuberculosis treatment for "taxpayers," while DIA might purchase treatment when beds were available. Not until public criticism of government policy by a Saskatoon newspaper was director Dr Harold McGill moved to authorize treatment for a "a limited number of tuberculous Indians."[47] Physicians' keen surveillance and authority to enforce middle-class notions of sexual propriety and acceptable gender roles exposed medicine's collusion in the colonizing project. Mary died at the sanatorium four years later.[48] As a rule, and while there were white citizens awaiting entry to their institutions, sanatorium directors felt no obligation to treat Aboriginal people. Instead, through their Canadian Tuberculosis Association, they joined with provincial bureaucrats to pressure the federal government to establish racially segregated institutions.

The extent of tuberculosis on reserves remained the subject of much speculation. Manitoba's Dr David Stewart boldly claimed that in the western provinces the "death rate among Indians [is] ten to twenty times as great as that among white people, and over 30 percent of the total deaths from tuberculosis occur among the Indians, who comprise less than three percent of the total population."[49] Moreover, the statistical picture of Indian tuberculosis also illustrated a satisfying decline in the white death rate. As Stewart explained in 1932, the official death rate in Manitoba per 100,000, "if Indian deaths were dropped ... would become 40, and if the half-breed deaths were dropped, a non-Indian rate of 34/100,000 would emerge." Stewart's statistics became considerably muddled when he conceded that "half-breed deaths" were only an estimate because they were counted in the census "according to the white racial mixture, as French, Scotch or English." In a more candid moment he allowed that since so few Aboriginal patients were attended by physicians, "there is some doubt about the accuracy of death causes of Indians ... and there is the strong tendency to put down an Indian as dying of tuberculosis. The poor fellow scarcely is allowed to die of anything else."[50] Moreover, white tuberculosis deaths were not always recorded as such. With the disease's social stigma and its associations with poor living conditions and low income, many physicians cloaked tuberculosis deaths in euphemisms, further obscuring the statistical picture.[51] In white communities, as Wherrett admitted in his history of tuberculosis in Canada, "doctors did not always report the disease. Doctors avoided disclosure on death certificates."[52] Furthermore, those presenting themselves at tuberculosis case-finding clinics in white communities did so voluntarily; when such clinics began on reserves residents were routinely denied their Treaty annuity payments until they submitted to X-ray and examination.[53] Thus, despite the seeming isolation of many Aboriginal communities, the medical surveillance would become far more complete.[54] There are good reasons to question the oft-cited statistic that the tuberculosis death rate in Aboriginal communities was ten times the white rate.

The practice of keeping separate statistics for Indian tuberculosis rates and "white" (provincial or national) rates became routine, highlighting the source of danger while simultaneously emphasizing the good work accomplished by the sanatoria. Much of the tuberculosis statistic making,[55] intended as it was to emphasize the threat of "Indian tuberculosis" and prod the federal government to assume greater responsibility for treatment, tended to over- rather than underestimate the threat. This is not to argue that tuberculosis was not a problem, but those creating the statistics had reasons to construct Aboriginal people as "tuberculosis-soaked," according to Stewart.[56] As John O'Neil argues, the practice also constructed knowledge that reinforced unequal power relations: "an image of sick, disorganized communities can be used to justify paternalism and dependency."[57] While the threat of Indian tuberculosis was made clear, limited access to reserve communities frustrated a more thorough knowledge of the "Indian problem," which would have to await the bureaucratic regulation that the Indian hospitals afforded. In the meantime, efforts increasingly focused on the much more accessible residential schoolchildren and Aboriginal infants.

In 1933 Dr Ferguson, director of Saskatchewan's Fort Qu'Appelle Sanatorium, began an experimental trial of the controversial tuberculosis vaccine BCG (bacillus-Calmette-Guerin) on Aboriginal infants. He lived at the sanatorium, which was literally surrounded by reserves and the threat of contagion. Funded by the CTA and the National Research

Council, Ferguson's trial – premised on the understanding that "primitive" peoples were more vulnerable to tuberculosis and that resistance could not be acquired except on a evolutionary time scale – hoped to prove that BCG could provide effective resistance in "less evolved races."[58] The BCG vaccine, developed at the Pasteur Institute in Lille, France, found greater acceptance in Europe and especially in French colonies than in North America, where its use before the 1930s was limited to Montreal's working classes. But Ferguson's BCG trial required newborns who had never been exposed to the disease, that is, born in hospital; his unvaccinated controls were born at home on reserves. The nearby File Hills Indian Hospital, built in 1914 as the centrepiece of File Hills Farm Colony, which was intended to illustrate to dignitaries and foreign visitors the government's successful management of residential school graduates, was a fire hazard and severely overcrowded, with space for seventeen patients, but with a daily census of twenty-eight. Taking advantage of the federal government's Depression-era public works program in 1934, Indian Affairs secured $100,000 to build the Fort Qu'Appelle Indian Hospital, across Echo Lake from the provincial sanatorium.[59] Ferguson had the hospital he needed. His twelve-year BCG study was an apparent success: only six of the 306 children in the vaccinated group developed tuberculosis and two died; while 29 of the 303 in the control group developed tuberculosis and nine died. But Ferguson's research also revealed that 77 of the 609 children in the trial, or more than 12 per cent, died before their first birthday, while only four of these were tuberculosis deaths (two in each of the vaccinated and control groups.) In all, nearly one-fifth of the children in the trial died from other diseases, mostly gastro-enteritis and pneumonia.[60] Overcrowded housing, poor nutrition, and unclean water posed the greatest threat to children, but, unlike tuberculosis, did not spread to white communities.

The new Fort Qu'Appelle Indian Hospital, opened in 1936, was a dour three-storey brick building that shared none of the sanatorium architectural style's sleeping porches and expansive grounds (illustration 1.1). And while general hospitals rarely admitted tuberculosis patients for fear of cross-infection, the Fort Qu'Appelle Indian Hospital had no such qualms, keeping tuberculosis patients on the third floor, with maternity, medical, and paediatric patients on the second floor. By early 1938, of the hospital's sixty-five patients, fifty-one were treated for tuberculosis. The practice of isolating tuberculosis patients from the community, yet institutionalising them with non-infected patients, suggests that

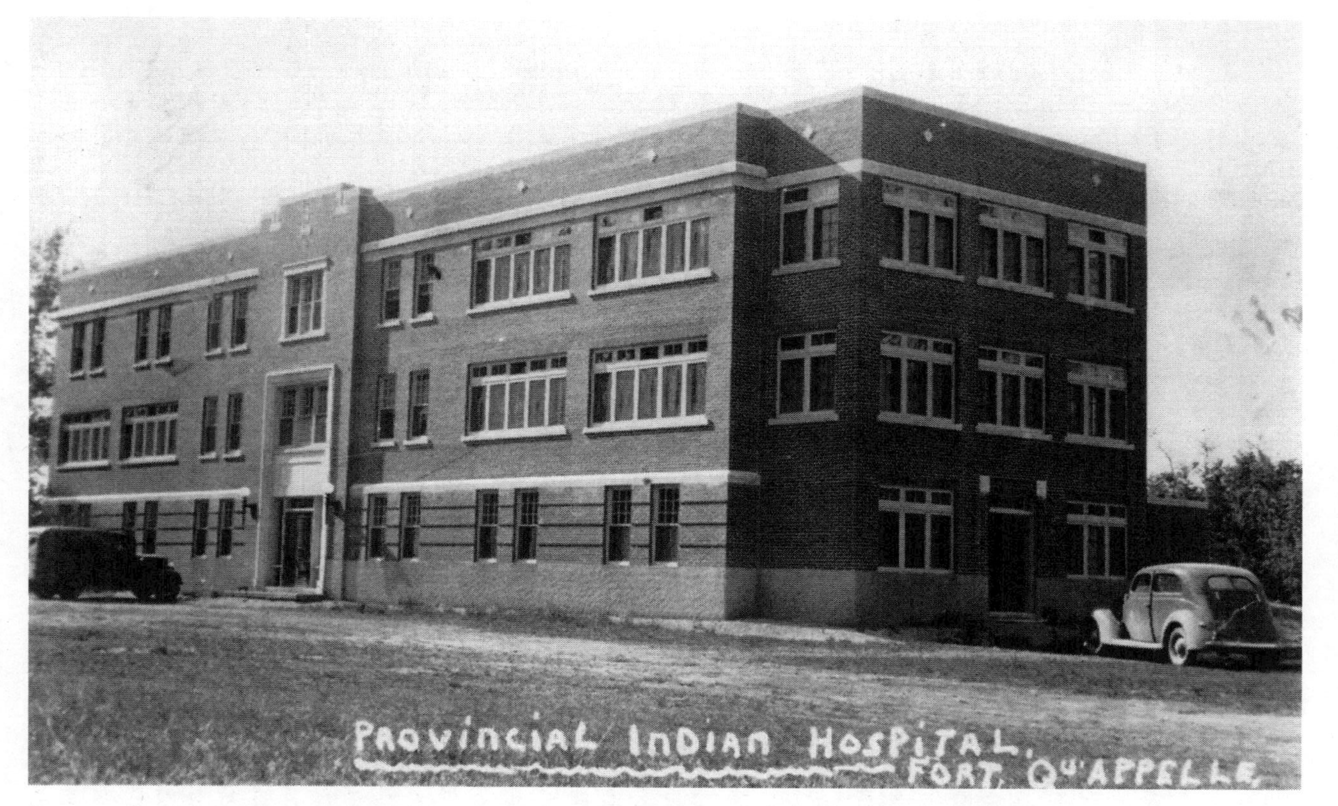

Illustration 1.1 Fort Qu'Appelle Indian Hospital. Built in 1936, the fifty-bed Fort Qu'Appelle Indian Hospital sat across Echo Lake from Saskatchewan's provincial sanatorium. It was the site of Dr R.G. Ferguson's BCG vaccine trial on Aboriginal infants in the 1930s and 1940s.

Source: Accession R96-472, Saskatchewan Archives Board.

their tuberculosis was seen as a threat only to the white community. As noted, the same year the hospital opened the Department of Indian Affairs became a branch of Mines and Resources, prompting director McGill's early 1937 directive mandating draconian cuts to all hospital treatment and explicitly ordering agents to remove patients from hospital. The bizarre logic of opening a new hospital while restricting hospital care cannot be explained without reference to the rationales for the hospital's creation: it emptied the forty-bed "Indian ward" that Ferguson's provincial sanatorium had been pressured by finances to maintain, while also providing facilities for his vaccine trial. BCG held great promise to control tuberculosis while leaving untouched the socio-economic conditions that led to its rise. The hospital was a success by the one standard that most mattered, as Indian Affairs branch director McGill enthused: "We have obviously a genuine sanatorium at this point which is taking care of these patients for almost exactly half what it costs to maintain a patient in a public institution." It is not clear how these savings were effected, but McGill added: "We have not had a single complaint of the treatment of patients."[61] The new Indian hospital, a tangible response to criticisms of state policies that left Indian tuberculosis untreated, came at the expense of medical care for Aboriginal people elsewhere, who, according to McGill's orders, were quietly removed from hospitals. Certainly Depression-era budget cuts adversely affected the chronically underfunded Indian Affairs, but endeavours like the Fort Qu'Appelle Indian Hospital suggest that expenditures were not necessarily or even primarily made in the Aboriginal people's interests.

In March 1936, the new Liberal minister of Indian Affairs, Thomas Crerar, agreed with the Catholic Archbishop of Winnipeg Alfred Sinnott that the department should contribute to a new hospital at Winnipegosis.[62] Despite Indian Health Service director Dr E.L. Stone's objection that it was not a suitable site since only 200 of the 1,200 residents were Aboriginal, Indian Affairs contributed nearly half of the $27,000 cost. The new Crerar Hospital, owned and operated by the Benedictine Sisters, opened in January 1937 with fourteen beds including a six-bed Indian ward. The hospital would be "freely open to sick Indians at such rates for maintenance as may be agreed upon from time to time," providing the Sisters with a small but steady income.[63] Though the Indian Affairs branch continued to contribute funds to finish the hospital, branch employees remained in the dark on many details since the minister and archbishop alone concluded the arrangements. In reporting on the newly opened building, Indian agent Waite and the departmental physician admitted their confusion: the Indian ward would treat tuberculosis, yet the new departmental policy prohibited the hospitalization of tuberculosis patients. The branch secretary replied: "I can give you no other answer in this connection than the instructions contained in the recent circulars on economy which have been sent to all Indian Agents."[64] It is not at all clear how many Aboriginal people were treated at the Crerar Hospital, despite the government's sizeable contributions in their name.

Reacting to the drastic cuts in Indian Affairs funding for tuberculosis treatment, the Canadian Tuberculosis Association warned that the "opinion has been expressed in some quarters that there is a higher incidence of the disease in communities adjacent to Indian reserves."[65] Physician and Liberal member of parliament Dr J.J. McCann cautioned the House of the threat of "Indian tuberculosis" during the 1937 debate on estimates of the Indian Affairs branch. Quoting from Dr Stewart's pamphlet, "The Red Man and the White Plague," McCann reminded MPs that falling white tuberculosis rates meant virtuous families – such as their own – with healthy, unexposed children were particularly vulnerable to "outside infection ... a spark in dry grass."[66] The CTA, representing sanatorium directors like Ferguson and Stewart, was the most powerful voice for racially segregated treatment. Established in 1901 by elites concerned with the economic impact of tuberculosis, the CTA exerted considerable influence on government policy. In a letter to the Manitoba premier, Stewart called the Aboriginal "dangerous neighbours," a "menace ... to the health of ordinary citizens," and an "uncontrolled nuisance."[67] At its 1935 annual meeting the CTA devoted a session to "Indian tuberculosis" and sent resolutions to the prime minister and minister of health, warning of the "menace of uncontrolled tuberculosis on Indian reserves to the surrounding white population" demanding more government action.

In June 1937 the CTA formed a joint committee of federal and provincial bureaucrats and sanatorium directors that met in Ottawa to consider how best to control the threat of Indian tuberculosis with the paltry $50,000 the Indian branch had at its disposal. IHS director Dr E.L. Stone opened the meeting by drawing a bold red line across the map of Canada from west to east that separated "those [Indians] to the south who are, generally speaking, in contact with and a menace to white populations, from those to the north, who ... are not."[68] Around 75,000 (of a total Aboriginal population of 115,000) lived in this "contact zone," representing just 0.6 per cent of the Canadian population of slightly more than eleven million. Despite their small number, Stone emphasized the threat: "Roughly two Indians out of three, are shown to be in contact with white people." Of the population in the "white contact areas" nine thousand were students living in sixty residential schools, but as Ferguson of Saskatchewan noted, the experience of the Tsuu T'ina reserve showed that schools were easily turned into sanatoria. Despite criticisms of residential schools, Ferguson claimed, "for the purpose of cleaning up tuberculosis among the children they are a wonderful institution." The irony that the schools, so clearly implicated in the spread of the disease, would now be the solution, seemed lost on Ferguson. But, as Dr Alexander, medical superintendent at Six Nations reserve near Brantford argued, adults were a greater threat: "I know of at least three families to whom an Indian maid has conveyed infection to the children." Though impossible to know, the source of infection seemed too obvious to be questioned. To stress the threat, the doctor lapsed into a telling military metaphor: Aboriginals were "an enemy in our midst, and while we have few guns trained on them there is no reason why we cannot attack them with such weapons as we have."[69]

The committee recommended dividing the $50,000 among the provinces based on a simple calculation of the number of "Indians in contact with white people (in the south) … and the probable amount of Tuberculosis among them."[70] Seventy per cent ($35,000) went to the four western provinces to establish "preventoria" in the schools that segregated children with "minimal lesions," and to pay the churches to provide sickly children with extra food and "one or two years better care than the rest."[71] Keeping infected and healthy children in the same institution likely only slowed the spread of disease within the schools. But, as Stone confided to his director, it might limit the spread from school to reserve, which posed a larger problem: "It would be hard to prove that the Residential Schools, as a group, are not agencies for the spread of tuberculosis."[72] Stone assured branch director McGill that he could keep ordinary annual medical costs to $10 per capita, or half the cost for white people, but more funds would be needed for medical officers and Indian tuberculosis sanatoria. Before it adjourned the conference also established an Indian Advisory Committee, essentially the management committee of the CTA, to keep the problem of Indian tuberculosis before the government and public.

The Indian Advisory Committee in 1937 recommended dramatically increased parliamentary appropriations for tuberculosis surveys in schools and reserves and an aggressive Indian hospital construction program. The CTA made clear that past efforts to ameliorate the predisposing causes of tuberculosis, diet and housing, only clouded the real problem that tuberculosis is a communicable disease, in the same way that "leprosy, typhoid fever, or smallpox are communicable diseases." Comparisons to historically frightening diseases emphasized the danger for those who remained complacent and implied the coercive measures that such diseases prompted. "Polluted with tuberculosis," Aboriginal people required a system of surveillance by medical personnel, as well as "training, supervision, treatment or segregation." Admitting that there was little understanding of the extent of disease on reserves, the CTA suggested that the elderly and "hopeless cases" should be segregated on reserves under the care of nurses, if any could be hired. But, the foundation of control efforts would be the confinement in special tuberculosis institutions of "young Indians ... [and] hopeful cases that can be cured, intelligent Indians whose education and sanitary habits will have some effect in raising the standards of the Indian generally." Such deserving hopeful cases might be trained to become healthy citizens.[73]

To satisfy curiosity about the extent of disease, in 1937 Drs Ross and Paine from Manitoba's Ninette Sanatorium surveyed reserves and residential schools in proximity to white population centres. They administered tuberculin injections that tested for exposure to tuberculosis (though not indicative of disease itself); they performed some physical examinations and attempted to take medical histories that were "usually meagre"; and, for good measure, took blood samples for the Wassermann test that indicated syphilitic infection. No treatment was offered. Their study, presented at the 1938 annual meeting of the CTA and subsequently published in the *Canadian Medical Association Journal*, proposed "to ascertain accurately the incidence of tuberculosis infection and disease ... there has been endless speculation but no statistical knowledge to temper the impression that the Indian was still overwhelmingly scourged by the disease." Hoping that their survey might be useful for a "future program" of treatment, the doctors found more than twice as much infection in reserve populations (11.6 per cent of 1,856 people) than in residential schools (4.2 per cent of 816 students), which is not surprising since it was common practice to remove ill schoolchildren for what was termed "observation at home." The house-to-house survey also provided ample opportunity to comment on living conditions – "uniformly poor, though in isolated cases quite good"; and on Indian character – "paradoxical" marked by stubborn superstitions, though "time and education" might correct these flaws. Surprised to find evidence of healed disease, given that it was generally conceded that the people had no natural resistance to tuberculosis, the physicians concluded: "If given the same opportunity as the white man, the Indian might respond to preventive and curative treatment measures almost as well." Marshalling more statistics for the cause, the Manitoba survey also provided a brighter side, diagnosing the Indian as "blessed with a natural indolence [that] should make him an ideal cure-chaser if he were not such an easy prey to periods of undisciplined activity."[74] The CTA needed little convincing of the threat to Canadians, and the solution would naturally be more institutional beds along the lines of the Fort Qu'Appelle Indian Hospital. For the government, the remarkable economy of that institution prompted McGill to advise his minister: "We have never wanted to go into building or operating of sanatoria, but if we can do so, as seems probable, on the standard of economy of the Qu'Appelle Indian Hospital, it is an open question whether we should not consider extension in the other provinces."[75] Unlike the purpose-built Fort Qu'Appelle Indian Hospital (and later the Moose Factory Hospital on James Bay), all subsequent Indian hospitals would be established in "borrowed buildings," slightly renovated military institutions and residential schools.

Naturally, the next Indian hospital to open was in Manitoba, home of minister responsible for Indian Affairs branch, Thomas Crerar. In 1939 the Anglican Church gladly sold its Dynevor Hospital, near Selkirk, to the government. The aging structure, built in the 1870s as a rectory for St Peter's parish and converted to an infirmary in the 1890s, became a fifty-bed Indian hospital managed for the government by the Sanatorium Board of Manitoba[76] (illustration 1.2). Friends of the government were no doubt pleased when the *New York Times* congratulated the government for its "steady progress" in the provision of hospitals for "sick Indians at a cost less than that of admitting them to public institutions."[77] The Dynevor Indian Hospital had its critics, however. Winnipeg's Catholic Archbishop Sinnott objected to its "Protestant" nature and demanded "a Catholic hospital for Catholic Indians." To that end he offered to sell the Catholic Crerar Hospital to the government; this time minister Crerar declined the archbishop's offer.[78] Dr J.D. Adamson of the Catholic St Boniface Sanatorium, which opened in 1931 in nearby St Vital and had recently added twenty beds to its Indian annex in anticipation of much-needed revenue from government patients,

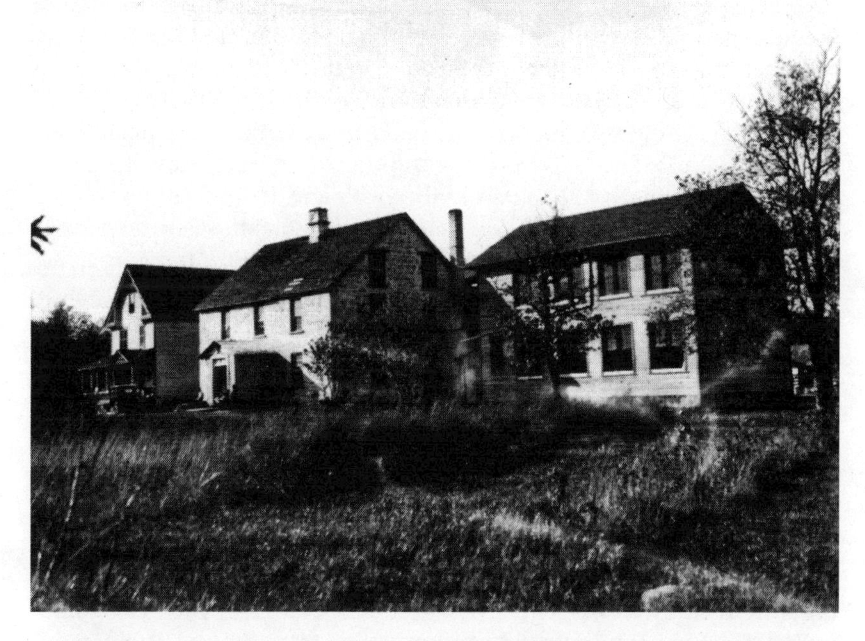

Illustration 1.2 Dynevor Indian Hospital, Manitoba. Built in the 1870s, the centre block was originally the rectory of St Peter's Parish, near Selkirk, Manitoba. Converted to an infirmary in the 1890s, the building was sold to the Indian branch in 1939 and opened as the Dynevor Indian Hospital managed by the Manitoba Sanatorium board.

Source: Rupert's Land 150, Archives of Manitoba.

claimed that the Dynevor Indian Hospital would mean an "enormous over-supply of beds."[79] But, explained Sanatorium Board's Dr E.L. Ross, Dynevor was not intended to be a "fully equipped sanatorium," but an inexpensive alternative providing rest and nursing care, well removed from white populations. Indeed, Dynevor made do without an X-ray machine when renovation costs exceeded the Indian branch budget.[80]

Because high death rates, the grim reality of tuberculosis treatment in any sanatorium, threatened to tarnish Dynevor's image, the dead were buried across the Red River at St Peter's Parish.[81] In its first year the hospital admitted sixty-seven patients, nearly half of whom were children removed from schools. The most common treatment at Dynevor was the painful pneumothorax "refills." Pneumothorax, or therapeutic lung collapse, was an extension of rest therapy surgically induced, but the lung naturally reinflated and a "refill" of gas injected into the pleural space maintained the lung collapse.[82] In its first year alone Dynevor performed more than 300 pneumothorax refills.[83] By its fifth year, 29 per cent of Dynevor's patients were dead, and another 12 per cent were "unimproved."[84] The efficacy of pneumothorax, the mainstay of surgical treatment in Canadian sanatoria in the 1930s and 1940s, is impossible to judge, but of the First World War veterans treated at the Central Alberta Sanatorium in Calgary, only half of the pneumothorax patients lived, and less than one-third improved.[85] Besides surgery, or often because of it, bed rest was strictly enforced. As in all sanatoria, some patients resisted the enforced idleness, strict routines, or the prospect of surgery, but Dynevor's physician suggested that "the philosophy of the Indian" made the problem more acute.[86] Police forcibly returned patients who "ran away" (left against medical advice) under the authority of the provincial Communicable Disease Control Act.[87] While all sanatoria faced recalcitrant patients, since much of the therapy was concerned with cultivating the proper attitudes of the hygienic self, patients were not held against their will. But Indian hospitals were different; as we shall see, the Indian Act was subsequently amended to compel medical examination, treatment, and hospitalization. Aside from the Indian hospitals operated by the Manitoba Sanatorium Board, IHS also operated its own Indian hospitals at Fort Alexander, Fisher River, and Norway House.

British Columbia had no sanatorium beds for Aboriginal people in the 1930s. Dr W.H. Hatfield, head of the province's tuberculosis program, warned their threat to health was more acute because they were not confined to reserves, but "free Indians" mixing with the white population and causing alarm.[88] In 1941 the Indian branch opened the Coqualeetza Indian Hospital near Chilliwack, British Columbia.[89] Founded as a Methodist mission school in 1889, it expanded in 1924 when the DIA built a larger 200-student residential school. A 1932 inspection found so much tuberculosis that the missionaries built a small preventorium for the most ill rather than send them home.[90] By 1938 the missionaries could no longer manage the school and turned it over to the government; three years later the 185-bed Coqualeetza Indian Hospital opened with six girls transferred from the preventorium. A 1948 fire destroyed much of the building; remarkably no one was killed, but conditions were far from ideal for the ninety-eight patients who remained in the undamaged wing, or for the twenty-two patients in "the converted hen house, known as the preventorium," which was rotting and in immediate danger of collapse.[91] Thus, the wartime increase in institutions of varying quality, a response to the CTA's campaign to expose the threat of Indian tuberculosis, also reflected Indian Affairs' constant search for economy.

At war's end attention turned to reconstruction, and, like Indian Affairs policy generally, the Indian Health Service undertook policy discussions in early 1945. Acting director Dr Percy Moore steered the policy deliberations. Moore got his start in Indian Affairs as a physician at the Fisher River Hospital in Manitoba after graduating from the University of Manitoba medical school in 1931. Appointed as assistant to director Dr E.L. Stone in Ottawa in 1937, Moore became acting director two years later while Stone served in the military. Moore subsequently became director in 1946 when the Indian Health Service was transferred to the newly created department of National Health and Welfare. He remained director for the next twenty years, until his retirement in 1965.[92]

An Order in Council established the Advisory Committee for the control and prevention of tuberculosis among the Indians, with a mandate to make recommendations to guide Indian Affairs' efforts. But the focus was entirely on the need for institutional care, repeating the recommendations of the 1937 Advisory Committee that advocated increased hospitalization and larger appropriations for tuberculosis control. The 1945 Advisory Committee, with its mandate that ten of the twelve members be nominated by the CTA, ensured that expert opinion – provincial health bureaucrats and sanatorium directors – would prevail over the federal bureaucracies that were limited to just two representatives, deputy minister and psychiatrist Dr Brock Chisholm from National Health and Welfare and Dr Percy Moore from Indian Affairs branch. Needless to say, no Aboriginal representatives were invited. Meeting for two days in May 1945, the committee concerned itself with establishing institutions for treatment of "Indian tuberculosis." While the extent of the disease was still unclear, committee chairman and executive secretary of the CTA, Dr G.J. Wherrett, made use of the available statistics to show a "satisfactory fall" in the white death rates and an increase in the death rate for the Aboriginal population, though he admitted that the Bureau of Statistics was "not quite satisfied" that the Aboriginal population figures were complete.[93] But the deliberations quickly widened from tuberculosis to a discussion of what was commonly referred to as the "Indian problem," or the place of Aboriginal people in society.

Moore stated the case bluntly: "Only a few years ago it was common, when one mentioned the Indians or the Indian problem, to have one shrugging his shoulders and say 'Oh, they are dying out, and the sooner the better.' Such is not the case. The Indians … have the largest annual increase of any racial group." To which Brock Chisholm, deputy minister of Health and Welfare, replied, "That is one good reason why they should become citizens."[94] The term "citizenship" implied many things, but foremost was what an earlier generation called assimilation, or the removal of cultural, linguistic, political, and legal differences with other Canadians. Alarmed by the threat posed by an increasing, and apparently increasingly diseased, population, the committee approached their task with a certain sense of urgency. Manitoba's Dr J.D. Adamson noted that Aboriginal soldiers carried on as citizens, but upon return to their reserves "degenerate immediately … we cannot do anything of a substantial nature until we endow them with the responsibility and dignity of full citizenship."[95] The discussion ranged widely from the need for Aboriginal people to embrace the values of Christian capitalist workers, to the value of education, indeed even higher education, to "raise up the Indian" to embrace the advantages and especially the responsibilities of citizenship. Only then might tuberculosis among them be defeated. An exasperated Moore successfully redirected the discussion back to the need for hospitals and a "direct attack" on tuberculosis, but the discourse made clear that until complete integration to citizenship there would be no solution of the "Indian problem." Ironically then, the deliberations focused almost exclusively on treatment in segregated institutions. For the committee, representing the interests of sanatorium directors and provincial bureaucrats, integration might be the desired goal, but it most certainly would not happen in their provincial institutions.

The Advisory Committee essentially mapped the program for postwar Indian Health Service. With representatives from all the provinces except Quebec, the committee agreed that it was an urgent national issue, though some provincial representatives feared threats from other racialized minorities. Nova Scotia's deputy minister of health Dr Peter Campbell admitted that he had no idea how much tuberculosis there was in the Aboriginal population, but the bigger problem was the province's "negroes." British Columbia's Dr Hatfield was more worried about the Chinese and Japanese, "and let me add that we hope we will not have the Japanese long."[96] Manitoba's contingent worried about "half-breeds." The acknowledged expert, Saskatchewan's

Dr R.G. Ferguson, whose twelve-year BCG vaccination experiment on Aboriginal infants was nearing completion, advocated a direct attack, including vaccination. And referring to the committee's earlier discussion about education and citizenship, "[it] made me wonder whether half the men in this room had ever seen an Indian." He thought the residential schools took fine care of the children and that the people on reserves were well nourished, if not overweight. The Indian agents were "loyal and hard-working men," and reserve houses were "pretty good for Indians." The problem, he continued, was not with living conditions, but with "genetics ... These Indians are born without any acquisitive instinct."[97] Reminding the committee that tuberculosis was an infectious disease, "something like typhoid or smallpox," Ferguson explained that the response should be to "vaccinate and segregate." As for higher education, Ferguson scoffed that they might be ready in "two hundred or possibly one hundred years." The young students who managed to get a high school education "go bad." Young women come home "in a pregnant condition, or a boy comes home as a useless smart Aleck." No, what was needed was a practical education along very simple lines "involving their learning to sweat and work."[98] At that, Brock Chisholm clarified his earlier comments regarding citizenship and education; he did not intend to suggest that Aboriginal people should be educated among whites, but their "method of living should be raised so that they would have their own schools, and train people in their own communities where they would provide their own education."[99] The rhetoric of integration aside, continued isolation clearly remained the prescription. As medical men they saw themselves as social experts, qualified to comment on all aspects of the "Indian problem," while demonstrating their understanding of race as a biological reality, if not a pathology requiring treatment. The ambiguity reflected in the committee's discussions – that integration to citizenship might be the goal, but segregation should remain the means – was ultimately incorporated into the emerging Indian hospital system.

The committee was clear that the strategy would be an expansion of institutional segregation and isolation in Indian hospitals. What was less clear was the extent of the disease. The most commonly cited figure, which fluctuated depending on the circumstances, was an Aboriginal death rate ten to twenty times the white rate. The statistics were badly flawed and extrapolated from very small surveys conducted in the 1920s and 1930s. But those surveys, to satisfy curiosity not to provide treatment, understandably outraged Aboriginal communities.

In Manitoba, an attempted repeat tuberculosis survey faced the ire of the community: "The chief and councilors nearly kicked us off the reserve. It took us three or four days to convince them to let us bring our x-ray machine ... because we had not done anything about it the first time."[100] As Saskatchewan's Ferguson told the committee: "If you survey a much greater area than you can treat, and just get the Indians on a waiting list, you discourage them. I think that is a rather serious thing."[101] Dr Barclay, DIA superintendent at Coqualeetza in British Columbia, admitted that there was little understanding of the extent of the disease, and to conduct surveys without offering treatment "they lose interest and you lose face."[102] Using a rough calculation of need – two treatment beds per tuberculosis death, three per death in areas near white populations – the committee recommended a focus on the western provinces, northern Ontario, and the Northwest Territories and Yukon. Brock Chisholm cautioned against modest proposals. Instead, the time was ripe for a rapid and substantial expansion of hospitals: "when reconstruction is on the map is the time to ask for what you want."[103] In addition to the hospitals already established, over the next few years two Indian hospitals were opened in British Columbia in redundant military facilities at Nanaimo and Miller Bay near Prince Rupert; two in Alberta, at Hobbema and in Edmonton, the largest institution, the Charles Camsell Indian Hospital in what had been the American military headquarters for its Northwest Command; one more in Saskatchewan at the Commonwealth air training camp at North Battleford airport; two more in Manitoba at the American military base at The Pas and the Brandon Military Hospital; the Moose Factory and Sioux Lookout Indian hospitals in Ontario; in Quebec City, tellingly, Inuit patients were held in the Parc Savard immigration and quarantine facility. But there were limits. In Halifax, the Rockhead quarantine and immigration hospital, a substantial building that had withstood the 1917 explosion and had recently been vacated by the Navy, was briefly considered for use as an Indian hospital. But, as the CTA's Dr Wherrett implied, it would be impossible to find white employees to work in such an environment, with the African-Canadian settlement, Africville, immediately in front of the hospital and the city jail to the rear. "Practically the only human activities to be seen from the hospital ... are those of colored people or jail inmates."[104] Nevertheless, by this expansion, in addition to the two band-owned hospitals – the Blackfoot Hospital in Alberta and the Lady Willingdon Hospital at Six Nations reserve – and other small cottage hospitals of one sort or another scattered across the country, there were twenty-two Indian hospitals by 1960.

The Advisory Committee meeting also considered what was, for the federal bureaucrats Moore and Chisholm, the principal reason for the meeting: sectarian hospitals. In what would be a fundamental shift in how health care for Aboriginal people had been delivered, Moore pressed for a recommendation that the Indian hospitals be strictly non-denominational. As he told the committee, the government was under considerable pressure from Christian churches to provide support for the expansion of religious hospitals connected to many residential schools, rather than establishing non-sectarian hospitals. While many committee members were loath to imply, for instance, that Catholic nuns were not competent to run a hospital, Brock Chisholm pressed for a resolution. It was not a question of religion or politics, Chisholm argued, but simply a medical matter; on that basis the committee was obliged to take a stand. "If this committee finds that the best medical care can be given by a sectarian hospital system, it should say so. If they believe ... that the best medical care can be produced by departmental control, and by the administration of non-sectarian hospitals, then it should say so."[105] Committee members bristled at being backed into a corner, arguing that it was not their remit to make the decision. Chisholm repeated the options. Calling the issue a "thorn in their side," Moore claimed that it had occupied more time and energy for ministers, deputy ministers, and everyone in the Indian Affairs branch "than has the consideration and treatment of tubercular Indians." After a prolonged discussion New Brunswick's Dr Charles MacMillan asked bluntly: "Would you like to run your own hospitals, Dr. Moore?" To which he answered, "Yes."[106] This was arguably one of the most important recommendations considered by the committee, marking the ascendancy of bureaucratic over missionary control of health care for Aboriginal people, while providing politicians with medical authority to face down the still powerful churches that resented interference in their work. It was a particularly vexing issue in the north, where government relied upon Christian denominations to provide all hospital care largely because the missionary societies themselves bore half the costs. As a result those northern hospitals were poorly equipped and understaffed. Committee chairman Wherrett's Arctic survey the previous year found deplorable health conditions among the Inuit, yet 150 of the Mackenzie Valley's 233 mission hospital beds were empty.[107] He urged the committee to recommend that Inuit patients be evacuated to southern government hospitals, since in the Northwest Territories they were "getting nothing more than board and room. You could not say that they are getting bed rest, because they [missionaries] do not keep them in bed."[108] To the argument that Inuit patients might be more comfortable hospitalized in the north, Moore reckoned that once they were removed from their communities it did not much matter if they were 10 or 1,000 kilometres from home. Tuberculosis control, and ultimately hospital care in general, could no longer be left in the hands of well-meaning but misguided missionaries.

Before the Advisory Committee adjourned, Moore wanted recommendations on two more issues that would come to define the institutions: staffing and the necessity of compulsory treatment. The Indian Health Service employed twenty-four full-time physicians, but Moore hoped to triple that number. The committee agreed that salaries would need to be competitive with provincial medical incomes or else "there is something peculiar" about anyone taking the job.[109] But physician salaries did not keep up with increasingly lucrative private practice after the war; staff turnover was a constant problem. As for Aboriginal medical staff, there was no consideration of Aboriginal doctors, though the committee agreed that young women might be trained as maids. With the poor academic achievement in residential schools, nurse training was impossible for most; Moore reckoned that throughout the country there were maybe four or five "Indian girls" in training. In a revealing comment that pointed to assumptions about the larger social purposes of the hospitals, Moore recalled that in his travels he could spot the "brighter" women right away. Surprised to find their homes well kept, he learned that they had either been sanatorium patients for a number of years or had worked as maids in the institutions.[110] Aside from their medical value, Indian hospitals would also provide valuable training in classed notions of respectability, as long as there was sufficient discipline and authority to keep patients institutionalized.

Finally, the committee was asked to recommend compulsory treatment. Moore stated frankly, "We certainly do not feel that our program should be left to the whims of an Indian, as to whether or not he will accept treatment."[111] The implication was that Aboriginal people would not voluntarily accept hospitalization, though the sanatorium directors on the committee knew all too well that beds in their institutions were reserved for provincial citizens. Nevertheless, Moore found the existing "Regulations for Medical Services" (1934) did not provide sufficient authority; indeed, the regulations were principally concerned with limiting medical officers' ability to incur expense by treating or hospitalizing Aboriginal people without departmental approval.[112] The regulations empowered an Indian agent to remove an individual with "acute communicable disease" for treatment, but there was nothing to compel the patient to stay in hospital. Moore explained: "We can ask the Mounted Police to pick up an Indian and take him to hospital, without taking him to court. Then if he refuses we can take him to court and sentence him to thirty days' imprisonment."[113] Provincial legislation was awkward and varied too much between jurisdictions. Compulsory treatment implied a detention cell or locked ward, and the committee's sanatorium directors were less supportive than Moore had hoped. Ferguson thought that detention wards in the hospital might sully the whole effort, unless it was carried out in a separate institution. Moore admitted that they had already built a detention ward in the hospital to be opened at The Pas. Manitoba's Dr Ross thought it easier to put a bed or two in a prison than to make a sanatorium into a jail. Moore persisted until the committee included a recommendation to Indian Affairs to revise the medical regulations to allow compulsory treatment and detention in Indian hospitals.[114] The next year he advised that the Indian Act be amended to include the authority to make regulations concerning compulsory treatment and hospitalization of venereal disease and tuberculosis, including detention in a sanatorium, and the compulsory return of patients who left against medical advice.[115] The 1951 revisions to the Indian Act's section 72 (1) that provided authority to make regulations was amended to include "compulsory hospitalization and treatment for infectious diseases," and, as we shall see, the subsequent Indian Health Regulations (1953) provided ample authority for coercion and compulsion. The Advisory Committee was allowed to adjourn having provided the state with the necessary medical expertise to manage the threat of Indian tuberculosis.

Overwhelmingly paternalistic, coercive in nature, and informed by the understanding of race as a biological reality that posed a threat to the nation's health, Indian hospitals were the mid-century answer to the failures of the past. Those who "graduated" from residential schools to Indian hospitals would no doubt recognize the institutional discipline and regulation. The lessons to be learned were individual self-control and the cultivation of healthy citizenship taught by the new medical experts. If they resisted they might well find themselves subject to the Indian Health Regulations and incarcerated in yet another state institution. The Indian Health Service also established nursing stations in remote areas, but its principal focus was Indian hospitals that would institutionalize and isolate not just tuberculosis but all Aboriginal patients.

Acknowledging the failure of past policies that left health care to poorly funded missionaries, the Indian Health Service was moved in 1945 from the Indian Affairs branch to the newly created Department of National Health and Welfare. A logical move in some respects, it obscured the links between poor health and its socio-economic causes while demonstrating faith in the power of biomedicine to cure the former while leaving the latter untouched. The move also alerted Canadians that a benevolent state, increasingly engaged in protecting and defining something called national health, would isolate the threat of Indian contagion while reserving community hospitals for citizens. The contradictions of the Indian hospitals' creation – isolating Aboriginal people while advocating for integration; segregating tuberculosis yet admitting all patients; coercing patients into hospital while characterizing the practice as humanitarian – point to the utility of the hospitals as economical institutions of confinement where surveillance, discipline, and surgery might cure the "Indian problem," or at least limit its spread.

Chapter Two

Neither Law nor Treaty

Neither law nor treaty impose an obligation on the Dominion government to establish a health service for the Indians and Eskimos, with the possible exception that in original treaties there is reference to the provision of "medicine chests." However, for humanitarian reasons and as very necessary protection to the rest of the population of Canada, it is essential to do everything possible to stamp out disease at its source where it may be within the confines of the country.[1]

– Brooke Claxton, minister of National Health and Welfare, 1946

Postwar expansion of the Indian Health Service took place within a larger reformulation of government policy reflecting an unprecedented public interest in Aboriginal people's place in Canadian society. As minister Claxton assured Canadians recently troubled by the "Indian problem," the creation of Indian hospitals was motivated not by quaintly vague treaty promises, but by the highest humanitarian ideals. From this moral and ethical high ground enlightened self-interest came into sharper focus, as did the threats to the nation's health posed by Aboriginal people. Moving the Indian Health Service to the larger Department of National Health and Welfare, the state demonstrated its commitment to include Aboriginal people in the calculations of national health, if only to keep them sufficiently isolated. Two months after the minister's pronouncement, in August 1946 Canada's vice-regal couple officially opened the 500-bed Charles Camsell Indian Hospital in Edmonton. Though Aboriginal communities were never consulted or afforded any input, many welcomed the postwar expansion of Indian hospitals as a belated acknowledgment of the state's responsibility for health care. The Charles Camsell Indian Hospital, the showcase of the expanding Indian Health Service, also demonstrated the fundamental contradictions at the core of racially segregated hospital care. Intended to check the spread of tuberculosis in particular, the hospitals removed and isolated sufferers from their own communities; at the same time, as inexpensive alternatives to community hospital care that would also protect the sensibilities of paying patients, Indian hospitals functioned as general hospitals, admitting all Aboriginal patients tubercular and otherwise. The costs of such contradictions were borne by patients whose care and safety became seriously compromised. Moreover, post-war changes in tuberculosis treatment, from lung collapse therapy and bed rest, to chemotherapy and aggressive chest surgery in the 1950s – innovations that led to the "miracle of the empty beds" in Canadian sanatoria – ensured, paradoxically that those beds would increasingly become occupied by Aboriginal patients.[2]

The abject failures of the state's policy of assimilation through residential schools and isolation on dwindling reserves, policies developed for a "dying race," had become glaringly obvious by the 1930s; and with Aboriginal populations growing, these were increasingly expensive failures. According to historian John Tobias, "aimlessness" marked Indian Affairs policy from the 1930s to war's end.[3] A less generous assessment of the Indian Affairs branch under the leadership of "Colonel" H.M. Jones (where civil servants were expected to stand when he entered the room) termed it "Colonel Jones' lost battalion."[4] And after 1945 the place of Aboriginal people in society troubled many Canadians. Prompted in part by their considerable contributions to the war effort, Aboriginal people came to the attention of concerned Canadians who wondered how, after fighting intolerance and racism abroad, Native people were still denied basic citizenship rights at home. An enthusiastic editorial in *Saturday Night* magazine, reflecting the biases of urban Torontonians whose experience with Aboriginal people was limited to summer vacations in cottage country, advocated for "the Indian." Their admirable record of wartime service proved "that they can work as well and endure discipline to as great an extent as their white brothers." Women worked in summer hotels "as chambermaids, kitchen girls, laundresses – jobs which entail hard work and an instinct for cleanliness. While they are doing these things, their men serve as guides, boatmen, and handymen ... these jobs they do well."[5] Canadians demanded a "new deal" for Aboriginal people so that they might integrate into society, albeit at the bottom rung, as normal working citizens. The government received petitions and resolutions from concerned citizens across the country: the Sudbury city council, the Army, Navy and Air Force Veterans' Association, the Sault Ste Marie city council, the Dock and Shipyard Workers' Union, the Alberta Teachers' Association, the Alberta Conference of the United Church, the Social Security Council of Canada, and "interested representative Canadian citizens" – a sociologist, an anthropologist, a police magistrate, and the director of Vancouver Folk Festivals.[6] The latter group, calling for a solution to the country's "vital question" through improved education and administration, also advocated for Indian hospitals on reserves. Though not the royal commission many called for, a special joint committee of the House of Commons and the Senate was struck in 1946 to enquire into the administration of Indian Affairs and to recommend revisions to the Indian Act.

For two years the Joint Committee heard from citizen, church, and professional groups and its deliberations were regularly reported in the press. But, as historian Hugh Shewell argues, the committee was a "tool of state propaganda" meant to elicit public consent to an agenda the state had already adopted.[7] Heavily influenced by the emerging social sciences, the committee's recommendations proposed that the "Indian problem" would only be solved when Aboriginal people became equal, normal citizens in a liberal view of the modern individual. In particular, they would receive services through their provincial governments, leading to reductions in the federal fiscal and legal responsibility for Aboriginal people. This certainly was not the message of the various Aboriginal organizations that submitted briefs to the Joint Committee in which they stressed the obligations that stemmed from their special relationship with the federal government. Nevertheless, the revised Indian Act (1951) removed some of its most repressive features while maintaining the earlier assimilation policy, which came to be termed integration for "citizenship."[8] To that end, the Indian Affairs branch was again moved in 1949, from the Department of Mines and Resources to the Department of Citizenship and Immigration, where, ironically, alongside immigrants, Aboriginal people could eventually become Canadian citizens.

Popular support for Aboriginal citizenship emerged within a broader climate of rising expectations for an activist and reformist state. In 1945 the Indian Health Service was transferred from Indian Affairs to the newly created Department of National Health and Welfare, the heart of the welfare state. Though severing the treatment of disease from its social and economic causes on reserves, medical men (the IHS bureaucracy was exclusively male) would direct health care. But the Liberal government's Green Book proposals for a comprehensive postwar welfare state, including universal health insurance, met concerted opposition, and by May 1946 Prime Minister Mackenzie King had lost the political will to carry out the reformist program.[9] One month later health minister Brooke Claxton addressed the Special Joint Committee. His submission, as we have seen, acknowledged federal responsibility for Aboriginal health care, though stressing a moral rather than legal obligation, a position successive governments maintained. While failing to deliver on the promise of universal health insurance, Claxton nevertheless reassured Canadians that an expanded IHS would protect the national health by doing "everything possible to stamp out disease at its source."[10] The new IHS, evidence of a vigilant yet generous state caring for the poorest of the poor, also marked Aboriginal people as a looming health threat. As one of its first acts the new bureaucracy took possession of the army's sprawling military complex in Edmonton that would become the Charles Camsell Indian Hospital, its showpiece institution.

Built in 1913 as a Jesuit college for boys, in 1942 the three-storey brick building became the headquarters of the American military's Northwest Command, when they added large California redwood frame buildings eventually covering three city blocks[11] (illustration 2.1). With the American withdrawal in 1944 the Canadian army purchased the facility but by 1945 deemed it redundant and eventually turned it over to IHS for use as an Indian hospital.[12] Local protests erupted as soon as residents learned that the "Jesuit College" would become an Indian hospital. Petitions from veterans groups, the mayor, local politicians, and the hospital's neighbours demanded the redwood buildings be used to relieve the local housing shortage, while the hospital itself should be reserved for veterans. According to the city's mayor, "tubercular Indians" posed a particularly dangerous threat.[13] A mass public meeting in late November attracted more than 300 angry citizens, along with at least one RCMP confidential informant sent to keep an eye on the supposed volatile combination of disgruntled veterans and leftist political activists.[14]

To reassure Edmontonians, the government clarified its rationales for segregation and isolation: the hospital would treat all conditions, not just tuberculosis, "and thus relieve the public wards of the Edmonton hospitals from treating Indians in these institutions." Moreover the

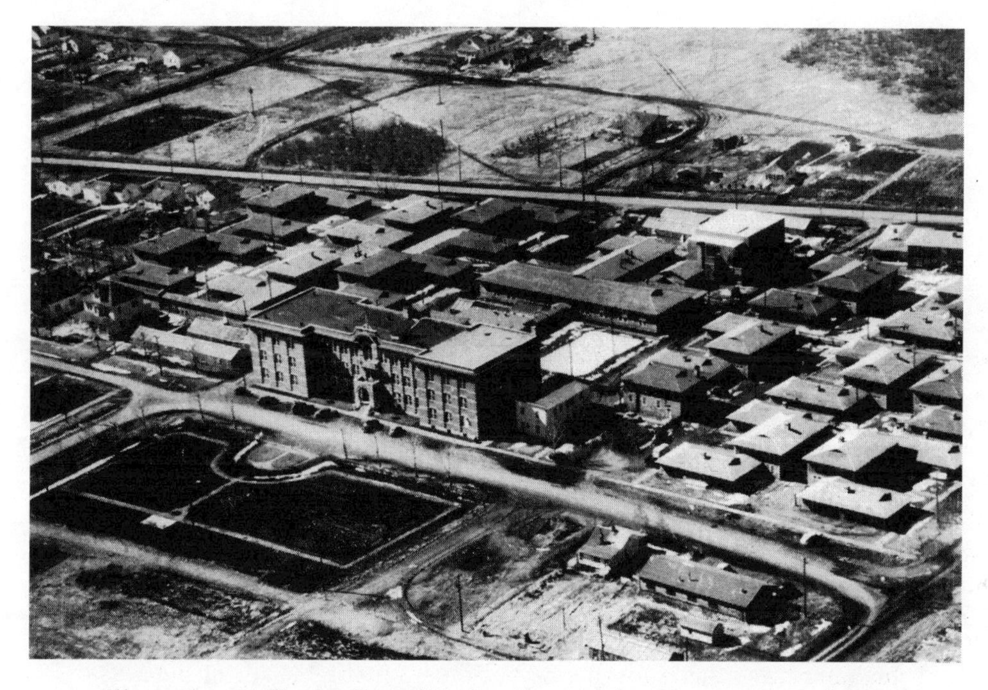

Illustration 2.1 Charles Camsell Indian Hospital Complex. The brick central building, originally a Jesuit college for boys, became the headquarters of the American military's Northwest Command in 1942, eventually covering three city blocks. Deemed redundant by the Canadian military at war's end, the warren of wooden buildings became the Indian hospital wards.

Source: PA-139304, LAC.

hospital's grounds would be fenced and patients completely confined in the institution, noting that it was better to have "these people under treatment than to have tuberculous Indians wandering about the streets of Edmonton ... spreading the disease."[15] Minister Brooke Claxton also reminded citizens of the hundreds of jobs the hospital would bring, and that "tuberculous Indians who are not in hospital are a danger to the community." Appealing to veterans, he noted that nearly 3,000 Indians (124 from Alberta) served in Canada's armed services during the war, and 167 made the ultimate sacrifice.[16] To appease the critics, 100 of the hospital's 500 beds were reserved for veterans until a new sanatorium for their use could be built. IHS, anxious to take control of the institution, quickly transferred fourteen Aboriginal patients from local Edmonton hospitals to the newly named Charles Camsell Indian Hospital.

The discursive practice of naming the pre-eminent IHS institution reflected the Canadian state's new interest in the resource-rich north, and thus honoured one of its sons. Charles Camsell (1876–1958), a geologist and deputy minister of Mines and Resources (at the time the bureaucratic home of Indian Affairs), was not the first name to be considered for the hospital, nor the second. Bureaucrats rejected some of the usual sources: "The Tweedsmuir Indian Hospital" for the late governor general, Sir John Buchan, 1st Baron Tweedsmuir of Elsfield, and "The Royal Tunis Hospital" for the current governor general's proud military career in the late war. "The Alexander Indian Hospital" would only cause confusion since Edmonton already had a Royal Alexandra Hospital. *Kapasowin*, Cree for "place of rest," was briefly considered, but Percy Moore warned that neither Cree nor Blackfoot names should be used for fear of provoking the supposed "great rivalry" between them, and besides, a Blackfoot name would be "difficult to spell and pronounce."[17]

Camsell was born at Fort Liard in the Northwest Territories, where his father was the Hudson's Bay Company's chief factor of the Mackenzie River District. As his autobiography claimed, he was a true *Son of the North*.[18] In 1884 the eight-year-old Camsell travelled to Winnipeg to begin his education. The trip by York boat, ox cart, river steamboat, wagon, and train, took three months, including a detour around the Saskatchewan Metis settlements that would descend into violence the following year.[19] Years later he noted approvingly that he flew from Winnipeg to his birthplace in less than three hours. His life spanned the era of technological and economic change captured by the term "opening the north." That Camsell was instrumental in those changes is not lost on the reader. His autobiography makes rare, yet harshly critical, mention of Aboriginal people: "The Indians were a miserable, dirty lot, always in a state of semi-starvation ... Like most of their race they were improvident, gorging themselves when food was plentiful and starving quite cheerfully when it was scarce."[20] Camsell's own experience of nearly starving in an unsuccessful attempt to reach the Klondike goldfields in 1897 was put down to bad luck, not improvidence. Indeed, as a commemorative history of the hospital explained, as a consequence of his experience Camsell "developed a strong, cheerful disposition, an even temperament, a splendid physique, as well as coordination and stamina."[21] As deputy minister of Mines and Resources he was also commissioner of the Northwest Territories, thus responsible for both the administrative and legislative functions of northern government, directly influencing Canadian policy. Camsell resisted territorial self-government and saw nothing inconsistent with administering the north from an office in Ottawa.[22] Camsell and his wife, along with other senior government officials, demonstrated their support for Indian Affairs' integration policy by employing young Aboriginal women as domestics in their tony Ottawa homes.[23] Interestingly, his autobiography does not mention that his mother was in fact Metis, which would not have been unusual given his family's involvement in the fur trade.[24] Camsell thoroughly embraced capitalist and Christian Euro-Canadian society, while deriding the backwardness of the north's Aboriginal people. A stint in the Charles Camsell Indian Hospital might inspire the Aboriginal sons and daughters of the north and west to admire, if not emulate, Camsell's life. Perhaps ultimately, this successful assimilation explained why he was honoured by the state. Camsell agreed to lend his name on the condition that it always be referred to as the *Charles* Camsell Indian Hospital. He was present at the opening ceremonies, which "pleased him greatly."[25]

The largest of the IHS institutions, the Charles Camsell Indian Hospital provided tuberculosis treatment for Aboriginal people from Alberta, northeast British Columbia, and the Territories as well as admitting patients for general hospital care in its obstetric, medical, surgical, and paediatric wards. The solid brick main building, the former Jesuit college, hid from view the maze of tinder-dry wooden buildings that became the hospital's wards and the covered wooden walkways that connected them. Deputy minister of health Brock Chisholm declared that the Indian hospitals would operate on two "cardinal policies." First, that "no effort or reasonable cost should be spared to give the patients the best hospital care attainable"; and second, that "Indian wards of the Government of Canada should have the highest priority in employment and that in particular the [Charles Camsell] hospital should become a training centre for Indian health workers."[26] Ultimately, the seeming generosity of his cardinal policies was quietly ignored, as patients were crowded into shoddy borrowed buildings. The second cardinal policy will be examined in detail in the next chapter, but suffice it to say that, but for a short-lived program to prepare young women to train elsewhere as ward aids, IHS undertook no formal health care training. Aside from a few graduate nurses who struggled to find schools to accept them, Aboriginal workers filled the least-skilled and lowest-paid positions in IHS hospitals.

The Charles Camsell Hospital's shortcomings were obvious when IHS took over the institution, and the centralized bureaucracy made resolution of seemingly simple maintenance problems time consuming and at times impossible. As Dr E.L. Stone, former IHS director and by 1945 Alberta regional superintendent, admitted on first inspecting the complex, "My worst misgiving is about the buildings. That the fire hazard is very serious goes without saying ... Sooner or later their settling will break gas mains to the heating units and they will burn."[27] The natural gas lines were so badly corroded that an inspector warned, "many gas leaks are almost certain to develop with the resultant hazard and danger of explosion."[28] The electrical wiring was defective and "a major fire hazard."[29] Worse yet, in case of fire, the water supply was not dependable because of badly damaged water lines throughout the institution. A ruptured sewer line under the main kitchen floor, first brought to the department's attention in January 1949, that smelled like "long-dead rats" was still festering eleven months later.[30] Without its own laundry the hospital relied on local commercial services, which refused to handle some of the most soiled hospital linens. In May 1946 surgeries were cancelled for a lack of clean sheets and surgical drapes; linens were instead sterilized and resterilized rather than washed. Patients' pyjamas and bedding went unchanged for weeks. A decade later the hospital finally got its own laundry.[31] The building's shortcomings certainly compromised the comfort and safety of both patients and staff, but there were no efforts to upgrade the facility for more than twenty years until it was rebuilt in 1967. As the IHS flagship, the Charles Camsell Indian Hospital was in better repair than other less visible Indian hospitals located in remote and isolated locations. But just as the pomp of its opening ceremony obscured the hospital's segregating and isolating impulse, the building's facade hid its many shortcomings. Passing by the Charles Camsell Indian Hospital though, citizens might be reminded of the threat lurking within while being reassured that theirs was a most economical humanitarianism.

The Camsell Hospital's first medical superintendent, thoracic surgeon Dr Herbert Meltzer, was appointed in 1945. Circumstance more than anything made Meltzer an ideal – indeed the only – candidate for the position. A thorough national search conducted by the Canadian Tuberculosis Association's George Wherrett found that Meltzer was the only chest surgeon with tuberculosis experience who would take the work at "anywhere near the [civil service] salary."[32] But a 1929 University of Manitoba graduate like Meltzer had few choices. Joining the staff of Manitoba's Ninette Sanatorium upon graduation, Meltzer left two years later in 1931 to open a private practice. However, like many physicians of his generation who subsequently landed in the IHS, he found private practice impossible during the Depression. After a year of postgraduate training in New York he returned to Ninette in 1935 as resident surgeon, and again resigned in 1941 to join the Army Medical Corps.[33] After his discharge in 1945, Meltzer accepted the offer as medical superintendent of the fledgling Camsell Indian Hospital, while also serving as chief of staff, radiologist, and thoracic surgeon. The new superintendent brought along his friend Dr Matthew Matas, also discharged from the medical corps, though there was concern that with these two the IHS might be criticized for having "too many Jewish people on staff."[34] Drs Margaret and William Barclay as well as much of the nursing staff were also recruited from the army, giving the hospital a distinctly military character.

William Barclay recalled that Meltzer administered the Camsell Hospital with the "discipline and chain of command" of an army hospital. Strict discipline for Aboriginal patients, deemed necessary if not beneficial in its own right, did little to inspire trust.[35] Meltzer, more comfortable giving orders than taking them, was an uneasy fit with the civil service. Demanding, tempestuous, and given to histrionics to get his way, he threatened resignation at least four times between February and March 1946 alone.[36] But more fundamentally, Meltzer disagreed with the unorthodox practice of combining tuberculosis and general hospital treatment in the same institution: "To me that is a very serious matter, and one that I cannot fit in with my conscience. As the Department insists that we look after these non-tuberculous cases, we must do something to increase the protection of these individuals from tuberculosis."[37] A month later Meltzer threatened to stop admitting non-tuberculous patients, instead referring them to the city's general hospitals, thereby undercutting the promise of Indian hospitals.[38] As Meltzer's direct superior Dr E.L. Stone put it, "The feeling in the city is that now we have an Indian hospital, why do we ask downtown hospitals to take Indians."[39]

Given that the hospitals were intended as alternatives to care in expensive community hospitals, economy and efficiency guided IHS efforts, from repurposing military barracks and residential schools, to keeping operating costs to a bare minimum. The logic of hospital efficiency, calculated as per diem cost per patient, meant that hospitals could maintain a low per diem rate by cutting costs or admitting more patients, or both. Since operating costs such as building maintenance and wages remained relatively constant regardless of occupancy levels, by definition a full – or overfull – hospital was an efficient hospital. Like the pre-war Fort Qu'Appelle Indian Hospital that operated at half the cost of admitting patients to local institutions, the Camsell Indian Hospital established maternity, paediatric, and medical wards alongside tuberculosis wards. But the former army hospital's large dormitory wards were completely inappropriate for a combined tuberculosis/general hospital treating men, women, and children, creating dangerous conditions. In a frank explanation for overcrowding Percy Moore rationalized the practice:

> I know the larger units of the hospital adapt themselves poorly to what would be an ideal for treatment, but sometimes we have to make a compromise. We have never had sufficient funds for a fully adequate program and I am anxious to do the maximum good with this institution to the maximum number of people possible ... The sooner we are operating to capacity, the sooner our high per diem rate will be reduced.[40]

Meltzer rightly questioned how the "maximum good" could be served by placing tuberculous patients in the same ward as the uninfected: "We already have one case of a little girl from Edmonton School who was investigated for diabetes. Exactly one month after her discharge, she was re-admitted with a Highly Positive Tuberculin [indicating exposure to tuberculosis], Erythema Nodosum [inflammation of the skin] and Pulmonary Lesion [tuberculosis]."[41] By 1950 Meltzer's services as the hospital's superintendent were no longer required. The bureaucracy was faced with the necessity of either discharging him or "making things so uncomfortable that he would [finally] resign."[42] They ultimately negotiated an agreement where Meltzer left the civil service for private practice, but continued as a consultant and the hospital's chief of surgery. Dr Lynn Falconer, another Manitoba medical school graduate who joined the IHS in 1938 and was Percy Moore's assistant by 1940, took over as superintendent, creating a clearer chain of command from Ottawa to Edmonton. Shuffling personnel eased some tensions at the hospital, but the abysmal infrastructure remained. Moreover, patient care and safety became seriously undermined in all the Indian hospitals by the self-serving and contradictory policies of their creation – segregating Aboriginal patients from expensive community hospitals while isolating tuberculosis patients from society to protect the national health. The central premise, indeed the promise of Indian hospitals, was that they would always be less expensive than provincial institutions.

More Indian hospitals opened in the late 1940s. Anxious to demonstrate their efficiency, Moore estimated that it cost between $8 and $10 per day to treat patients in general hospitals, while the per patient rates in the four largest Indian hospitals were half that: Camsell Hospital at $4.18, Miller Bay $4.66, Coqualeetza $3.91, and Brandon $3.99; at Nanaimo Indian Hospital on Vancouver Island, another former military institution, the $8.10 rate was temporarily anomalous because the institution was not yet full. As Moore's assistant made clear, "these figures are appreciably lower than the rates that can be obtained at even the smaller hospitals operated by communities or even religious orders and that we should be able to keep our institutions at full occupancy is a very appreciable saving of public funds."[43] But the repercussions of "full occupancy" did not go unnoticed by the Indian hospitals' constituency. The Indian Association of Alberta, though never asked for its input, regularly sent copies of its minutes to IHS. In 1949, after passing several resolutions praising the Camsell Indian Hospital's work, the Association voiced some concern: "We see old people in the same wards as TB patients and children playing in the same rooms where old people are lying sick. We fear there is great danger of infection spreading under such conditions."[44] Dr Falconer, as IHS regional superintendent, attended the Indian Association's annual meetings for a time, but as criticisms of policy and practice increased he charged the Association with encouraging "the malcontents on the various reserves ... a good sound sane well-meaning Indian does not take too much interest in it."[45] Many IHS physicians, not unaware of their peers' increasingly lucrative incomes in private practice, accepted that theirs was a higher calling as the embodiment of the institutions' humanitarianism. They would brook no criticism of their efforts, especially not from the recipients of the IHS largesse.

In the early 1950s the Camsell Hospital became seriously overcrowded with 560 patients in an institution with a capacity for 475.[46] Despite the strident rhetoric of "tuberculosis-soaked" reserves, in the Camsell Hospital's first full year of operation, 69 per cent of admissions were for some form of tuberculosis; in 1947 tuberculosis admissions dropped to 40 per cent, and the following year tuberculosis accounted for

36 per cent of admissions.[47] This is not to argue that tuberculosis was not a burden on Aboriginal communities, but it does suggest that it was neither the most burdensome nor the most likely reason for Aboriginal people to seek treatment. By the end of 1957, with all tuberculosis patients in Alberta and the Northwest Territories under care,[48] tuberculosis accounted for only 13 per cent of admissions to the hospital. A near equal number of admissions were of parturient women and their newborns (12 per cent). More than 60 per cent of patients admitted were children, and the single greatest cause was pneumonia or bronchopneumonia (30 per cent of all non-tuberculosis admissions).[49] Poor and overcrowded living conditions likely accounted for these admissions.

The overcrowded hospital quickly became a hazard. Initially, "Unit 3" served as a general and isolation ward, but it soon developed into "a conglomerate mass of women and children with every disease you would think of. It became more or less a pest house."[50] Nevertheless, Dr Falconer judged the "patients themselves were better off than in their primitive conditions at home and statistics would tend to substantiate this."[51] It is not clear to which statistics he referred, but patient care tended to be judged not against accepted hospital standards, but against perceived inadequate home conditions. On that basis, institutionalization itself, even in a "pest house," was seen as both necessary and therapeutic, regardless of the outcomes. But patients continued to be made more ill by their time in hospital. As Dr Matas admitted, "It is unusual for a child to be admitted with one condition and be discharged without having had some other infection or communicable disease. Isolation is carried out as far as possible and more so in surgical cases, but this does not seem to insure freedom from intercurrent diseases." For instance, an Inuit boy was admitted on 17 September 1957 for repair of an umbilical hernia, but "purulent otitis media" (acute inflammation of the middle ear with discharge) prevented surgery; shortly after the infection subsided, he developed, in turn chickenpox, measles, bronchopneumonia, rubella, and a recurrence of otitis media. He was finally discharged four and a half months later.[52]

According to Falconer the problem was not overcrowding as such, but the building, the staff, and, ultimately, the patients themselves. In a rather cryptic passage that pointed to the perceived need for strict patient discipline, he explained that the hospital needed first "proper facilities to control the patients with a firm hand and secondly better control of and more staff ... to properly run an isolation ward."[53] One staff member, Kathleen Steinhauer-Anderson, one of the very few Aboriginal nurses employed at the Camsell Hospital, recalled for historian Laurie Meijer Drees: "The conditions there [pediatric ward at the Camsell Hospital] were pretty bad. The babies were all dried with the same towel! I had to petition hard to get separate towels and towel racks for each baby patient. Some things were just improper."[54] Not surprisingly, "infectious hepatitis" (hepatitis A), a liver infection transmitted in food and water contaminated with infected fecal matter, frequently spread among staff and patients. From four cases in 1951, to thirty cases in late 1954, and ten more in the first three months of 1955, it was deemed an "epidemic," though it might have been more properly termed an endemic condition in the hospital.[55]

More troubling, discharged patients became vectors of disease transmission to their home communities. An Inuit woman, discharged from the Camsell Hospital to her home at Bathurst Inlet in the high Arctic, developed measles and pneumonia a week later. She was flown to Yellowknife, but not before spreading measles to others, resulting in three or four deaths. Making a virtue out of necessity, Falconer advised: "It is felt particularly with natives that we should not isolate them from measles but rather let them have the infection while in the hospital where they can be looked after with a better chance of survival."[56] Certainly the hospital attempted to protect the most vulnerable patients, especially children. With a particularly dangerous measles epidemic raging in the hospital, an infant from the Arctic with cleft palate spent three and a half months in the community hospital at nearby Cold Lake before he could be transferred to Camsell Hospital for surgery. Yet director Moore considered this a "virtual waste of money."[57] As the costs of community hospital care continued to climb throughout the 1950s Moore hoped to further increase the bed capacity at Charles Camsell Indian Hospital: "It is becoming more and more necessary to avoid prolonged hospitalizations in non-departmental institutions whenever possible."[58] But institutionalization had its limits. Filled to capacity and beyond, the hospital found it necessary to transfer some of the chronically ill and severely handicapped to Indian hospitals in other provinces, or, ironically, to northern mission hospitals that would take a "boarder" rate of as little as $2.50 day. This, according to Moore, "would appear to be a very good chance to unload a few bodies from our hospitals." Patients' families, however, were rarely informed about where their loved ones might be sent.[59]

Aside from concerns for efficiency, IHS motivations for moving chronically ill patients from the Camsell Indian Hospital was to make room for "problem cases" or patients with medically interesting conditions. As Moore explained to the hospital's superintendent, "Charles Camsell is a very large hospital and with outstanding diagnostic and consultant facilities and should be used as such rather than as a boarding home ... Vigorous action must be taken to make it possible to use Camsell as a consultant hospital."[60] From the outset IHS had intended that the Camsell Hospital would be associated with the University of Alberta's medical school. A close relationship certainly made the hospital a good medical neighbour in Edmonton, offering up interesting cases for medical students and researchers, while taking advantage of specialists' services. And despite its otherwise overwhelming concern for economy, IHS directed the superintendent at the hospital's opening: "Regardless of the extra costs involved and in order to become affiliated with the medical school university professors are to be consulted in genitourinary, orthopaedics, ear, eye, nose and throat, obstetrics and gynecology, to give them direct access to the hospital's interesting material."[61] Many of these patients, the "interesting material," were subjected to intense medical scrutiny and photographed before their deaths, adding to the hospital's macabre image archive of patients suffering from gross deformities and far advanced diseases. The hospital also kept a museum of pathological specimens of various organs of the body infected with tuberculosis.[62] But in order to become a teaching hospital for intern and graduate training the Camsell Hospital needed accreditation, a voluntary process of peer review to maintain minimum standards. IHS hoped too that accreditation would "add prestige" to the Camsell Hospital and "ease some of our difficulties in the recruitment of top drawer staff."[63]

Never a terribly rigorous process, hospital accreditation emerged from the realization that "if the health professionals don't police themselves, somebody else will."[64] More self-study than critical evaluation, accreditation required hospitals to complete a questionnaire and (with ample advanced notice) undergo an inspection. The American College of Surgeons conducted hospital accreditation in Canada until 1951, when a joint Canadian and American commission took over inspections. Not until 1959 did organized medicine (Canadian Medical Association, Royal College of Physicians and Surgeons, Association des médecins de langue française du Canada) and the Canadian Hospital Association establish the Canadian Council on Hospital Accreditation. Described as a "low-key enterprise" with only seven staff by the 1970s, the Council had no mechanism for enforcement. As the executive director noted, "We can say 'there's your trouble boys' – and they'll do everything they can to put it right."[65] But accreditation also required hospitals to keep extensive medical records; draft by-laws and regulations for medical staff; hold monthly staff conferences attended by at least 75 per cent of the medical staff; conduct regular nursing staff conferences; and employ registered X-ray and laboratory technicians.[66] But, as Moore well knew, most IHS hospitals fell far short of having enough trained staff for minimal patient care, much less for attending to increased administrative duties.[67] Presumably, though, it was the very absence of administrative and technical departments and employees that allowed the Indian hospitals to operate at half the per diem rates of other hospitals. Acknowledging the futility of attempting to receive accreditation in the other Indian hospitals, IHS agreed that the Camsell Hospital alone would apply for accreditation as a "pilot project."[68] In 1956 Camsell Hospital received a one-year provisional accreditation, and subsequently a three-year accreditation, principally because of its affiliation with the university's medical school, but the Joint Commission warned that it would not again accredit the hospital "unless radical renovations are made eliminating the present fire hazards or a new hospital constructed."[69] By 1958 the Canadian Medical Association recognized it as an approved hospital for postgraduate training in thoracic surgery.[70]

Interns and residents at the Camsell Hospital studied under former superintendent and, after 1950, surgical consultant Dr Herbert Meltzer. As noted, the doctor's stormy relationship with IHS bureaucrats stemmed in part from his concerns over hospital policy. And as a surgeon, Meltzer also clashed with his peers over therapy at a time of profound shifts in how tuberculosis was understood and treated. The "conquest" of tuberculosis is often told as a linear and progressive story, from the early days of long sanatorium stays focused on bed rest, to surgical collapse therapy, and finally to ultimate victory in the advent of effective chemotherapy, but there were no such certainties in Canada in the 1940s and 1950s.[71] From the hospital's opening in 1946, Meltzer as a thoracic surgeon wanted "selective cases": otherwise strong, young, and minimally infected patients who stood a good chance of surviving chest surgery. His immediate superior, Dr E.L. Stone, thought otherwise:

> I would do away with most of the tuberculosis surgery and emphasize the function of the hospital as a place of isolation, that is use it as a means of controlling infection rather than as a place where a few

> selected patients get highly specialized treatment. I am not sure whether the chief result of chest surgery for Indians isn't to produce surgical cripples and eternal dependents … cut down the cost on everything but nursing and feeding.[72]

William Barclay, who performed all the autopsies, "of which there were many," recalled that other doctors on staff were equally troubled by the surgical treatments undertaken "with little or no evidence as to their effectiveness."[73] Nevertheless, chest surgery became fundamental to tuberculosis treatment at the Camsell Hospital. But Meltzer's careful approach, keeping patients in hospital for at least a year after surgery, put him at odds with the hospital superintendent, who pressed Meltzer to perform more surgeries and perform them more quickly once patients were admitted to hospital. Falconer complained that patients were spending too much time in hospital: "This, at present rates, indirectly costs thousands of dollars a year and of course keeps the individual patient occupying a bed longer than can be justified … I do feel that if the surgery service were stepped up, in a year or more we would have more beds available for patients."[74] For his part Meltzer criticized the practice of admitting "chronic bone cases and older-age-group cases" (not suitable for surgery) and filling half the beds with "a permanent population … I maintain, that to use the Camsell as a surgical hospital, it cannot be crowded – let alone overcrowded."[75] But overcrowding was not the only threat to the surgical program.

In 1953 the source of "serious" infections in surgical patients was traced to the practice of keeping the doors open between the hospital's laboratory and the adjacent operating room. Cultures obtained from the air during an operation showed "staphylococci in rather profuse growth."[76] Increasingly frustrated, in 1954 Falconer withdrew from the hospital's administration and replaced Stone, who had retired as IHS superintendent of the Foothills region (Alberta and Northwest Territories). Meltzer's friend and Camsell physician, Dr Matthew Matas, succeeded Falconer as hospital superintendent. With the mild-mannered Matas as hospital superintendent Meltzer declared himself "much happier" and continued to direct the hospital's focus on surgery, though he complained that his meagre consultant's salary was "ridiculous in comparison with the volume of surgery I do."[77] By early 1960 Meltzer, despite his resentment at being overworked and underpaid, would not relinquish his position as chief of surgery at the hospital.[78]

In 1953 Meltzer undertook major chest surgery on 105 of the 350 patients with pulmonary tuberculosis, 68 per cent of all surgeries in the hospital.[79] The most common chest surgery, performed on eighty-seven patients that year, was thoracoplasty, a surgically induced "rest cure" where several ribs were removed to collapse the diseased lung and paraffin wax (plombage) inserted to maintain the collapse and prop up the chest wall. The procedure usually required the removal of seven or eight ribs, but surgeons were reluctant to remove more than two or three at a time, so patients endured several excruciating procedures. By 1953 Meltzer reported that he changed his technique from a two- or three-stage thoracoplasty to a single operation: "As a result, with some increase in our tempo of surgery, we are completing surgery on exactly twice as many patients."[80] Performed under local anaesthesia, the operation was "painful and deforming" according to Dr Barclay.[81] Local rather than general anaesthesia was deemed necessary to maintain the patient's cough reflex to prevent aspiration and the possibility of infecting the other lung. As for the terrified patient, awake and aware of the saw cutting into their ribs, Meltzer claimed, "the argument that patients suffer mental torture under local anesthesia cannot be entertained. Mild hypnosis counteracts mental strain almost completely."[82]

In the five years from July 1949 to August 1954 Meltzer performed thoracoplasty with plombage on 324 patients, reporting "good results after a short follow up" in 314 patients (96.9 per cent); 9 patients were deemed "improved"; 4 patients "relapsed after discharge"; 70 were still in hospital, and 253 were "at home." There were no "early" deaths (as a direct result of the surgery) and only five "late mortalities." As the surgeon explained, "The proof of the pudding is in the eating, and the proof of good results similarly depends on how they are maintained after discharge and under adverse home conditions ... I feel these results justify continuing our present principles of therapy."[83] But with collapse therapy, as Dr E.L. Ross, the longtime medical superintendent of the Sanatorium Board of Manitoba noted in 1953, "about one-third of our patients died, about one-third *half recovered*, and about one-third became cured."[84] Surgery left long, disfiguring scars, the plombage often migrated from its original site creating infection, and patients were left with limited lung function and lifelong deformity – "surgical cripples" as Dr Stone put it.

Admitted to Camsell Hospital as a sixteen-year-old in 1956, Dave Melting Tallow from Siksika (Blackfoot) reserve east of Calgary spent three years on bed rest and antimicrobial medication and, in 1959, underwent lung resection, or the surgical removal of a part of his lung:

> They removed three ribs, and scraped three. And they removed part of my lung. I think that was to access my lung, I'm not sure. But for some reason they took three ribs. Now I've got these stumps in my back on my left side and no ribs there. And the rest of them were scraped. They cut a part of my lung out and I think they put wax in there to hold it together until it healed shut.
>
> They used a saw. I was awake and I could hear the saw. They got part way and then they told me, now we're breaking the ribs off. They said, get ready, then they broke the ribs off. When they did that it felt like somebody hit you inside the chest. And they did that three times. When they broke it off that's when it hurt. Felt like somebody hit me with a fist inside my chest. I just heard the saw buzzing away and cutting stuff. I could hear it inside me, but there was no pain really until they broke them off. And I didn't even really feel them taking a part of my lung off. That's what they said they did. I didn't feel any of that.[85]

He recovered from his surgery, and at seventy years of age in 2010 reported only occasional shortness of breath, but he was particularly bothered by the suggestion made by a physician who examined him years later that perhaps he had been the subject of medical experimentation, a disturbingly frequent charge made by former Aboriginal patients that will be examined in greater detail later. As a thoracic surgeon, Meltzer continued to cut into chests to treat pulmonary tuberculosis precisely because effective antibiotics ensured greater success in surgically excising even the smallest area of infection.[86]

Another elder – Roy Little Chief, also from Siksika – after twelve years at residential school suffered a haemorrhage in 1956 and was admitted to Charles Camsell Hospital. He spent nearly a year in hospital and understood that the only way out of the hospital was to have surgery: "So this was my life in there for eleven and half months. And what we were told there by the other patients was, the only way you'd get out of the hospital is for you to have surgery." His surgery was performed under local anaesthetic "I got on the operating table and then they started putting needles in me. Probably to freeze my back and I remember coming to, I was facing down and I felt … when they were cutting it open and then I felt hot water on my back. It must have been the blood coming out. And I heard the doctors say, there's blood."[87]

For IHS physicians, surgery seemed to offer certainty in the uncertain world outside the hospital: patients could be returned to their still-impoverished homes with less chance of relapse; or they might be encouraged to integrate into society as cured (with the scars to prove it), posing little threat to the public. Dave Melting Tallow chose neither. After a brief rehabilitation attending school in Edmonton, he left for the United States, travelling, working, and enjoying freedom from the surveillance of Indian agents, police, teachers, and physicians in a society that chose instead to isolate and segregate African Americans.

Thoracic surgery, made more daring and heroic with effective antibiotics in the 1940s and 1950s, did not easily give way to the new chemotherapy regime, particularly for Aboriginal patients. In Manitoba IHS contracted with the private corporation Sanatorium Board of Manitoba to provide tuberculosis treatment for Aboriginal patients in three segregated institutions: Dynevor Indian Hospital near Winnipeg, the former American military hospital at Clearwater Lake at The Pas in northern Manitoba, and the redundant Brandon Military Hospital.[88] The arrangement relieved IHS of providing tuberculosis treatment while providing the Sanatorium Board with a steady income of more than $800,000 annually.[89] Treatment at Dynevor and Clearwater Lake Indian hospitals consisted of bed rest, while patients requiring surgery were transferred to what became known as the Brandon Indian Hospital. Dr Arthur Povah, a 1945 medical graduate who contracted tuberculosis and spent a year in Ninette Sanatorium as a patient, continued his association with tuberculosis as chest surgeon at Brandon.[90] The 260-bed hospital, owned by the Department of Health and Welfare, but operated by the Sanatorium Board, treated Manitoba Aboriginal people and, increasingly after 1950, Inuit patients. By 1953 Povah noted that in his practice "pulmonary resection [surgical removal of a section of lung or the complete organ] has pretty well replaced other surgical procedures for the treatment of tuberculosis and arrangements have been made to do three of these operations every two weeks."[91] And though antibiotic treatment at Brandon increased by 1956, the rate of chest surgery increased nearly threefold, from six surgeries per month in 1953 to sixteen pulmonary resections per month three years later.[92] By 1959 Brandon Indian Hospital's patients were transferred to the once exclusively white Manitoba Sanatorium (Ninette) for surgery, and the former Indian hospital, renamed the Assiniboine Hospital, was renovated for the chronic care of white patients "of slightly more refined tastes" by adding new beds, dressers, night tables, and curtains.[93]

Canada only slowly followed the trend in other jurisdictions away from surgery towards a greater reliance on chemotherapy alone. The "tuberculosis trade" was reluctant to change. As Sanatorium Board of Manitoba's Dr E.L. Ross put it, "tuberculosis is an aggressive disease and demands aggressive and bold measures to combat it. Antimicrobial therapy has opened the door for definitive (excisional) therapy [surgery] and in a few years we will, no doubt, have a much better understanding of what should be excised and what can be safely left."[94] By 1956, American sanatoria, or at least those represented at Wisconsin's Pembine Conference, embraced chemotherapy to a much greater extent than Manitoba practice, which continued to rely on surgery. Ross admitted that the Sanatorium Board was not continuing drug treatment long enough: "We need to accept the fact that post-sanatorium chemotherapy is a phase of the overall treatment program, but, of course, not a substitute for sanatorium ... our indications for resection are fairly aggressive [compared to American practice]."[95] In 1959, British specialist Dr P.E. Baldry from Middlesex toured Canadian sanatoria, where he found a disturbing number of surgeries because, he said, there was not the "same confidence placed in long term chemotherapy" in Canada. He expressed surprise at the continued practice of lung resections for small foci of infection, while noting with approval that most sanatoria undertook far less surgery than in previous years. Baldry also noted that Canadian sanatorium doctors have "little faith in their patients and by British standards separate them from their homes for rather long periods."[96] And an increasing number of patients in sanatoria were Aboriginal.

For instance, in Saskatchewan in 1953 the superintendent of nurses at the Prince Albert Sanatorium noted the institution was filled to capacity with 270 to 280 patients daily, "a little less than one quarter of these being white people, which is further proof that we are winning our battle against tuberculosis among the whites." The other patients were Aboriginal.[97] The Mountain Sanatorium in Hamilton, Ontario, with 753 beds (126 vacant) in 1956 was home to 332 Inuit patients; a year later there were only Aboriginal patients in the institution.[98] As the unfortunately named Dr A.L. Paine, medical superintendent at Manitoba Sanatorium, explained, "More white patients with residual minimal lesions are being treated conservatively, though resection is still favoured to prevent relapse in those of Indian blood."[99] Paine undertook what he called "salvage surgery," or lung resections to reduce the perceived risk of relapse once Aboriginal patients returned home.[100] In Canada generally, surgical treatment for tuberculosis outpaced both American and British practice, while Aboriginal patients underwent chest surgery to a greater extent than other Canadians. As patients who continued to be viewed as careless in their own health, posing an ongoing threat to the national health, and subject to relapse in their "adverse home conditions," Aboriginal patients underwent more aggressive treatment.

Long-term hospitalization in sanatoria continued even after Aboriginal patients received the benefits of chemotherapy treatment. For most non-Aboriginal patients outpatient chemotherapy treatment was increasingly the norm in the 1950s, leading to what the Canadian Tuberculosis Association called the "miracle of the empty beds." As inpatient populations fell, costs per patient rose, prompting many sanatoria to close and transfer patients to centralized institutions. In Manitoba the Sanatorium Board closed the segregated Indian hospitals at Dynevor in 1957, Brandon in 1959, and Clearwater Lake in 1965, transferring all patients to the Manitoba Sanatorium. In 1956 the medical superintendent at Ontario's Fort William Sanatorium, facing falling patient populations and rising costs, wondered if some Aboriginal patients from Manitoba could be transferred to his institution, but with more than 500 available beds, Manitoba refused.[101] At the same time, IHS policy was "not to treat Indian tuberculous patients on an out-patient basis in view of the fact that we cannot supervise their activities very closely while they are at home and in the majority of cases their medication would not be taken regularly. The Indian people, at the present time, do not have the educational background for home therapy of active tuberculosis."[102] In Saskatchewan, after 1965 the Anti-TB League that operated the provincial sanatoria assumed treatment for Aboriginal patients. As the League's general superintendent reported in that year, the average length of treatment for non-Aboriginal patients decreased from the previous year, from 10.11 months to 8.63 months; for Indian patients the average length of treatment increased from 14.41 months in 1964 to 17.93 months in 1965. "As the proportion of Indian patients increase the average length of treatment in Sanatorium will increase, as we normally treat Indian patients longer in Sanatorium in order to ensure that they receive adequate chemotherapy."[103]

Manitoba maintained a similar policy. The Sanatorium Board's Dr Paine explained in 1967: "Until recently patients of native extraction were kept in sanatorium for the entire period of drug taking [one to two years]."[104] At the same time, with the advent of national hospital insurance in the late 1950s, IHS was attempting to close many of its Indian hospitals and "get out of the hospital business."[105] With empty beds to fill, and patients with little power to influence their own treatment, sanatoria continued to institutionalize Aboriginal patients far from their homes and families. Moreover, the practice aided considerably the Sanatorium Board's financial health. In 1965 it received $680,730 from IHS for the treatment of Aboriginal patients.[106] Interestingly, Paine reckoned that treatment policy changed because of an altered "native psychology" and a "more responsible attitude" from a "fatalistic acquiescence of this situation to active demand for earlier discharge to drugs at home as is commonly practiced in white patients."[107] While Aboriginal demands for a voice in treatment predate the late 1960s, home treatment was certainly prompted by the desire to close the increasingly dilapidated and expensive institutions. Sanatoria across the country closed in the late 1960s; the province closed the Manitoba Sanatorium in 1972 and put it up for sale the next year.[108]

Treatment for Aboriginal people was determined by medical perceptions of an essentialized "Indian" patient as irresponsible and reckless, requiring the surveillance and discipline that institutions provided. Meanwhile, the appalling conditions on many reserves – overcrowded homes and inadequate infrastructure that bred much disease – were allowed to remain essentially unchanged (though ex-patients were sometimes provided with extra food rations for six months after discharge.) Indeed, these "adverse home conditions" justified institutionalization in dangerously crowded wards while surgeons, emboldened by antibiotics, continued to open Aboriginal chests as the price to be paid in order to leave the institutions and no longer pose a threat to the national health. As a humanitarian effort to extend the benefits of modern medical care, there could be little room for criticism or complaint. There were clear parallels to residential schools, where, despite the acknowledged poor conditions and worse treatment, children were presumed to be better off than under the care of their purportedly unfit parents in unfit homes. Many students in residential schools, "agencies for the spread of tuberculosis," graduated to Indian hospitals.[109] Institutions of confinement, increasingly seen as necessary and a normal environment for Aboriginal people, continued to damage families and communities. But Indian hospitals also promised to become "training centres for Indian health workers," according to the deputy minister, and while Aboriginal employees became integral to the operation of the institutions, they rarely rose above the least-skilled and most poorly paid positions.

Chapter Three

Everyone in Their Place: Labour in the Indian Hospitals

It is proposed to make every effort to train Indians as doctors, nurses and sick attendants wherever possible. It is felt that the true interests of the Indian will best be served when they are taking an active part in looking after their own people. This may be taken as a necessary part of the development, which is essential to the well being of the Indians. What must be done is to encourage their natural pride in their own race and customs while at the same time learning the ways of life, which will enable them to live in association with the white man.[1]

– Brooke Claxton, minister of National Health and Welfare, 1946

The Indian hospitals' first "cardinal policy" – that no effort or reasonable cost should be spared to give patients the best hospital care – was, as we have seen, rather loosely interpreted. The second cardinal policy, that the hospitals should function as a training ground for Aboriginal health workers, was never seriously pursued. Minister Claxton's qualified promise in 1946 to make "every effort" to train Aboriginal health workers rang hollow from the outset. While some Aboriginal registered nurses and aides who trained elsewhere found employment in the hospitals, most workers, without formal training, struggled to advance beyond the least-skilled and lowest-paid positions, yet this Aboriginal staff made up a significant segment of IHS support personnel. The professional ranks were initially dominated by an enthusiastic group of Canadian-born male physicians and female nurses whose careers had been interrupted by Depression and war, and managed by a small bureaucracy of their physician peers. But soon enough, doctors found few opportunities for career advancement outside of the quickly growing IHS bureaucracy itself. Moreover, as state investment in national hospital infrastructure and health care increased exponentially in the postwar years, nurses and other staff were drawn to better positions elsewhere. However, state investment in IHS failed to keep pace, creating constant turmoil in staffing the Indian hospitals. Some European refugee physicians, so-called "DP doctors" (displaced persons) found temporary work, but IHS professional staff was overrepresented by those either at the beginning or near the end of their careers. Patient care was seriously compromised by often dedicated, but poorly trained, underpaid, and overworked staff.

In 1946, Dr Stone, regional IHS superintendent, advised the medical director at Charles Camsell Hospital that support staff recruiting should begin with recovered patients, specifically, "a reliable middle aged Indian woman" who might form the nucleus of the Indian staff, but, he warned, "do *not* try to use recent graduates of Indian Residential schools. They are too young." He might well have mentioned that female residential school graduates rarely had more than a grade eight education, and of course no medical training. Though Stone thought the Camsell Hospital might eventually establish a graduate nurse-training program, it never materialized.[2] The few Aboriginal registered nurses (RN) who worked in the Indian hospitals took their training in accredited programs at provincial institutions, despite very limited support from Indian Affairs and discrimination in the educational system and society generally.[3] Many Aboriginal nursing students entered training specifically to work in their own communities but were often passed over for the positions since Indian agents fretted that by returning women to reserves they would undergo a cultural regression when faced with supposedly perilous social influences. After all, the state policy of integration presumed that Aboriginal RNs would take their skills and fade into the urban Canadian landscape, not return to reserves. As historian Mary Jane McCallum argues, "It was assumed that medical services for Aboriginal people would be delivered by those same agents who also provided the army, the police, the education system, the missions and in many ways regulated the lives of Aboriginal people – the State and the Church."[4] IHS preferred instead to hire non-Aboriginal registered nurses, and when few applied, they recruited overseas. Historian Laurie Meijer Drees argues that IHS "did little to encourage or recruit" Aboriginal people into formal health care roles providing instead sporadic on the job training for service positions.[5] Though the Indian hospitals failed to offer training, many Aboriginal women enrolled in provincial Registered Nurse Assistant and Licensed Practical Nurse programs and found work with IHS. These programs, requiring a grade eight education, appealed to Indian Affairs policies of low academic standards with a focus on manual or vocational training for Aboriginal people. Two programs in the west provided courses specifically for Aboriginal women that required candidates to take a preliminary two-month training period in IHS hospitals to determine their "fitness and aptitude" for the course.[6] Training Aboriginal workers for semi-skilled and low-paying positions rather than for professional or para-professional careers resulted in part from the state's limited commitment to health care, which it characterized as a moral rather than a legal obligation. Despite pledges to do so, the IHS would not commit to the long-term investment that formal career training required.[7] It is also clear, however, that the hierarchical, paternalistic, and physician-dominated IHS bureaucracy perceived Aboriginal participation as limited to the role of patient or ex-patient, such as Stone's "reliable middle aged Indian woman." It is safe to say that those who rose above service roles in the hospitals did so in spite of, not because of, IHS policies.

Scholars of colonialism and medicine, examining local participation, especially the role of "subordinates and intermediaries" in the health work of empire, draw attention to their significance in translating across language and cultural barriers.[8] Working as aides, maids, domestics, kitchen help, orderlies, drivers, and janitors, Aboriginal employees acted as unpaid translators and cultural brokers, providing comfort and support for patients.[9] But hospital employees, women trained to wash and scrub, were also assumed to carry the benefits of Western medicine back to their communities, which were still supposedly mired in "backward" and "superstitious" notions of health care. Percy Moore observed that in his travels he found that women who had been patients or maids in hospitals lived in the best-kept reserve homes.[10] Moreover, IHS deemed the labour itself as valuable instruction in self-discipline and self-improvement. Vocational training as X-ray and laboratory assistants was also most often provided in terms of rehabilitation.[11] Indeed, as IHS claimed, "as soon as our patients are able, they engage in rehabilitation employment around the hospital."[12] The discourse of employment as improvement and rehabilitation also served to justify low wages.[13]

Minnie Aodla Freeman, born in 1936 in an Inuit community on Cape Hope Island in James Bay, worked for a time in a hospital in Fort George. After she became ill herself, she was sent to Moose Factory

Indian hospital on the James Bay shore, then to Hamilton's Mountain Sanatorium. "No preparation, no warning, no choice, and no reason given why [we] had to go so far away to be cured. One afternoon we boarded the train to Hamilton."[14] Though she was on strict bed rest for a "spot" on her left lung, with her knowledge of English she was quickly recruited as a translator for the staff. She resented being "shipped like cargo and meant to behave like cargo."[15] In 1952, after a year in hospital sixteen-year-old Freeman expected to be released, but instead she was offered work at the Mountain Sanatorium as a translator. Living in the nurses' residence, she was put to work on the children's ward and once a week read anatomy texts with a nurse, but she was expected to drop everything when she was needed as a translator. "The nurses and doctors spoke to me only when they needed a translator. Otherwise I was different and strange to them ... I saw and I heard. I never made known my feelings or frustrations."[16] She left after two years. Back in Moose Factory, Freeman hoped to find a job, and since the Hudson's Bay Company did not hire Aboriginal people, she applied at the Indian hospital. "I went to see the administrator, who had no manners whatever and not one polite word. I could see that he felt very important with himself and was eager to impress the natives with his high and mighty job. He hated his job because there was no one there who understood his importance. He was not listening when I introduced myself."[17] Freeman explained she could type forty words a minute and was also interested in nursing at the hospital. Instead she was offered a position as a live-in domestic for one of the hospital's secretaries. Freeman eventually accepted a position with Indian Affairs as a translator, and in 1957 she was sent to Edmonton to visit and translate for Inuit patients at Charles Camsell Indian Hospital, though no one thought to enquire if she spoke the same dialect. "It was very sad to see all these Inuit. Some had children in the North from whom they had not heard since they arrived. So many worries ... I had never heard the Inuit language of the western Arctic. I tried to speak with some but could not understand. They didn't understand when I spoke to them and yet they seemed so happy to see me. All I could do was return my Inuk smile to let them know that I felt for them."[18] Freeman found herself in the "middle," expected to explain *qallunaat* (non-Inuit) culture to the Inuit, and Inuit culture to the *qallunaat*.[19]

Women from Carry the Kettle First Nation east of Regina recall working as aides in the Fort Qu'Appelle Indian Hospital, where they helped patients navigate the rigid hospital routine: bringing food trays to hungry patients between meal times; visiting with lonely patients despite hospital policy; accepting an elder's choice not to take their medications.[20] Grace Anderson from Fairford Reserve (Pinaymootang) worked as a nurse's aide at Clearwater Lake Indian Hospital at The Pas, Manitoba, in the early 1960s. Anderson, struck by the rigid social and professional hierarchies among the staff, recollected that the British doctor and head nurse remained completely aloof from the Aboriginal aides. "These people [non-Aboriginal staff] were just functioning from day to day, same thing day in and day out. There were no pictures on the wall, there were no plants anywhere, nothing to give you a feeling of anything pleasant. It was, as they use the word, sterile and foreign, uncaring to put it plainly."[21] The strict racial divisions among staff had not changed much from the hospital's early postwar years when "white girls" employed as aides refused to room with young Aboriginal staff. The hospital built cubicles in the army barracks for the "Indian girls," reserving the maids' quarters for white staff.[22] The patients, by the 1960s almost exclusively Inuit, struggled to communicate with anyone in the hospital, though a Cree nurse's aide managed to interpret to a limited extent. Anderson worked in the seventy-two-bed women's ward where patients kept busy sewing mukluks from duffel, no doubt destined for federal employees in the north. Never allowed outside, the mostly Catholic Inuit patients' grim existence was relieved by Sunday prayers. An old accordion provided some entertainment, Anderson recalled, "But the other nurses wouldn't allow them, but when I was in charge working evenings I allowed them to dance ... And they did square dancing and that was the high, very great thing. They would come and hug me."[23] The women arrived at the hospital with nothing beyond the clothes on their backs, Anderson recalled, without toiletries and only a few combs for the whole ward to share, yet each patient was provided with a clock, so they might learn the value of time. Aboriginal employees, like Anderson, aided and also resisted IHS plans while creating a healthy space in the institutions that eased anxious and vulnerable patients. A significant if rarely acknowledged fact in the Indian hospitals was that Aboriginal workers accounted for up to 15 per cent of the IHS workforce by the 1960s.[24] Racialized and professional hierarchies rendered them all but invisible in the documentary record.[25] Despite the limitations and low expectations placed on Aboriginal workers, they were fundamental to the hospitals' operations while rendering Indian hospitals less foreign for patients.

The hospitals also provided workers with a relatively stable though meagre income. As a teenager Frank Malloway spent nearly three years at Coqualeetza Indian Hospital at Sardis, British Columbia, with pleurisy, misdiagnosed as tuberculosis. He returned to the hospital in 1954 and trained to be a nursing orderly; he worked for four years on shiftwork and six more years on permanent night shift. He recalled that it was "a good place to work. There was a lot of Natives working there ... All the medical staff that I remember were white people. There was no Indian nurses. They had Indian ward aides, there was no Indian nurses." He met his wife, who also worked at the hospital, and when they started a family he worked the night shift, which allowed him to spend time with his children during the day.[26] In 1964 Frank left hospital work for better wages as a logger.

At the Fort Qu'Appelle Indian Hospital, Agnes Cyr worked in the laundry and the sewing room for more than twenty-five years until her retirement in 1977. Born in 1912, she had attended Lebret School for only two and a half years when she was sent home to the Pasqua reserve to care for her blind mother and younger siblings. Her early life spent managing a household and farm during the Depression taught her hard work and disappointment, as she planted gardens only to watch them blow away in the dustbowl. As a parent she made "darned sure" that her children got an education. Her daughter trained as a registered nurse in Saskatoon and worked in Toronto; her son trained as an X-ray and laboratory technician. At the hospital Cyr worked in the laundry and as a seamstress turning huge bolts of flannelette into baby clothes, diapers, "little dresses, lots of things, little vests for newborns." It was clean and quiet work, "the best part of my life when I was there. We always enjoyed each other's company. And the staff – the nursing staff – well in fact everybody was really good. We all got along." She admitted that the wages were never very good and that much of her income was spent on car payments "so I could get to work. I made sure it [the car] was brand new. I enjoyed them. If I wanted to go somewhere I'd just get in the car and go" (she gave up driving at the age of 93). In the evening her husband then drove to Regina for his night shift as a heavy-duty mechanic.[27] Their long service suggests that, for these workers, caring for community members even in a restricted capacity was meaningful and rewarding work. Though a valuable source of waged work, the hospitals might have been the means to develop Aboriginal professionals and administrators to interpret and control the delivery of health care. But, despite the minister's qualified 1946 promise to provide training "wherever possible," it was obvious to IHS medical bureaucrats that only they could know what was "essential to the well-being of the Indians."

All the Indian hospitals struggled to maintain even the most basic nursing service in the 1950s. A rapidly increasing national demand for health care, and specifically hospital services, and a 40 per cent increase in patient loads from 1950 to 1955 alone, resulted in serious nursing shortages across the country. The strong demand for their services allowed registered nurses and their provincial associations to press for improved wages and working conditions. In 1947, for instance, the Manitoba Association of Registered Nurses advised that nursing shortages in hospitals resulted from "instability" in nurses' employment, or staff turnover. Hospitals, it recommended, should improve nurses' living quarters, which were often just small bedrooms in the hospital building itself; reduce hours of work from the common 48 hours to 44 hours per week; provide regular, scheduled time off; and increase salaries. "A satisfied staff is a stable staff." The Manitoba association reported that hospital nurses were often underpaid and that salaries should be adequate to provide security and "commensurate with the value of her service to the community."[28] It was a competitive market for nurses' services and the IHS, in the interests of efficiency, hired fewer registered nurses and relied increasingly on the cheaper labour of ward aides and inexperienced "Indian maids" to staff the hospitals. Faced with persistent staff turnover, hospital superintendents – civil servants with limited autonomy in a highly centralized bureaucracy – could do little but plead for improvements in salaries and working conditions. All Indian hospitals struggled with "instability" in their professional staff, but some were worse than others.

Miller Bay Indian Hospital, an air force hospital on British Columbia's north coast thirteen kilometres from Prince Rupert, was hastily built in anticipation of a long Pacific war but was never used, and became redundant before war's end. Certainly the influx of wartime American and Canadian military personnel disrupted Aboriginal communities throughout the northwest through the severe epidemics of infectious disease that followed the building of the Alaska Highway and the Canol pipeline.[29] But the urgent necessity for an Indian hospital in the Prince Rupert area stemmed from the apparent threat that local Aboriginal people posed to citizens and the troops. A 1944 petition from the Prince Rupert board of health and concerned citizens, calling themselves the Community Council Association, demanded protection from "infected natives [that] act as a reservoir of infection for other people."[30] Local hospitals refused to admit active cases of tuberculosis or venereal disease, and were already full. Claiming that tuberculosis went untreated, and that "80 per cent of alleged sources of venereal disease reported to local health authorities in 1943 were native women," the petitioners urged the federal government to open an Indian hospital at Miller Bay. Citing the petition, the minister responsible for Indian Affairs, Thomas Crerar, explained to minister of National Defence J.L. Ralston the danger of untreated tuberculosis: "More urgent still, there are some 28 Indian women who have been reported as sources of venereal disease. This is a distinct hazard to troops in the area."[31] Crerar had in mind the vacant and fully equipped seventy-five-bed army hospital across the street from the Prince Rupert General Hospital. Instead, the more remote and unequipped Miller Bay Hospital became available.

At the hospital's official opening in September 1946, local dignitaries, politicians, and the press toured the institution, hailing it as the "most modern tubercular unit in the Dominion." Aboriginal leaders such as Mr and Mrs Henry McKay of Greenville (Laxgalts'sp), Leonard Leighton of Metlakatla, and Henry Kelly, councillor for the Tsimshian at Port Simpson (Lax Kw'alaams), attended the opening. Kelly spoke of the hospital as a "milestone along the road of progress in the new deal promised by the government of Canada for my people."[32] Long excluded from local hospitals and left without treatment, Aboriginal communities welcomed the prospect of improved health care. But the government's extension of medical services cannot be separated from its larger colonializing project to isolate Native people in the interests of settler society. Dr W.S. Barclay, inspecting local conditions for IHS, recommended the Miller Bay institution, noting that it would "go a long way to quieting any criticism and of course would provide a certain amount of supervision and actual hospital care."[33] This neat summary of the institution's usefulness, in order of importance, reflected the broader IHS raison d'être, where community and national safety required the close surveillance and "actual care" of Aboriginal bodies. The bureaucracy's wildly uncharacteristic alacrity in establishing the hospital signalled the intensity of danger that Aboriginal illness suddenly posed to national health and military vigour; the enemy was already among them. Regardless, with its promise of renewed health for Aboriginal communities and a tangible recognition of government responsibility for health care, the hospital was welcomed, as Kelly put it, as "the new deal promised."

A one-storey flat-roofed olive green building, the hospital was perched on rocky terrain surrounded by muskeg soil. Staff residences in adjacent buildings contained small bedrooms for nurses and larger dormitories for Aboriginal maids. With its brown battleship linoleum and light green walls, the institution retained a distinctly drab military appearance (illustration 3.1). For patients, whose families and friends found it difficult to visit, it was dreary if not a dangerous place. Most of the hospital's beds were in two large dormitory wards, each with one nurse to care for seventy-five patients, ranging from children to adults. Not unexpectedly, it became difficult to find nurses to work in such conditions for the same wages that they could demand in city hospitals, a situation predicted during the hospital's hurried planning stages. As Barclay had warned, the hospital would require trained nurses to carry out the separate technique for hospitalized venereal disease, as "this could not be delegated even to ward aides."[34] By 1949 the hospital superintendent complained that poor IHS salaries resulted in "a large proportion of inferior nurses who for lack of provincial registration are unable to secure positions elsewhere." Better wages and working conditions might attract "a better type of nurse."[35] The alternatives seemed clear enough: either reduce patient admissions or increase nurses' salaries to attract qualified candidates. But Miller Bay, already one of the least efficient of the larger Indian hospitals, judging by its $4.88 per patient per day costs, could ill afford to close beds. It was clear to director Percy Moore and to all Indian hospital medical superintendents that "considerable use will have to be made of "Practical Nurses" if patient strength is to be kept high."[36] Indeed, the next year the hospital increased its capacity from 158 to 172 beds, further reducing its per diem costs.[37]

The staffing problems only increased. Advocating in 1951 for a special living allowance to attract nurses, Miller Bay's medical superintendent Dr J.D. Galbraith suggested that few nurses were interested in tuberculosis nursing, fewer still in nursing Indians, though he allowed that Nanaimo Indian Hospital on Vancouver Island did not suffer the same shortages as Miller Bay. Increasingly frustrated, he pleaded with Ottawa: "We simply have to get some more graduate nurses immediately." Later that year, after two more nurses resigned, the situation was described as "desperate."[38] Of twenty registered nurse positions, eight were filled by RNs, five by ward aides, and seven remained vacant. Moreover, labour shortages in service positions, principally Aboriginal maids and janitors, occurred regularly as the local canneries'

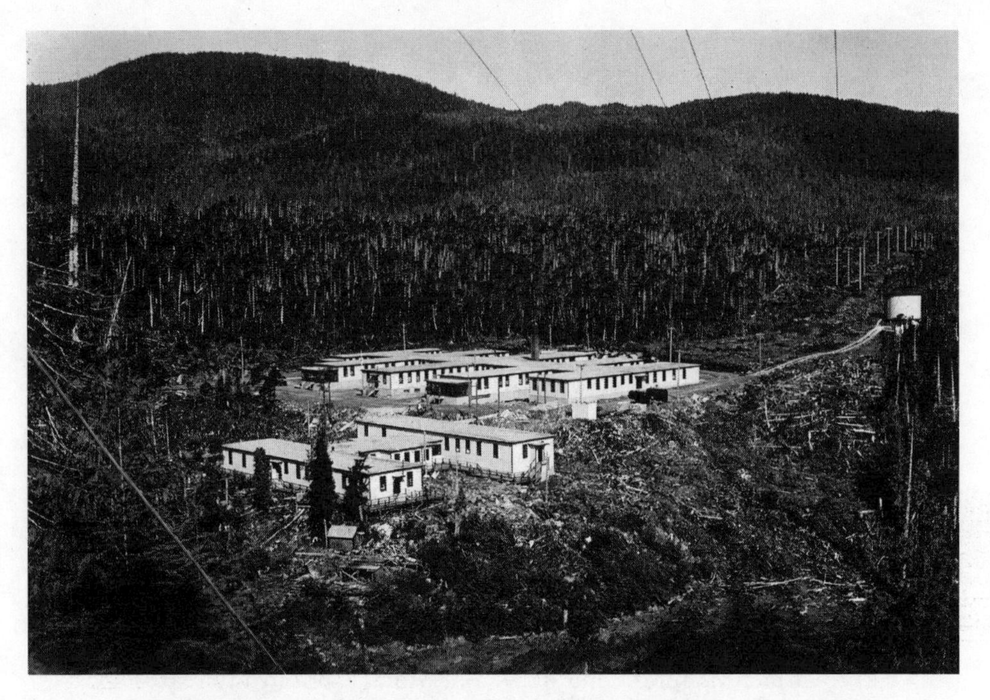

Illustration 3.1 Miller Bay Indian Hospital, near Prince Rupert, BC, 1947. Carved out of the bush thirteen kilometres from Prince Rupert, Miller Bay Indian Hospital's isolation made life difficult for patients and staff.

Source: Prince Rupert City & Regional Archives & Museum of Northern B.C.; Wrathall collection, JRW1267 acc WP1998-071-17552.

better wages drew workers from the hospital. Low salaries and grim living conditions in the hospital's staff residences, thirteen kilometres from town and without regular transportation, did nothing to encourage staff to remain. Recreation was limited to drinking parties in staff residences. Galbraith worried about the influence such parties would have on the maids "Indian and white," but the hospital's matron (and ex-army nurse) defended the practice, pointing out that the residences were in fact their homes, and "we did it in the army." More worrying was the use of liquor by male staff who lived in one wing of the hospital.[39] When the superintendent prohibited liquor in junior staff residences, they travelled to Prince Rupert's "beer parlours and other questionable spots in the red light district." This was a problem "especially for our Indian maids ... almost every week some of them are jailed." Their crime – drinking in a bar – applied only to Aboriginal workers. As the superintendent complained, the situation not only gave the hospital a bad name, "but leaves us short of staff."[40] A standard RCAF-issue recreation hall was quickly moved to the Miller Bay Hospital grounds and minister of Health and Welfare Paul Martin sent his congratulations on the new facility's opening as a "tangible expression" of the department's sincere appreciation for the staff's "devoted service."[41] Staff might have appreciated higher wages and better working conditions as a more tangible expression of IHS gratitude. Nevertheless, medical superintendent J.D. Galbraith, who left Miller Bay for Coqualeetza Indian Hospital shortly thereafter, suggested that staff discontent seriously impeded hospital operations, translating into a "lack of discipline among the patients."[42]

Discipline, self-imposed or administered by staff when deemed necessary, was considered essential to tuberculosis treatment. Though they were in fact hybrid institutions that included tuberculosis care, Indian hospitals nevertheless operated very much as sanatoria. Graduated degrees of enforced idleness, called "routines" or "classes," from absolute bed rest to limited activity such as walking to the bathroom, to increased movement about the wards, defined classic sanatorium treatment. Patients participated in their own cure, learning self-control, by following the strict rules. Closely regulated, patients followed rigid schedules for bathing, sleeping, and eating; they were told when to cough and how to spit. One sanatorium director put it succinctly: "Everything which is not expressly allowed is forbidden."[43] As historian Alison Bashford argues, the sanatorium was a disciplinary institution, but also instructional – "highly policed but aiming to produce self-policing subjects."[44] In Indian hospitals the disciplinary function predominated since Aboriginal people were deemed to lack the capacity for self-discipline, independence, prudence, and foresight – the attributes of healthy citizenship. Indeed, Indian hospitals as segregated institutions were seen as necessary precisely because Native people were not deemed sufficiently "advanced" to benefit from the sanatorium cure among whites. Prolonged hospitalization and bed rest, even when treatment also included surgery and antibiotics, continued to define the Indian hospitals, where the attributes of self-discipline might be learned. In the highly patriarchal, gendered, and racialized structure of Indian hospitals, the medical superintendent as the authority figure was aided by the nurse matron, who managed the graded ranks of mostly female staff, who in turn tended to patient care and domestic duties. Smooth operation of what historian Kathryn McPherson termed the "hospital household" depended on the firm authority of the medical superintendent.[45] Lack of "patient discipline," engendered by staff turnover, was thus a central preoccupation of Miller Bay's superintendents.

Dr G.R. Howell, himself a former sanatorium patient, replaced Galbraith and in 1954 undertook an investigation into the apparent breakdown in patient discipline, particularly in the women's ward, which, he said, was characterized by "sullenness, lack of co-operation with staff, rule breaking, rudeness," leading to further staff discontent. Wards were overcrowded, with the women's thirty-three-bed Ward B adjoined to the large children's Ward C. Unlike male patients, women were not allowed outside for walks; windows did not operate properly so they were kept shut; there were no privacy screens around beds for patients having bed baths or using bedpans; the whole ward was disciplined if one patient broke the rules; and patients required a note from the medical superintendent to visit one another if they were not close relatives.[46] For the twenty-six boys in Ward A there was one toilet in a bathroom with no window, and, without bedpan sterilizers in the children's wards, infectious hepatitis became a problem.[47] Some minor improvements resulted from Howell's investigation: Wards B and C were divided into two administrative units; privacy curtains were installed in the large adult wards; women were allowed supervised walks on fine days; new patients were to be instructed in hospital rules, especially the use of Kleenex and the importance of bed rest; four nurses were transferred from the women's ward and one resigned. Howell imagined the enquiry itself was cathartic and improved morale.[48] But the superficial reforms did little to improve care for the hospital's 175 patients or the living and working conditions for its 147 employees. One nurse at Miller Bay called the working conditions "extremely primitive."[49]

Continued operational problems prompted another inspection in 1956 that found serious shortages of medical and service staff. On a seasonal basis, local canneries and the fishery continued to attract workers with consistently better wages. The hospital's matron attempted to operate the pharmacy, supervise the kitchen staff, arrange schedules, recruit personnel, and file the endless paperwork required by the centralized IHS bureaucracy, all of which left her with little time to manage the staff. Moreover, with too few trained RNs, ward aides performed nursing duties, and untrained maids acted as ward aides. Howell's deteriorating health meant he was often at home in Prince Rupert while three staff medical officers provided care for 175 patients. One of the officers handled the laboratory work as well as ward duties, though, as the inspector noted, he was "not licensed to practice medicine and probably will not be able to obtain a license."[50] Low staff morale, seen as both cause and consequence of high turnover especially among RNs, made the mood at Miller Bay as gloomy as the wet, grey weather. But, as much as IHS bureaucrats portrayed Miller Bay's problems as a combination of poor patient discipline and even worse management, it is clear that in order to keep patient day costs as low as possible, capable employees were pushed to take on work that was often well beyond the scope of their training. Moreover, patient care would certainly have suffered at the hands of overworked and disgruntled staff. And while IHS accepted the situation as inevitable, the provincial nurses associations did not.

Among the workers at Miller Bay (and in all Indian hospitals) were a number of nurses who could not or would not write the necessary examinations to become registered with the provincial nursing associations. Some had trained at small non-accredited hospitals; others trained at European centres, while others trained at mental hospitals. None were considered qualified for registration. They did the work of hospital RNs, administering medications, inserting catheters, assisting doctors with procedures, and supervising other nurses, while being paid as ward aides or "practical nurses" whose normal duties, while similar to RNs, excluded assisting doctors and inserting anything into patients' bodies.[51] According to the Canadian Nurses Association a ward aide was to be at least eighteen years of age with a grade eight education and have a training course of six to nine months.[52] IHS drew censure from the Canadian Nurses Association for employing ward aides to do the work of RNs, for hiring nurses who could not register in Canada, and, particularly at Miller Bay, for putting ward aides in supervisory positions.[53] The British Columbia Nurses Association stressed its recommendation that "at no time shall a non-registered nurse be placed in the position of supervision or authority over registered nurses."

Throughout the west the IHS was heavily criticized for its employment practices, and in British Columbia, the Nurses Association advised its members against taking positions in IHS hospitals.[54] By 1958, in an effort to appease the nurses associations, IHS in British Columbia deducted $20 from nurses' salaries if they did not maintain their registration. Regional superintendent Dr W.S. Barclay judged that IHS's "reputation as an employing agency has gradually improved" by respecting the provincial nursing standards, but director Percy Moore would not commit to a policy requiring registration in the nursing service: "As far as actual standards of nursing service are concerned it is believed that it can be demonstrated that our sights are high. Also it is believed that comparison with organizations doing similar work is favourable ... within reason, we must and shall do our best to comply with local association requirements."[55] Nevertheless, the following spring the hospital advertised for ten ward aides, "senior high school students and/or other suitable female personnel," to cover registered nurses and ward aide positions vacant because of shortages and summer vacations.[56] Not until the 1960s did the Miller Bay Indian Hospital attempt to provide a training program for Aboriginal women. The six-week course for "Indian girls" who lacked the grade eight education required by schools for ward aide training, aimed to improve the "quality of work done by such applicants, and gives them a valuable insight into hospital ethics and nursing staff procedures."[57]

Saskatchewan fared little better in its attempts to recruit and retain qualified employees at IHS wages. Fort Qu'Appelle Indian Hospital in southern Saskatchewan, further restricted by an unwritten agreement with the bishop that its hospital matron (nurse supervisor) must always be Roman Catholic, did without a supervisor when no acceptable candidates could be found.[58] By July 1952, and without a matron for some time, the hospital hired an experienced (though Protestant) candidate. As the past vice-president of the Saskatchewan Registered Nurses Association, she was seen as "invaluable" in rehabilitating somewhat the IHS's reputation as an employer.[59] Percy Moore conceded that the other federal agency operating hospitals, the Department of Veterans Affairs, required nurses to maintain registration, calling it a "good policy," yet "we are not prepared to say that any nurse entering Indian Health Services must have registration."[60] Moreover, IHS required its staff to work forty-eight hours a week while the norm by 1949 was a forty-four-hour week.[61] Refusing to work under such conditions, Fort Qu'Appelle Indian Hospital's matron resigned after just three months, prompting the medical superintendent to plead, "As she is the only registered nurse on the staff, the matter of obtaining an acting matron of any grade is quite urgent."[62] Three months later the medical superintendent also resigned, leaving the sixty-bed institution without a matron, any RNs, or even a physician. Instead, the provincial sanatorium across Echo

Lake sent a doctor to the Indian hospital "for an hour or two occasionally."[63] IHS hospitals earned a reputation as an employer that ignored professional nursing standards and ethics, and where low wages and long hours taxed a poorly trained and ever-changing staff.

Indian hospitals were not immune to the dramatic increases in health care costs in the postwar decades. Across the country hospital expenditures soared, increasing an astonishing 275 per cent between 1945 and 1954.[64] Indeed, Canadians continued to demand modern hospital care though fewer and fewer could afford the ballooning costs, prompting the Department of National Health and Welfare to establish the 1948 National Health Grants program that matched provincial investments, subsidizing health care for "patients of moderate means." But the same bureaucracy continued to limit the funds available to IHS and Indian hospitals, which simply could not meet the increased costs for labour and services. Patient care, indeed patient safety, in Indian hospitals suffered in the interests of the national health.

The North Battleford Indian Hospital in central Saskatchewan, opened in redundant RCAF barracks at the airport in 1949 with sixty beds, had by 1955 an average daily occupancy of sixty-five patients. In that year IHS director Dr Percy Moore cut hospital staff. According to the Saskatchewan Registered Nurses Association's recommendations, adult patients required 3.2 nursing hours per twenty-four-hour period, while the ratio of registered nurses to non-professional employees (ward aides, nurse's aides, and orderlies) should be 67 per cent to 33 per cent. By those standards the North Battleford Indian Hospital needed thirty-seven staff (twenty-five RNs and twelve non-professionals), yet its already inadequate staff of twenty-four was to be reduced to twenty, including just seven RNs. Matron Jessie Morton advised that the forty pre-school children in the hospital required specialized nursing care that ward aides simply could not perform.[65] Medical superintendent Dr P.W. Head did not see how the hospital could manage its surgical, medical, obstetrical, paediatric, and tuberculosis patients with fewer than eleven RNs.[66] Tragically, but perhaps inevitably, a four-month old baby, admitted with "severe bronchopneumonia," but whose condition according to the physician "could be described as fairly good," was found dead in his crib the next day. With one RN and one aide on the ward of fourteen seriously ill infants, there was neither the time nor the hands to care adequately for the patients. The attending physician reported, "No reasonable explanation could be obtained as to why this baby should die unnoticed." Though he decided there was "a certain amount of negligence on the part of the nurses evidently," he advised that "since most of the babies are very ill the staff in the nurseries is totally inadequate."[67] He recommended two more ward aide positions for the hospital. The matron reported that with a patient increase to seventy, including forty to forty-five infants, "the nursing services are very inadequate" since seriously ill infants required at least five hours of nursing yet with the current staff they were only able to provide two hours each.[68] There is no evidence in the documentary record of any repercussions in the wake of this infant's death. Further, it would be naive to think that this was the only victim of the ruthless economizing at IHS. But aside from replacing the medical superintendent at the hospital, little changed.

Dr Thomas Orford, the new superintendent and a long-serving employee who began his career with IHS during the Depression, bluntly stated that with the staff allotted to the institution, "it is impossible to provide nursing care approaching requirements considered adequate by the American Hospital Association." The minimum standard for all paediatric care was 4.6 hours, while the North Battleford Hospital could barely provide 2.5 hours. Nurses and aides, Orford continued, "are overworked, tired, hurried and tend to become careless. Cross infection is a problem and some of the staff themselves are picking up staphylococcal lesions." To provide a minimum standard of care, the hospital needed at least two more nurses and four more aides, though Orford recognized that nothing would be done in the current year, and "to ask for four more Aide positions would be barking at the moon."[69] Director Moore, using his own formula that he acknowledged was "much more moderate than those generally accepted," calculated that Indian hospitals need only provide 3.2 hours of nursing care; that the ratio of RNs to non-professional staff should be 52 to 48 per cent; and that North Battleford had only sixty beds when in reality there were seventy. And though IHS had acceded to the forty-four-hour workweek, the industry standard was by this time a forty-hour week. On that basis Moore reckoned that North Battleford should have eighteen RNs and seventeen ward aides, or seven new nursing positions and two more aides. But, as he put it, "it is appreciated that it is not possible to obtain all of the positions," and that an attempt should be made to "move toward" filling the vacancies.[70] IHS, however, was allotted a limited number of civil service posts, and any expansion required time-consuming and often fruitless applications to Treasury Board while the civil service commission did the actual hiring. Instead, increasing staff strength in one Indian hospital came at the expense of other hospitals. Staff positions were "borrowed" from one hospital and "lent" to another. Seven years later, by 1965, North Battleford Indian Hospital continued to operate without adequate staff. Borrowing positions from Charles Camsell Hospital in Edmonton and diverting nurses from public health work to the hospital's wards temporarily papered over the problem, but the nursing shortages were chronic and it was obvious to all that poor wages and working conditions continued to hamper recruitment.[71] But by this time IHS, actively working to exit the hospital field altogether by inducing local hospitals to accept Aboriginal patients, began closing wards at North Battleford in response to the labour shortage. That the local community refused to allow the closure, recognizing it as an attempt to abrogate the treaty right to health care, came as unexpected and unwelcome interference in IHS plans, but that story will be treated later.

The same factors that drew nurses away from Indian hospitals – the soaring patient demand for hospital care and the substantial and growing federal interest and investment in national health – created even greater opportunities for physicians in postwar Canada. In 1945 Indian Affairs employed twenty-four full time physicians who became the core group as IHS moved to the Department of National Health and Welfare. It was obvious, however, that in the past Indian Affairs had struggled to attract a full complement of capable physicians; further compounding the problem, it refused to consider women physicians in the service. "Lady doctors are unsuited for dealing with Indian patients and it has never proved satisfactory where we have employed one."[72] Moreover, the 1930s budget cuts had completely discouraged some incumbents. The Edmonton-area reserve physician, described as "wholly useless," diagnosed patients from his car "without as much as going into the house to see the sick person."[73] Though Dr Stone recommended a "clean sweep" to remove some of the worst offenders, the market for ambitious young physicians did not favour IHS. With war's end veterans of the military's medical corps offered better prospects for IHS recruitment, especially with the so-called veteran's preference in civil service employment. But IHS was not the first choice for medical officers and nurses who also had preference for positions at Veterans Affairs and the newly created Department of National Health and Welfare itself. Stone advised that IHS concentrate its efforts on attracting veterans who had never established a private practice and therefore had "nothing to lose" by working in the civil service.[74] As a result, Indian hospitals took on a decidedly military cast, both in personnel and the actual buildings. This cadre of IHS physicians – male, white, and Canadian born; some former Indian Affairs employees and others from the military – rose through the ranks of the new bureaucracy. Creating positions for themselves as they went, the administrative side of the IHS inevitably grew from a string of Indian hospitals with a limited central office to an extensive system of zones and regions that all needed superintendents. But the medical bureaucrats found it increasingly difficult to recruit their own replacements for actual clinical work. Young graduates took positions in IHS hospitals for a year or two, just until they could establish themselves in the booming postwar marketplace for physicians in private practice and modern hospitals. The regional superintendent in British Columbia stated bluntly, "There appears to be little change in the situation here as to the supply of medical men. Experienced doctors are not interested in salaried positions."[75] In his study of the Sioux Lookout Hospital, T. Kue Young observed that there were two kinds of people who worked in Indian hospitals, those looking for a new experience, often with a missionary zeal, and those who could not find employment elsewhere.[76]

Of the latter group, Central European refugee physicians, so-called "DP doctors," could not work in Canada after the Canadian Medical Association refused to recognize their foreign medical credentials. But IHS, increasingly desperate for physicians, took advantage of the opportunity to hire a number of the émigré physicians. At Charles Camsell Hospital, Dr Meltzer proposed that the men be paid as orderlies and the women as ward aides at $150 and $100 per month respectively, though they performed the duties of medical officers.[77] Interestingly, the concerns that occupied IHS administrators were that by having the "DPs occupying positions as orderlies and ward aides, the rights and privileges of Canadian workers might be infringed."[78] However, deputy minister of National Health and Welfare Dr G.D.W. Cameron thought it important to make a distinction between "allowing medically trained persons to use their position of orderly to brush up their medicine and prepare to take qualifying examinations, and employing them as orderlys [*sic*] and using this as a device to get cheap doctors." How such a distinction might be made was not at all clear. Cameron did not think his department could be criticized for doing the former, but "I certainly think we would be putting ourselves in a bad position if we use them to do medical work ordinarily done by a doctor unless it is impossible for us to secure the services of a Canadian doctor."[79]

A year later eight émigrés (along with a woman doctor and a Korean) remained employed at Charles Camsell Hospital; though now deemed medical officers, they were all paid on a "voucher" or casual basis at rates well below the lowest pay grade. Administrators continued to worry that organized medicine might censure the practice of hiring "displaced persons who probably sought entry to Canada on grounds other than their medical qualifications," but recognized that "we get good value for our money in such cases." So long as the positions with IHS remained casual and carried no security of employment for the doctors, the Canadian Medical Association looked the other way.[80]

Unlicensed doctors shouldered much of the medical work in IHS hospitals. At Miller Bay Indian Hospital in 1951 medical superintendent JD Galbraith struggled to provide care to 175 patients. With "two displaced doctors and myself, the matter of medical coverage is spread as thin as it can possibly go." Admitting that considerable medical work was not done at all, Galbraith also pointed out that with "two DP medical doctors, a DP dentist, and a DP eye specialist here at the present moment, it is pretty evident that professional staff simply can't be attracted to this hospital at present salary rates." But aside from low salaries, tuberculosis work did not attract many professionals after the war. "They [interns] consider it to be a very limited specialty which most people seem to want to avoid."[81] Galbraith continued to press for "a fully qualified Canadian doctor" at Miller Bay, complaining, "We have just about reached the saturation point with DP's; they are so very helpless when it comes to dealing with behaviour and discipline problems on the wards."[82] Recall how Miller Bay, also beset by staff problems for placing ward aides in supervisory nursing positions, identified patient discipline problems as both cause and consequence of its seemingly chronic "low morale." Not surprisingly, most of the émigré professionals left the service as soon as they qualified for Canadian licences. By 1953, and with only one physician to help him, Galbraith admitted that medical work had all but stopped; even the laboratory closed when the "DP doctor," paid as a "lab boy," left.[83] And yet, even given the serious shortages of medical help, fully qualified women doctors were still denied consideration.

As Moore explained regarding an application to Miller Bay in 1955, "We are not anxious to take female doctors on for continuous employment but if [a female physician] were to be available for two or three months she might be useful."[84] IHS also employed unlicensed doctors to provide care on reserves and small communities. One physician, though "not qualified," was a "very able man and is willing to go on any special duties required of him."[85] Despite the impact on patient care, the arrangement was mutually beneficial: IHS exploited the labour of unlicensed doctors for much less than the market demanded, while at least some of the unqualified physicians earned a modest income while learning English and preparing for licensing examinations. But displaced persons were not the only unqualified medical men working for IHS. Well into the 1960s, an unqualified anaesthetist working at Charles Camsell Hospital "demonstrated an incompetence in administering the modern type of controlled anaesthesia." Dr Meltzer attributed at least two anaesthetic deaths at the Camsell Hospital to the unqualified doctor, calling him a "very great and unnecessary hazard."[86]

When the superintendent of Charles Camsell Indian Hospital described the staffing situation as "not healthy" he referred not to patient care, but to the impact of surging private practice incomes on IHS physicians. Dr Falconer judged that senior medical officers, not willing to lose the benefits of superannuation, "see and hear of medical officers younger than themselves making two and three times their salary in private practice ... so in all it is not a healthy situation [and] ... leads to a feeling of frustration and results in the classic picture of a Civil Servant who watches the clock and looks forward to his holidays."[87] Moreover, given the great opportunities in private medical practice, IHS bureaucrats viewed with deep suspicion the motivations of any well-qualified applicants to its service. Falconer wondered about one young surgical intern recommended to him. "From bitter past experience we are a bit skeptical of referred medical officers with high qualifications who are recommended to this region. We would like to question why, if he has a Fellowship, is he seeking employment in government service when it is understood they can do so much better in private practice, particularly when he is apparently presently in private practice."[88]

At a time when most non-Aboriginal patients with pulmonary tuberculosis underwent chemotherapy treatment alone, Charles Camsell Hospital's continued program of chest surgery seemed to offer opportunities for surgical interns not available elsewhere. While he received a number of letters of enquiry from candidates, Falconer complained that most were only interested in surgical work. He reluctantly recommended applications from non-citizens, in particular, "a Chinese boy ... I think we must make the best of a bad situation and try and employ people who are available."[89] Though patient care was surely compromised, only rare references to negligence, or worse, exist in the documentary record.

At the Lady Willingdon Hospital on the Six Nations reserve unlicensed physicians created dangerous situations for patients. The two-storey, twenty-bed institution built with band funds in 1927, was expanded to fifty-four beds in 1954. Six Nations continued to pay the doctor's salary until this mid-century expansion when IHS took over all costs and medical direction. The long-serving superintendent, Dr Walter Davis, graduated from University of Toronto medical school, and in 1914 began work at the Six Nations reserve, staying thirty-five years until his retirement in 1950. Not Aboriginal, but raised on the reserve after his parents abandoned him as an infant on the doorstep of a Six Nations family, Davis was a popular, respected, and active community member. Describing Davis in 1966, reserve residents told anthropologist Sally Weaver: "People didn't consider him a white man. He was one of us."[90] His reputation as an esteemed community resident arose from his respect for the traditional medical and cultural beliefs of the Longhouse people. Encouraging a medical syncretism, the doctor often advised patients to combine Indigenous and Western medicine.[91] With Davis's retirement in 1950, hospital expansion, and closer IHS control of medical operations, the community became increasingly critical of the quality of IHS physicians and the medicine they practised. The stability of Davis's tenure ended abruptly as no less than twenty-nine different physicians served the reserve in the next sixteen years, nineteen of whom were born and trained outside of Canada. Reserve residents, aware that some of the doctors were unlicensed, understood that the physicians were "second rate" and would not be allowed to work in white hospitals. Weaver found "the not infrequently expressed belief that the physicians are using the Indian people as 'guinea pigs.'"[92] Writing in 1967, the anthropologist accepted uncritically the IHS position that community criticisms of the quality of care stemmed not from inadequately trained personnel, but from the people's inability to adapt to, or understand, changed medical practices. However, Dr Davis's replacement as medical superintendent, Dr J.H. Wiebe, also expressed, in confidence, deep concerns about the quality of the hospital's medical officers well before a 1954 incident of negligence causing death.

In June 1953 Wiebe called the need for "fully qualified" medical officers "urgent." He complained that his current staff needed supervision at every step, and their difficulty with the (English) language caused "undesirable repercussions" among the reserve residents. Wiebe recommended to director Moore the need for young medical officers rather than older men who had failed at private practice, a necessary sacrifice of experience for enthusiasm. Under no circumstances, he explained, should the "burned out man, regardless of age, who has shifted from position to position over the years and is looking for a soft 'berth' be considered."[93] Wiebe needed help with surgery, someone interested in administering anaesthesia, and a radiologist. Of the new graduates who applied, two men would consider moving to the Lady Willingdon Hospital only if they could work together. Also expressing concern about another candidate's "handicap," Wiebe noted that "our experience has been uniformly unpleasant and unsatisfactory with people of this type." While never naming the particular handicap, Wiebe suggested it "is closely associated with inadequacies which reflect adversely on the work of the individual and the welfare of our institution." He did agree that "these people do have a right to an opportunity to rehabilitate themselves," and, if necessary, he would welcome the particular physician at Lady Willingdon Indian Hospital.[94]

Tragically, the following May 1954 Wiebe reported a woman's death by cardiac arrest on the operating table as she underwent a hernia repair: "This unfortunate episode again points out very specifically the urgent need for well-qualified medical staff. We were fortunate in having a coroner with an *unbiased mind*, otherwise an inquest might have resulted in undesirable publicity concerning an unqualified anesthetist. An autopsy was performed and no cause could be determined to which the cardiac arrest could be attributed."[95] The people's concerns about the quality of care seemed more than justified, but with collusion between IHS officials and an "unbiased" coroner, the appalling affair never came to light. Wiebe's frank report, blaming the unqualified anaesthetist, drew attention to the consequences of IHS hiring policy. But as hospital superintendent and the surgeon responsible, he might well have been motivated by self-preservation.

Wiebe went on to "strongly recommend" that IHS hire fully qualified medical officers. "It is clear that we are attracting medical officers, many of whom have been failures elsewhere, or who have handicaps which militate against a successful ordinary practice."[96] Nevertheless, given the widespread use of unqualified physicians, it is doubtful that this "unfortunate episode" was a rare occurrence. While death in hospital was, and is, hardly unusual, death by negligent treatment documented by autopsy should have been cause for fundamental changes in the IHS system. That it was not suggests a deep bureaucratic cynicism, one shared by Six Nations, who understood that the care at the hospital was "good enough for Indians."[97]

One year later, Wiebe still did not have the help he needed at Lady Willingdon Hospital. With one unqualified medical assistant for all the outpatient work in a community of more than five thousand residents, and the often overcrowded fifty-four-bed hospital, the medical superintendent outlined some of the disadvantages of unlicensed doctors, "aside from the very precarious legal and ethical situations in which we find ourselves so frequently involved." His medical assistant could not work alone without "constantly having to be bailed out of awkward, embarrassing, and dangerous situations," not to mention the "frequently prodigious amount of mental and physical effort which this type of assistant exerts in order to achieve inadequacy."[98] By 1957 Wiebe left the hospital to take up a promotion to regional superintendent. The unlicensed anaesthetist remained at Lady Willingdon Hospital, however.

In June 1960 Six Nations Council passed a resolution requesting the removal of this particular physician for his "negligent medical attention to out-patients." It is clear, however, that the community remained unaware of the anaesthetist's role in the 1954 death. The Council resolution also threatened the hospital's other doctors with removal if they were found to be neglecting their duty to "give attentive and proper medical attention to patients."[99] The medical superintendent, Dr Hayward, clarified for his superior (Dr Wiebe) that the resolution did not actually accuse the physician of negligence, but Council complained that the doctor was inaccessible when he was most needed. Wiebe then interpreted the resolution for his superiors, calling the Six Nations people "somewhat unreasonable." Suggesting that the Council itself be censured for not fostering more responsibility, Wiebe did not think it "to the advantage of the Indians or the [Indian Health] Service if they are allowed to hold our medical and hospital staff under threat."[100] Six Nations Council, however, considered it "their" hospital and its physicians should answer to the people. Beyond the specific grievances over care and accessibility, Six Nations residents were anxious about IHS continued efforts to have individuals pay for medical services directly or indirectly through a group health insurance plan, despite repeated Council rejections of all such schemes.[101] At the same time, after 1961, IHS began redirecting medical care away from the reserve hospital to surrounding communities in keeping with its plans to shut the hospital and retreat from health services generally.

Not coincidentally, complaints of medical negligence, if not malpractice, increased steadily until Six Nations Council demanded a meeting with hospital personnel and regional superintendent Wiebe. When the meeting was not forthcoming Council took their concerns to the local press, which drew the immediate attention of bureaucrats, and a conference was quickly arranged.[102] In a confidential report to Director Moore, Wiebe described the specific complaints raised by Council. He found in one case that "the patient would have benefitted by hospitalization and a more vigorous form of therapy"; in the next case, the physician's treatment was judged "entirely adequate"; in another he found "an error in judgment re the gravity of the situation and the method of treatment"; in yet another, "the method of treatment would find general acceptance by the medical profession." In sum, Wiebe found "errors in judgment," but "no evidence suggesting gross neglect."[103] Finding little fault with the quality of care, Wiebe suggested the complaints arose from "the lack of rapport" between doctor and patient, and from the lack of free choice of physician. However, director Moore, in a letter to his minister, instead reported that the Six Nations Council regretted the publicity, and stated that "many of the complaints were indeed irresponsible."[104] That IHS medical bureaucrats investigated their own colleagues was not lost on Council, and according to anthropologist Weaver's informants in 1966, Wiebe's conclusion that there was no evidence of malpractice "did not rest easily with the Council, nor does it still among some Council members."[105] While their criticisms of the quality of care were dismissed as unreasonable and irresponsible, they were soon shared by a most unlikely source.

A 1962 Royal Commission enquiring into government services, headed by the accountant and prominent businessman Grant Glassco, found the quality of care in Indian hospitals "not comparable" with community hospitals. The facilities were old, ill equipped, and inadequately staffed. Of the 117 physicians who joined the department of national health since the mid 1950s, 47 per cent were graduates of foreign medical schools. "Many of them have not passed their Canadian licensing examinations and are therefore not qualified for private practice." Of the Canadian physicians who joined the service in the same period, their average age was forty. "The great majority of these have left private practice." The Commission also noted that the department found it difficult to attract suitable personnel at all ranks, while medical graduates avoided the IHS "because of the remoteness of places of employment, the ill equipped hospitals, and limited opportunities for career development." The Commission report recommended, among other things, "the rapid transfer of Indian health care to normal community facilities." The Commission supposed that with the introduction of national hospital insurance, and available insurance plans for physician services, medical care should be relatively simple to arrange.[106] Of course, the accountant-led Commission overlooked several critical realities: the reluctance of provincial hospitals to accept Aboriginal patients and the increasingly vocal Aboriginal communities' demands that the federal government increase its commitment to health care and improve, not abandon, its facilities. In any case, the Glassco Commission's findings did not come as any surprise to IHS bureaucrats, who were well aware of the deficiencies.

Indian hospitals, as the minister pledged in 1946, might have served a most beneficial function as a training ground for Aboriginal health workers – nurses, doctors, and administrators – as was accomplished in similar circumstances elsewhere.[107] Yet, IHS provided only the most basic instruction for Aboriginal workers to fill the lowest ranks as support personnel. Indeed, it was difficult for Aboriginal RNs, for instance, to find work in their own communities. More than representing a benign "opportunity lost," the refusal to use the hospitals as training centres exposes the work of the disciplines, medical and social, in maintaining hierarchies and colour lines in the health care professions and Canadian society generally. That patients suffered and died at the hands of the overworked, the unqualified, and the negligent suggests a deep cynicism most clearly articulated by IHS director Moore himself in 1962 in reference to the inadequacies of professional staff: "Today we are stuck with what we have allowed ourselves to be satisfied with."[108] Indian hospitals, continuing the colonizing work of reserves and residential schools, kept people in their places: some as patients and poorly paid labourers; others as physician bureaucrats managing doctors who could not find work elsewhere. Yet, the presence of the intermediaries and cultural brokers – the Aboriginal RNs, nurse's aides, and orderlies – eased somewhat the hospitals' harsh conditions.

Chapter Four

Life and Death in an Indian Hospital

"Never were there photographs that showed the truth about my people's lives."[1]
– Minnie Aodla Freeman

Patient experiences – life and death – in Indian Hospitals varied tremendously, making any description partial and incomplete. Hospitalization, anytime and anyplace, would be nothing less than traumatic – endured certainly not enjoyed. And many patients, if not most, became well in the institutions, where, by the early 1950s, effective antibiotics saved lives. But patient narratives, some as remembered childhood experiences and others gleaned from the archival record, rarely refer positively to the institutions, the caregivers, or medicine itself. Working at the Camsell Indian Hospital, Aboriginal RN from Saddle Lake, Kathleen Steinhauer-Anderson observed: "Most of the patients demonstrated that sense of despairing resignation so evident at a residential school … Gaols seem to elicit somewhat the same response from native people familiar with such institutions."[2] Linking these sites of isolation and discipline, she points to a persistent reality in the lives of many Aboriginal people. Though individuals experienced hospitalization differently, given Indian Health Service's centralized bureaucracy and its hierarchical and paternalistic structure, patients faced common circumstances. The most common of all was coercion, which was in keeping with the state's broader colonizing agenda to control, regulate, and assimilate Aboriginal people. Compulsion informed most interactions with IHS even though individuals and communities had pleaded for medical attention. They welcomed Indian hospitals, sought employment with IHS, and took an active interest in negotiating for better facilities and improved treatment. Despite evidence to the contrary, for IHS the existence of coercive policies was made to imply their necessity. In a 1945 warning of things to come, Percy Moore boldly stated, "We certainly do not feel that our program should be left to the whims of an Indian, as to whether or not he will accept treatment."[3] From mass annual X-rays to mass BCG vaccination, from forced relocation to forced institutionalization, from lost patients to lost graves, patients felt the objectifying reality of Indian hospitals.

In the decade before 1945, with limited budgets and few beds, admission to an Indian hospital was highly selective. The best candidates were those most likely to be "cured," a pragmatism not unknown to hospital and sanatorium directors everywhere who were concerned to create public confidence in their institutions, but a practice that left the most ill with tuberculosis in the community.[4] Indian hospitals initially preferred two groups in particular: tuberculous schoolchildren, easily controlled and an acknowledged threat to the larger civilizing mission of the schools, and pregnant women. The physician at Manitoba's Fisher River Indian Hospital, where Moore got his start in the 1930s, called it an "unholy combination."[5] The putative social value of the hospital, to teach the superiority of Western medicine, clearly trumped the medical, but pregnant women may well have chosen a hospital birth for its more prosaic appeal – running water and a warm building in winter. Nevertheless, the postwar expansion of institutions and treatment beds allowed for more extensive and aggressive medical surveillance of communities that often began with a chest X-ray. At times partnered with provincial tuberculosis associations, at other times with their own X-ray equipment, IHS undertook annual surveys of schools and reserve communities.

Mass X-ray surveys, a significant aspect of tuberculosis campaigns in non-Aboriginal communities in the 1940s and early 1950s, were made possible by the military's development of the portable X-ray machine. The new technology, actually a fluoroscope fitted with a camera to capture the image, was easily transported by truck or airplane and made it possible, and economically feasible, to X-ray whole communities, indeed whole provinces.[6] These "travelling clinics," preceded by much media fanfare, relied on enthusiastic service club volunteers to encourage neighbours to be "tuberculosis conscious" and line up for their chest X-ray, creating an opportunity to demonstrate responsible, healthy citizenship to friends and strangers. Organizers understood, however, that the "improvident and careless" would never present themselves for X-ray; neither would older elite men and ex-servicemen, those whose credentials as responsible citizens could not be questioned.[7] Portable fluoroscope machines made province-wide campaigns (of mostly healthy people) feasible, but they also involved a significantly higher radiation dose than radiographs using a full-size film.[8] As fewer and fewer cases of tuberculosis were discovered in the surveys, and especially once the dangers of exposure to ionizing radiation became widely understood by the mid-1950s, the enthusiasm for mass surveys quickly faded. By 1957 tuberculosis authorities in British Columbia, concerned about the hazards to children in particular, instructed that *"no person 15 years or under should have a routine or admission chest x-ray unless he has shown a positive tuberculin reaction."*[9] But, while citizens might line up for a chest X-ray, would they submit to a much more invasive tuberculin test? A 1957 survey of the white and Aboriginal population of Manitoulin Island in Ontario studied the participation rate in a community survey that added tuberculin testing to its usual X-ray examinations. It concluded that there was no reason to expose to X-ray those not infected with tubercle bacilli. Tuberculin testing could easily identify positive reactors, and only they needed an X-ray.[10] The study also emphasized the marginally higher infection rates among whites living in close proximity to Aboriginal communities, highlighting the presumed source of infection. But, at the outset the researchers eliminated from their study 348 people (presumably Aboriginal) who, having been previously vaccinated with BCG, would show a positive tuberculin reaction. Beginning in 1946 the widespread use of the BCG vaccine in Aboriginal communities, while conferring some protection against tuberculosis, also rendered the tuberculin test useless, making frequent X-rays necessary despite the recognized dangers.

Most provincial health authorities, except Quebec, rejected systematic BCG vaccination because of persistent concerns about its efficacy and potential risks, particularly because it interfered with the tuberculin test. Alberta and British Columbia refused to consider its use, while other provinces employed it selectively for nurses and others routinely exposed to tuberculosis.[11] Yet R.G. Ferguson's Qu'Appelle BCG trial on infants, completed in 1945, convinced IHS of the utility and economy of the vaccine for Aboriginal communities. In Manitoba, IHS initiated BCG vaccination in 1948 in southern reserves and schools, and four years later in the north. In an admittedly "unscientific" study from 1948 to 1954, morbidity and mortality dropped steadily, though the role of BCG could not be determined with any accuracy. Nevertheless, fewer vaccinated children developed active disease, prompting the conclusion: "We know it [BCG] is safe ... We will continue to use it as extensively as possible."[12]

But it was not always safe. The protection offered by BCG diminished after two years, making revaccination necessary. Armand Frappier, director of Montreal's Institute of Microbiology and Hygiene and the driving force behind BCG production and distribution in Canada, advised that only newborns or those never exposed to the disease (verified by a negative tuberculin test) should receive BCG.[13] The tuberculin skin test, however, took one to three days to develop a reaction, a waste of time for hurried survey crews that spent as little time in Aboriginal communities as possible. Frappier instead devised a simpler scratch test to gauge sensitivity using a diluted dose of BCG that produced an immediate reaction. The Manitoba study's recommendation of mass testing of "all Indians under 16" by the BCG skin test at least every two years and an X-ray every year, appears to have been taken up by IHS nationwide.[14] But when two schoolgirls were admitted to Sioux Lookout Indian Hospital with tuberculous lymphadenitis (tuberculosis of the lymph nodes) after revaccination with BCG, there was considerable consternation. While director Moore thought it an interesting case report that might be published in the medical press, his superior, deputy minister of health Dr G.D.W. Cameron, found it "disturbing ... The clear inference is that our people are being careless about their sensitivity testing whether it is the standard mantoux or Frappier's own test using diluted BCG." In order to keep the "confidence and goodwill of the Indians," he advised against publishing anything that would lead to questions of what went wrong, "was it the BCG or was the job improperly done?"[15] Despite Cameron's personal concerns about the safety of the BCG skin test, its use continued in Aboriginal communities in conjunction with annual X-ray examinations.[16]

As late as 1966, IHS continued to vaccinate with BCG without first determining a negative reaction through tuberculin testing. Dr Matthew Matas, then regional superintendent for Alberta and the Northwest Territories, assured the joint meeting of the Department of National Health and Welfare and the CTA that IHS continued to encourage BCG vaccination "without being too concerned about tuberculin sensitivity, fully realizing that some severe local reactions may occur ... The risk of an Indian or Eskimo contracting tuberculosis is infinitely greater than any risk of his developing a serious reaction to BCG vaccination."[17] Another risk IHS was willing to take was annual X-ray examinations.

Conceding that a biennial X-ray survey would likely suffice, Matas explained that communities were conditioned, "brainwashed," to the yearly visit of the X-ray team. "If the survey were conducted less frequently, less cooperation might be received as fewer visits might be interpreted as indicating that there was no problem."[18] In areas where tuberculosis infection remained high, X-ray surveys were undertaken two or three times a year.[19] The damage caused by "serious BCG reactions" and the long-term impact of thirty to forty or more years of (at least) annual X-rays beginning in early childhood may never be known, though the risks to white Canadians were deemed too great.[20] Indeed, by IHS calculations, iatrogenic injury to Aboriginal bodies was the price to be paid to contain tuberculosis infection in Aboriginal communities and, ultimately, to protect an increasingly tuberculin-negative Canadian public.

Mass X-ray surveys of Aboriginal communities usually accompanied the treaty party: Indian agent, police, and doctor. Treaty time in summer was an occasion for often widely scattered hunting and trapping bands to reunite for wedding celebrations, to renew friendships, and to discuss issues and concerns with each other and the Indian agent. While tuberculosis surveys in towns and cities relied on citizens to voluntarily present themselves for examination, reserve communities were not allowed the same autonomy. A convenient, if disreputable, practice of withholding treaty annuity payments until every family member consented to X-ray examination allowed for far more thorough surveillance than was possible in white communities.[21] As CTA's Dr Wherrett put it, "The Indians and Eskimos were easy to screen because they were congregated on reserves and in small communities."[22] In the summer of 1949 the treaty party and X-ray crew flew into remote Manitoba communities. At Shamatawa, 176 people were X-rayed; Dr Yule pulled teeth, while the RCMP constable and Indian agent (as magistrate) dispensed justice. They fined a trapper for taking a beaver out of season, though the treaty party, including the constable, later dined on illegally caught sturgeon. In the evening's soccer match, "natives against whites," the X-ray technologist recalled that Chief Beardy called out to his players in Cree "telling his boys to go easy on us. Thank goodness, for they still nearly ran us to death!"[23] It was a very public demonstration of a healthy and vital community. Likewise when the survey crew arrived at Nelson House reserve (Nisichawayasihk Cree Nation) treaty day celebrations were underway with ball games, contests of strength and stamina, canoe races, and a dance in the evening. These were not the diseased and decaying communities they expected to find. The survey party took 7,038 X-rays that summer, though many were never interpreted since the 158-bed Clearwater Lake Indian Hospital at The Pas was full.[24] The surveillance of Aboriginal communities continued apace with schoolchildren and whole communities X-rayed at least annually from the early 1940s until the late 1960s, creating a detailed archive of personal information on thousands of people.[25]

Much depended on the X-ray findings, but the gains in machine portability and economy were often lost in accuracy. Detail was less clear than on a full-sized chest X-ray, and any slight movement caused a blurred image. Ten per cent of abnormalities were not recognizable on the miniature films, though more advanced tuberculosis could be detected.[26] In the rough conditions of field surveys, and especially the hurried shipboard examinations that brought many Inuit from the eastern Arctic to southern hospitals, the opportunities for misdiagnosis were manifest. A skill learned through long practice, X-ray interpretation was an inexact science at the best of times. As visiting British physician P.E. Baldry reminded Canadian colleagues, "large numbers of Eskimos are radiographed and in each case a decision has to be made on a single film whether or not there is an abnormality which requires the individual to be brought out for treatment. It is obviously not always easy to be certain on a single radiograph whether a shadow is due to active tuberculosis. Nevertheless in view of the fact that once patients have been evacuated some of them cannot be returned home until the ship makes another journey the next year it is obviously important to make the correct interpretation."[27] Baldry's caution, while recognizing the significant disruption in patients' lives by an incorrect diagnosis, also points to the acknowledged subjectivity in X-ray interpretation: survey crews expected to find tuberculosis. In her study of the changing cultural meanings of tuberculosis and its treatments, historian Katherine Ott notes how subjectivity influenced physicians' judgments. A 1951 study found that physicians' and radiologists' interpretation of 150 X-ray exams differed one-third of the time, and when shown the same X-ray twice (without their knowledge) their own readings differed one-fifth of the time.[28]

Though tuberculosis was the principal focus of the surveys, potential patients were screened for any signs of disease. Inuit, identified by their disk number and sometimes their name, were boarded on the annual patrol ship, which they termed "*Matavik*" or "where you strip" in Inuktitut.[29] They were moved through the shipboard medical examination

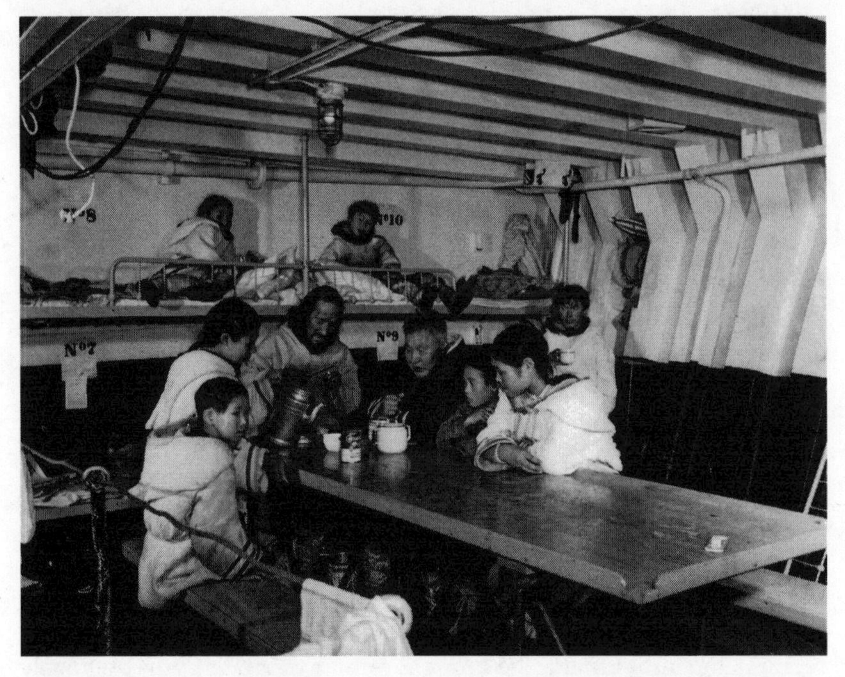

Illustration 4.1 Inuit on-board ship heading south. This carefully constructed image did not reflect reality for many Inuit relocated to southern hospitals. It would have been unusual for families to travel together as this image implies. Children were often sent alone and unaccompanied by family members.

Source: PA-176873, LAC.

process with a serial number written on their left hand: "X-P-D-I" denoting X-ray, physician, dentist, and immunization. An arrow drawn under the letters meant they were free of disease and could go home, but "TB" written on the hand meant evacuation to a southern hospital. They were kept on-board until the ship sailed with no chance to bid goodbye to family and friends.[30] Without proper interpreters and treated as so much cargo, Inuit patients were numbered and stowed aboard, with no opportunity to question their diagnosis or their fate. Their bodies literally inscribed with the colonizers' diagnosis and marked for relocation, patients felt the disciplining power of Western medicine[31] (illustration 4.1).

It is not possible to generalize about the experience of life in an Indian hospital. The *Camsell Mosaic*, a 1985 celebratory history edited and published by former Camsell Indian Hospital employees, includes a triumphantly alliterative chapter "Moccasins, Mukluks and Miracles" in which grateful ex-patients recall the kind and caring ministrations of nurses and physicians. Patient narratives could hardly be otherwise in a progressive history, "a tale worth preserving," told by those who placed themselves at the centre of nothing less than "one of the more notable successes in recent medical history – the conquering of a killer disease."[32] Nevertheless, individual encounters with the hospitals varied tremendously. Some patients spent years in the institutions, and some a short time; some were treated with kindness and compassion, and some with indifference and disdain; some were young and quickly adapted, while older patients worried constantly about families at home; some lived to tell about it, and some did not. George Manuel, born in 1921 in the Secwepemc territory of the Shuswap people in British Columbia, and by 1970 the chief of the fledgling National Indian Brotherhood, recalled his teenage years in the Coqualeetza Indian Hospital in the 1940s. Diagnosed with tuberculosis of the hipbone, he entered hospital from the Kamloops Residential School, where the children were made to carry fifty-pound packs of cordwood a mile and a half up the riverbank to the school under the watchful eye of adult overseers who berated them. "Hunger is both the first and the last thing I can remember about that school. I was hungry from the day I went into that school until they took me to the hospital two and a half years later. Not just me. Every Indian student smelled of hunger." But in the hospital, he recalled, the nurses brought him the books and games he never saw at school. They taught him to read and to make the best use of his years of enforced quiet. He remembered "the baths and towels, meals, and beds, which were all warm and plentiful." He honoured the nurses for "rekindling the imagination of my childhood" and for keeping him alive "as though they were grandmothers of our own nation."[33] Manuel's sharply juxtaposed residential school and hospital experiences highlight the abusive treatment in the former institution and, despite his illness, the relatively positive experience in the latter.

In her collection of former patients' experiences, historian Laurie Meijer Drees found some common themes: tedium, boredom, loneliness, and emotional and physical harm. But patients also stressed more positive experiences, often recounted with a good deal of humour: a determination to get well, close friendships forged with other patients, and opportunities for growth through education and rehabilitation. Significantly, few patients recounted positive relationships with medical staff.[34] These and other narratives transcribed in the last decade are predominantly the stories of childhood or adolescence that reflect the vulnerability of youth but also acknowledge their hospital experience as an episode in the continuum of lived reality. Dave Melting Tallow, when asked about his hospital experience, replied: "It wouldn't be sad, and it wouldn't be a happy story. It would be just a story but it wasn't sad; it wasn't a good time. But then I had the operation [chest surgery]. Except for that time, the only really bad time I had was when I think they experimented on me. I don't know if they did or not."[35] Far different in tone and emphasis from the *Camsell Mosaic* narratives, these accounts also highlight another essential reality – survival – in spite or because of treatment. William Tagoona, a five-year-old in the mid-1950s, spent eighteen months in the Clearwater Lake Indian Hospital in Manitoba. He recalled that when nurses read them bedtime stories the children were told to keep their eyes on the nurse's face. If they looked away and were caught, "she'd take her belt off and hit you with it." The goodnight kiss was another strictly enforced duty. "If a child turned his head away from the nurse, then you'd get it again." Tagoona recalled vomiting in his plate of macaroni, "The nurse got really angry and mixed up the macaroni and vomit and force fed it to me."[36] Survivors' stories anchor bureaucratic policy and shifting medical discourse to the embodied experience of the Indian hospitals. Vulnerable but never completely victimized, patients, with the help of families and communities, resisted where they could and attempted to shape the institutions for their own purposes.

Access to hospital care, which in the past had been carefully mediated by Indian agents and departmental physicians, was understood in many communities as a long-promised government obligation that was finally fulfilled with the advent of Indian hospitals. The close association of medical care and treaty payments served to reaffirm the understanding that health care was a treaty right, a claim that IHS continued to deny, despite its practice. At the grand opening of Miller Bay Indian Hospital, as noted earlier, Henry Kelly, councillor for the Tsimshian, characterized it as fundamental to the "new deal promised" by the government of Canada.[37] The leadership of the Hobbema agency reserves toured the newly opened Charles Camsell Indian Hospital and presented the administration with a cash donation to demonstrate their support.[38] In the early 1950s the elderly Sweetgrass Chief Sam Swimmer spent his final years at Saskatchewan's North Battleford Indian Hospital and rarely missed an opportunity to link the hospital to the treaty right to health care. As he put it, "The Fort Carlton Treaty was made between God, the Queen, the White Man and the Indians. God remains with us. We have a Queen on the throne. The Treaty must never be broken."[39] Elders today agree with Chief Swimmer that, aside from a treaty entitlement, "their" hospital was a valuable community institution. Gordon Albert remarked: "I feel it was a very important part in the lives of Indian people that utilized the facility – not only because it was called an Indian hospital but they could identify with their own people who were in there and utilized that facility. They felt at home ... A lot of old people utilized that facility and it was to their liking."[40] Rose Atimoyoo recalled, "I was really impressed when I had my baby there because I felt right at home. The cleaning ladies were all native and I heard that language a lot there too. It was home to me and that is how I think mostly everybody felt, especially the old people."[41] Indian hospitals, particularly those situated close to reserves and increasingly staffed by Aboriginal workers, became tangible manifestations of a treaty or legal right, and community leaders took a proprietary interest in their operations.

Shortly after the Clearwater Lake Indian Hospital opened in northern Manitoba in 1947, Chief Cornelius Bignell and councillors of the local Pas Band (Opaskwayak Cree Nation) felt compelled to advise that "steps be taken to improve the conditions in the San so that people will gladly go there." Patients needed fresh air and requested permission to walk outside on warm days. There was not enough staff to comfort dying patients, who called out for water "until death claims them." Injections were administered too roughly and patients had severe reactions to the medications. A man working at the cemetery found out only later that he had buried his own wife. The chief and council questioned superintendent Dr Ridge's management: "Too many persons have died, and are dying too fast in such a short time. Very few leave the San cured." High death rates and few cures, a disturbing reality in the early years of IHS hospitals, reflected not only the limitations of tuberculosis treatment in the pre-antibiotic era, but also the practice of admitting the very ill in order to limit the spread of disease. It was a sharp departure from an earlier protocol that left the terminally ill, especially the elderly, in the community to spare hospital reputations. As Chief Bignell put it, "Now we wish to ask the Department to do its utmost to make the poor people feel happy and proud to go to this Sanatorium."[42] The implication was that if the hospital was met with non-cooperation, it was for good reason.

In response to the complaints, Dr E.L. Ross, medical superintendent of the Manitoba Sanatorium Board that operated the Clearwater Hospital for IHS, inspected the institution and, not surprisingly, found himself "very satisfied" with the medical treatment and the cleanliness of the wards. Ross admitted, however, that staff shortages were a serious problem, with Dr Ridge and only the assistance of a "DP doctor," just two graduate nurses, five practical nurses, and eight ward aides to care for 158 patients. Dr Ridge and Indian Agent Low agreed that the chief's statements "were grossly exaggerated and almost entirely unjustified."[43] While community concerns were not entirely ignored, the Indian agent assured IHS that the chief later "regretted" his complaint. IHS, explicitly rejecting claims that the hospitals represented any obligation more than humanitarian concern, dismissed community criticism as unwarranted and ungrateful grousing. Community involvement and activism only increased, particularly after government attempts in the mid-1960s to close the hospitals, which was interpreted as an abrogation of treaty responsibilities (a phase of the Indian hospitals that will be examined in depth in the next chapter). Reserve leaders were limited in their ability to act as patient advocates by the vastly uneven power relations, especially since IHS bureaucrats investigated community concerns and complaints about their own colleagues.

Patients also attempted to influence their own experience, often with limited success. The nature of tuberculosis care, premised on the rest cure to allow the body to heal, involved elaborate "routines" from complete bed rest to graduated degrees of activity that often took years to accomplish. This medical paradigm readily incorporated surgical lung collapse and only slowly shifted with the advent of antibiotic drug treatment. Patients quickly learned that discipline, self-imposed or administered, defined their lives in hospital while they underwent monthly chest X-rays and had their sputum regularly tested to gauge their progress. Minnie Aodla Freeman, from the Inuit community on Cape Hope Island in James Bay, recalling her treatment in the Moose Factory Indian Hospital, illustrates the essential helplessness of patients:

> Every week we had different faces catering to us. The doctors and nurses were all imported from the south. The ward I was in became very fond of one particular nurse and so did I. She had such a gentle face and nature … When she was on duty, we behaved for her, her pleasantness kept us pleasant. When she was off duty, we were just the opposite. We wore long faces like the ones that were on duty. We sneaked around behind their backs.

We ran to the windows to look out. They treated us like children, so we acted like children.[44]

After her transfer to Mountain Sanatorium in Hamilton in 1951, the fifteen-year-old Freeman, who had learned English in school, was quickly put to work translating for staff and Inuit patients. Suspecting that her language skills were the sole reason for her hospitalization, she inquired about her treatment and shortly thereafter began to get injections (likely streptomycin). "I dreaded them. Some nurses did not hurt, but others gave needles that sent pain all the way down my leg. We began to recognize which ones were not painful and which ones were."[45]

Children were often physically restrained to teach the discipline of bed rest. At Miller Bay Hospital younger children, tied in their beds, soon learned to untie their restraints.[46] The staff at Charles Camsell Hospital jokingly referred to a condition they called "cantstayinbeditis," which was followed by "castitis," in which patients were immobilized by plaster casts on both legs with a bar connecting the casts. Patients who struggled free of the leg casts were fitted with body casts extending up to the chest. The "condition" resolved itself when the "victim is convinced of the necessity for cooperation in the cure of his disease."[47] Agnes Bruno recalled how as a child in the Camsell Hospital all the girls on her ward were put in casts as punishment for misbehaving.[48] At Fort Qu'Appelle Indian Hospital disobedient children were restrained in straitjackets.[49] A former non-Aboriginal RN recalled her less restrictive, but perhaps more insidiously coercive, method of controlling young children at Camsell Hospital. "They [young boys] liked to call me 'Momma' and most days before afternoon rest period, as a special treat, I would carry each one to look out the window. Punishment for misbehaviour was withdrawal of these privileges."[50] Adult male patients had their pajama bottoms taken away to keep them in bed, or isolated within the hospital. Dave Melting Tallow recalled, as punishment for getting out of bed, being moved onto a ward with Inuit patients with whom he could not communicate.[51] The therapeutic value of highly regimented "routines" was extended to include patients who were hospitalized for conditions other than tuberculosis; all were seen to require the strict institutional discipline that for many began in residential school. "Up patients" at Camsell Hospital, identified by red armbands on their dressing gowns, were allowed to attend Friday evening movies in the recreation hall. However, if anyone took liberties to go elsewhere the privilege was withdrawn for all patients.[52]

Adult patients worried about families and children at home. "George," a twenty-eight-year-old father of four sons who spent a year in the Fort Qu'Appelle Indian Hospital in the 1950s, recalled his frustration at lying around idle, unable to help his young family who were struggling to put food on the table.[53] Minnie Freeman, who was hospitalized with older female relatives, recalled their anxieties: "My aunts talked about the cold weather at home, wondering how their families were, and how they were coping with their clothes for the winter."[54] After her discharge from hospital Freeman worked as a translator for Indian Affairs, and recalled meeting a group of adult Inuit patients at Brandon:

> Most of these patients were mothers and fathers. How were their homes managed with all the work that had to be done, especially the provision of food and clothing? Some of them had been in hospital for two years, some for one year and others for six months. Some had heard nothing of their relatives for a long time. Some did, and had had bad news about loved ones who had died.
>
> Our next visit was to a hostel. There we met people who were waiting to go home. The house ... had the smell of a human who has not washed for years. The Inuit looked as if they had not been out for months. They were so pale, not like the skin I am used to seeing on Inuit – wind-burned and sun-tanned. Their lavatory was horribly messy, dirty and smelly. And these were the people who were waiting to go home after hospital care. It would be no wonder if they went right back to the hospital.[55]

By the early 1960s Inuit patients began writing letters in syllabics to translators in the northern administration's welfare division ("Eskimology section") hoping to make contact with family at home, and to ask for help with their hospital experience. Anna wrote to ask when she would be released. She reassured "Bobby" (likely Robert Williamson, welfare section anthropologist and translator) that "we are fine, we Eskimos," though she expressed concerns that all the doctors in the hospital were "bearded ones ... when they talk they are not understandable. I really want to go home." The letters usually included expressions of gratitude for their treatment, which may have been a formality since patients understood they were writing to a government agency. One patient was thankful for his treatment and being "fed every day" though it was white man's food. Tommy, frustrated that there was no interpreter at the hospital, and worried about his wife and blind mother at home, wanted to leave even though he was not completely cured: "Even if I am made to stay here a long time yet I'm not likely to be made immortal." He closed with: "Go ahead and translate my words. Write them in English. The hospital is disgusting – awful." Lucy thought the nurses were rough: "being pushed by them is very miserable … please tell the doctors that we are being treated badly … I'm telling the truth." Leah expressed her gratitude, but she was lonesome: "Sometimes happiness can't reach me."[56] In larger hospitals with many long-stay patients, Indian Affairs provided funds for rudimentary education and occupational therapy programs where patients relieved their boredom and anxiety by producing crafts, clothing, and sculpture.[57] However, the programs were the exception rather than the rule.

Miller Bay Indian Hospital's isolated location, drab buildings, and poor management made patients' lives even more dismal. The perennial problems of staff shortages and high turnover (see chapter 3) were deemed by administration to stem from patients themselves. "Poor patient discipline," or discord with nursing staff and sullenness, was a particular concern on the women's Ward B. In a highly unusual step the hospital asked the patients for their feedback in a written questionnaire (which may have left out many patients): "I just haven't talked to [nurse] since she told me to shut up and mind my own business, when I told her not to force [a patient] to eat. I just told her in a polite way. Just not talking in case she makes me feel bad again." Another patient noted: "If we are good patients they are good to us but if we don't do as they tell us, sure mean." Patients complained about the food, asking for something other than jam sandwiches and cake. "Can't we afford a dietician?" one patient asked. Aside from concerns about hospital operations, patients also expressed their loneliness and frustration with their long-term hospitalization: "I am getting so tired of this hospital life and I am getting so lonely too." Feeling well yet not released from hospital, another patient wrote, "I am complaining of not being sick and you doctors had to keep me here for nothing. You doctors left me laying in my bed worried about my little girl at home."[58]

A newly hired social worker in 1955 suggested that an organized body to represent patient interests might improve hospital discipline and morale. A fairly common device in sanatoria where "self-policing" was the goal, patient committees were rare in Indian hospitals. Charles Camsell Hospital established a health committee in 1958, but, dominated by medical staff, it focused on teaching the five patient representatives about tuberculosis, general health rules, and parliamentary procedure for conducting meetings.[59] With slightly more autonomy, the Miller Bay Hospital's patient committee elected representatives for president, secretary and two councillors from each of the men's and women's wards. Informed that it was to concern itself solely with patient recreation, the committee, however, quickly extended its authority by issuing directives and recommending staff changes. To superintendent Howell's dismay, "they desired, indeed, to participate in the operation of the hospital." Within the year the committee pursued its interests more directly. Changing its name from "The Patients' Recreation Committee" to the "Miller Bay Indian Hospital Native Council," it shifted identity and focus from patient recreation to advocacy and expanded its mandate to include grievance and food committees. The superintendent viewed the Native Council as having some value "in the process of integration with the rest of the population," but warned again, "they should never be permitted to pass from an advisory stage to a stage in which they participate in the actual operation of the hospital."[60] Howell's concern that an organized patient voice might presume to adjust the hospital's power relationships points to deeper anxieties that patients and their supporters might indeed know and articulate their own health care interests that challenged IHS.

Patients in the men's ward at Fort Qu'Appelle Indian Hospital in 1962 bypassed the bureaucrats and appealed directly to the prime minister. The frustrated petitioners reminded John Diefenbaker of their special relationship, quoting the treaty promise that "the ears of the Queen's government will forever be opened to our complaints and wishes." They also appealed to the government that had not only recently granted Indians a measure of legal equality with the vote, but was also preparing the first Canadian bill of rights. Yet, they said, they were still treated as "children or a flock of sheep." They wanted the same respect and to be granted the same privileges – longer visiting hours and hospital leaves – accorded to white tuberculosis patients in the provincial sanatorium on the other side of Echo Lake. They appealed to the prime minister to stop the staff from opening and searching parcels that were sent to them in the hospital; they wanted to wear their clothes, not pyjamas, outside for their one hour of exercise in the small yard behind the hospital; visiting hours were too short and staff turned away their relatives who had travelled long distances. The petition might be read as reflecting little more than an understandable impatience with the banality of institutional life and its everyday indignities, if not for their final plea to the prime minister to protect them from retaliation.[61] That the petition was found in IHS files suggests that it missed its intended recipient, though the hospital was no doubt informed of the petitioners' identities and complaints.

Many patients recognized the strict discipline and rigid routine in hospital as a continuation of their residential school experiences. Indeed, many became ill in school and were moved from one institution to the other and back again, as students, patients, and, for some, workers.[62] A teenaged patient at Camsell Hospital in the 1950s, Roy Little Chief from Siksika recalled, "Well, I guess at that time we were well trained in the residential school, we followed authority. In the Camsell we could have been rebellious, but we learned to sneak around; run around during rest period."[63] Kathleen Steinhauer, from Saddle Lake reserve in Alberta, a nurse's aide and later an RN at Camsell Hospital in the 1950s, likened patients' "despairing resignation" with the residential school experience.[64] For some, though, the comparison was not apt. Dave Melting Tallow, who attended Crowfoot School at the Blackfoot reserve and was later hospitalized at the Camsell Hospital, recalled: "It wasn't like school at all. In school you were getting hit all the time, getting beat up, and hit all the time by the nuns. They punched like a priest. Those things happened in school. School was bad. Over there [Camsell Hospital] you could get visitors any time you wanted a visitor. They'd come and visit you and they didn't beat you up."[65] Frank Malloway from Sto:lo Nation at Sardis, British Columbia, a child patient in the Coqualeetza Indian Hospital in the late 1940s, witnessed what he only later understood to be the sexual abuse of another child in the hospital.[66] Patient narratives linking the experiences of residential schools and Indian hospitals point to the continuities of institutionalization as government policy. The terrible legacy of removing children from the supposed deleterious influences of families and communities, putting them in the hands of teachers, nurses, doctors and social workers who were deemed to know the children's best interests continues to damage individuals, their families, and indeed the nation itself.[67]

Another disturbingly common theme in patient narratives was the suspicion that they were subjected to medical experimentation; such mistrust of the motives of medical personnel was not without foundation. In the 1940s and 1950s Percy Moore, using IHS hospitals and in cooperation with Indian Affairs and leading national and international scientists, conducted a series of experiments in the then cutting-edge research into vitamins and malnutrition. They found ideal subjects in hungry, if not starving, Cree communities in northern Manitoba and James Bay, as well as in a number of residential schools. In the initial reporting of the Manitoba research the investigators noted:

> It is not unlikely that many characteristics such as shiftlessness, indolence, improvidence and inertia, so long regarded as inherent or hereditary traits in the Indian race, may, at the root, be really the manifestations of malnutrition. Furthermore, it is probable that the Indians' great susceptibility to many diseases, paramount amongst which is tuberculosis, may be attributable among other causes, to their high degree of malnutrition arising from lack of proper foods.[68]

"Shiftlessness and indolence," or the "Indian problem" needed the expert management of Indian hospitals and scientific study. The study, widely quoted in the press, was submitted as evidence to the 1946 Special Joint Committee of the House of Commons, and the Senate struck to recommend revisions to the Indian Act.[69] Historian Ian Mosby argues that the research resulted in little amelioration of the conditions in communities or schools that led to the people's hunger and malnourishment. While the bureaucrats and scientists recognized the connections between disease and malnutrition, they also "came to view Aboriginal bodies as 'experimental materials' and residential schools and Aboriginal communities as kinds of 'laboratories' that they could use to pursue a number of different political and professional interests."[70]

Indian hospitals also provided ample experimental material. As Aboriginal RN Kathleen Steinhauer told historian Laurie Meijer Drees in 2004:

> There is the thought that the hospitals were used for medical experiments. Occasionally new treatments for tuberculosis emerged and it seemed to many people, including patients and staff, that these treatments were pioneered on patients in the Indian Hospital system. When patients consented to treatment, I believe they often did not fully understand what was being asked of them.[71]

Several of Meijer Drees's other informants raised similar concerns, as did Frank Malloway and Dave Melting Tallow.[72] Elders from Piikuni (Peigan) and Kainai (Blood) First Nations in Alberta, and Carry the Kettle First Nation in southern Saskatchewan likewise expressed apprehensions about the medical care in Indian hospitals, suggesting patients were used as "guinea pigs."[73] Certainly, R.G. Ferguson's BCG vaccine trial in the 1930s and 1940s conducted on Cree and Assiniboine (Nakoda Oyadebi) infants in the Fort Qu'Appelle Indian Hospital was experimental (not unlike the 1950s trial of isoniazid [INH] on the Navajo at Many Farms, Arizona).[74] Residential school principals, not parents, consented to BCG, smallpox, and diphtheria vaccinations for schoolchildren, though as early as 1921 Ferguson sought parental consent to tuberculin test non-Aboriginal children.[75] In Indian hospitals tuberculin-negative patients under twenty-one years of age were routinely given BCG vaccination since signed hospital admission forms were deemed to cover all hospital treatments. As late as 1966 the Saskatchewan Anti-TB League vaccinated children with BCG without parental consent because the consent forms were awkward and time consuming, and besides, "it was good for them."[76] While white hospital employees were asked to sign a voluntary consent form for BCG vaccination, Aboriginal employees' consent was simply assumed. The assistant director advised hospital superintendents "not to stress this point [BCG vaccination] and suggest that you carry on as if it were a normal routine procedure and take it for granted that they do consent to vaccination." While admitting that there was no way to enforce vaccination if an employee refused, Moore's assistant did suggest that an Aboriginal employee should willingly cooperate "if he wishes to retain his job in the hospital."[77] IHS Indian hospitals' paternalistic and authoritarian structure, where medical personnel presumed to know what was best for them, left little room for patients, or Aboriginal employees, to question or indeed consent to treatment.

Moreover, patients with little experience of the frightening world of hospitals would find the cultural and language differences intimidating at the very least. The use of untrained interpreters who were often young domestic workers or patients with little understanding of medical terms and procedures created further confusion. Even patients who understood English found themselves distressingly vulnerable. Minnie Freeman, who was left for weeks to wonder what treatment she might receive, recalled: "My culture told me not to ask, that in this situation I might cause the people who were taking care of me to alter their behaviour completely, that I should accept what was happening and not force the hands that held my destiny. I figured they would tell me when they were ready."[78] Medical staff interpreted such culturally appropriate behaviour as an inherent Inuit stoicism, and as consent.

At Camsell Hospital, for instance, staff presumed that Aboriginal people had a "high pain threshold" and required minimal sedation, but, remarked a former nurse in retrospect, "they do have the same pain as other people."[79] Inuit patient Joanasie Salomanie suspected that he was part of "a medicine experiment using different things on us. I'm sure they were practicing on us because there were so many patients there." But author Pat Sandiford Grygier disregarded his informant's concerns, suggesting instead that medical personnel were "not sure of the correct dosages or applications of the new drugs just coming in, but were probably eager to use anything that offered an improvement."[80] Indeed, the treatment for tuberculosis shifted quickly in the 1950s, but patients' suspicions stemmed not just from an imperfect understanding of medical culture.

The difference between medical research's clinical trials and human experimentation is patient consent.[81] Given the very unequal power relationships between medical staff and patients, coupled with often perplexing language barriers, and the widespread perception that many Aboriginal people would not willingly accept treatment, patient consent for treatment was often simply taken for granted. Camsell Hospital, from its founding, developed a close relationship with the University of Alberta medical school, which offered specialist consultants to the hospital, while the hospital's patients provided interesting teaching and research "material" for the medical school.[82] In a statement intended to demonstrate the Camsell Hospital's successes, IHS claimed that in the late 1940s it was "one of the first hospitals to experiment with the use of streptomycin and to achieve a breakthrough in tuberculosis treatment."[83] The Camsell Hospital also undertook a 1956 trial of various different preparations of the common anti-tuberculosis drug para-aminosalicylic acid (PAS) on "Indian and Eskimo" patients. The experiment, which involved forty-eight patients, required five daily blood samples to be taken by vein puncture.[84] The blood of Inuit patients was of particular interest to researchers conducting metabolic tests for the Defence Research Board.[85] Blood samples were taken from "nearly two dozen hospitalized Eskimo patients" for an American researcher studying "widely separated ethnic and geographic racial groups." Consultant Allan Edwards conducted clinical trials of TSH (thyroid-stimulating hormone) from drug maker Nordic Pharmaceuticals for his study of hypothyroidism in "Native races."[86] He proposed to bring in another university consultant and, with grants from pharmaceutical companies Bristol Laboratories or Ayerst McKenna

Harrison, run trials of new antibiotics for treatment of pneumonia and renal infections. As he noted, the hospital had "adequate clinical material" and it had long been recognized that "patient treatment is very likely to benefit when a clinical study is being conducted." But IHS director Moore did not think it would be "politic" to accept grants from drug companies. Instead the studies could be performed by hospital staff using the hospital laboratory and would be a legitimate expense of public funds. But, he continued, if the drug companies wanted to "give us some 'samples' to use in the study, or if, because of our interest and theirs, they wished to offer us a special price on a batch of drugs to be used in the study, that is quite a different matter."[87] By the 1970s the department became more diligent in securing consent, especially for sexual sterilization, but not without controversy.[88] The ubiquity in patient narratives of distrust of medical personnel not only reflects the reality of life in an Indian hospital, it also points to a wider suspicion of the intentions of the colonizing state's myriad policies and its institutions intended to eliminate their languages and cultures.

Patient narratives also highlight resistance. Challenging their incarceration, and rejecting the treatment regime of the strictly controlled environment, some patients left hospital. The recalcitrant patient was a common problem in sanatoria, but in the pre-antibiotic era when treatment relied on bed rest and the cultivation of self-discipline, where cures were rare and wards were full, patients were not kept against their will. But Indian hospitals were not sanatoria. Certainly patient narratives of resistance that emphasize survival and the strength of the people, individually and collectively, are an important counterweight to persistent images of dependence and victimization.[89] But it is important that historical interpretations that stress the people's agency through narratives also provide the historical context of the coercive nature of IHS policies and its close collaborations with police and courts lest they imply that resistance and resiliency somehow mitigated the damage done to communities and individuals.[90] For example, in Manitoba, in a most single-minded search for the contagious, medical superintendents made liberal use of the provincial public health act, sending the police to return patients to hospital. In 1946 "George Hamilton" from a northern reserve presented himself at the Dynevor Indian Hospital for treatment, and after two months he was allowed to go home to tend to family matters. When he did not return to hospital the medical superintendent, Dr Campbell, swore out a warrant and the local RCMP arrested Hamilton and escorted him back to Dynevor Hospital. Dr Campbell hoped to operate and remove some of his ribs, and though Hamilton refused that treatment, he remained in hospital. In his absence, Hamilton's family had no means of support, but only after two of his young children died did Indian Affairs finally arrange for a $10 monthly ration and a wood supply to keep the rest of the family alive. Hamilton was kept in hospital. When community members complained to Indian Agent McPherson about Hamilton's plight, he "informed the Indians that any person with T.B. could be arrested." McPherson reported the appalling case to his superiors only because, as he warned, "these Indians have a habit of going to some outside white people preferably Lawyers and Politicians in whose hands they will put this matter."[91] The details of Hamilton's experience are exceptional in the archival record, but the files are replete with RCMP reports documenting the arrest of "Indians" and their usual one-year sentence to hospital.[92] Historical interpretations that foreground resistance as survival, without inquiring into its wider social, political, and economic contexts, relieve us from confronting the conditions that made resistance necessary. While Manitoba was especially vigilant in bringing the ill to justice, it is clear that white Manitobans were not likewise subject to arrest.

One can only imagine the distress of patients such as the two Inuk women who walked out of Parc Savard Hospital in Quebec City in February 1952. Dressed only in bathrobes and slippers, the women walked a considerable distance before they were brought back to hospital. They had been in Parc Savard for four years, and with no one on staff who could speak their language they likely assumed they would remain there, forgotten indefinitely. Leo Manning, former Hudson's Bay Company manager and by the early 1950s one of a very few Inuktitut speakers working for the northern administration, acted as interpreter and visited the hospital in 1952. At the time there were ninety Inuit patients (fifty-five adults and thirty-five children) as well as immigrants requiring medical care, ill mariners, and a few veterans in the hospital. Some Inuit men kept busy with wood carving, while women knitted socks and sweaters and produced beadwork for slippers for a local firm that paid them $2 per dozen. Manning found Inuit patients' morale "very low" and in his three-day visit recorded patient messages to be broadcast by CBC Northern Message Service out of Winnipeg.[93]

Parc Savard (see illustration 4.2), originally built at the turn of the century as a quarantine hospital for immigrants, began accepting Inuit patients in the late 1940s and by 1956 operated as a general hospital with surgery, obstetrics, gynaecology, paediatrics, orthopaedics, cardiology,

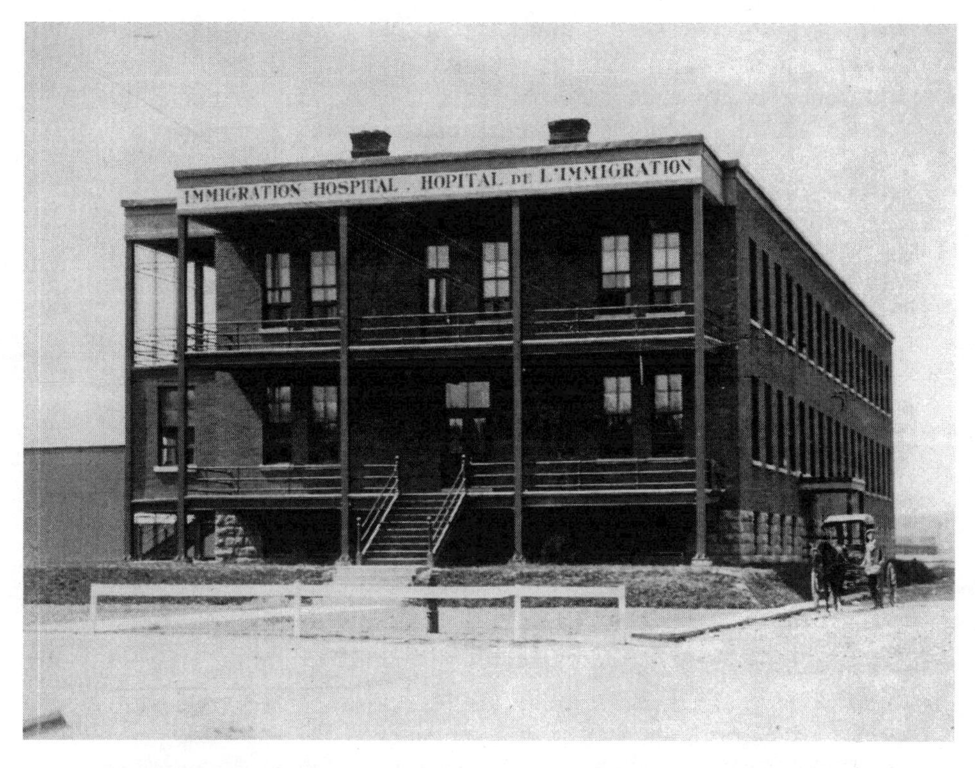

Illustration 4.2 Parc Savard Immigration Hospital, later Parc Savard Indian Hospital. A quarantine hospital for immigrants, Parc Savard at Quebec City also accepted Inuit patients by the 1940s. The insect- and rodent-infested building had 198 general hospital beds.

Source: PA-117288, LAC.

and diagnostic radiology with a daily average of 198 patients. Hospital superintendent J.E. Labrecque complained that he had only three physicians on staff; the buildings were literally crumbling; the heating and lighting were inadequate; in Ward D, which had twenty-eight beds, there were only three toilets and one bathtub; and the hospital was infested with cockroaches, fleas, bedbugs, mice, and rats. Worse yet, the slum adjacent to the hospital property was home to a factory that repaired old mattresses. "Needless to say that it is a nest for rats which are causing us great inconvenience."[94] It is not clear where the two Inuk women hoped to go when they left the hospital in bedclothes in February, but they could be forgiven for thinking they would be better off elsewhere.

Generally, provincial sanatoria did not keep patients against their will. Certainly public health legislation provided the authority to remove the infectious to sanatorium but rarely the power to keep them there. Sanatorium directors worried that to treat patients as criminals risked losing public confidence in the institutions. The ill might avoid medical treatment for fear they would be incarcerated.[95] In most jurisdictions citizens' civil liberties were not sacrificed for the public good. Public health bureaucrats in Saskatchewan contemplated compulsory detention for the "incorrigible open case of tuberculosis," but when the Anti-TB League that operated the provincial sanatoria refused to provide a locked ward, the matter rested.[96] The exception, however, was Nova Scotia, where amendments to the provincial public health act in 1948 provided the authority for detention and compulsory treatment of patients with "open" pulmonary tuberculosis who would not conduct themselves responsibly, though the "intelligent and co-operative" could carry on safely at home. Class and race most often marked the difference between the "irresponsible" and the "co-operative." By 1954, as J.E. Hiltz, medical superintendent of the Nova Scotia Sanatorium in Kentville, told the readers of the *Canadian Medical Association Journal*, fifty-two patients (including five "Indians") were convicted and sent to the detention unit, 200 kilometres away on the grounds of the Roseway Hospital in Shelburne. The locked ward was a "fireproof and escape-proof" concrete bunker situated far from hospital buildings so "the noise" did not disturb others.[97] But not all provincial jurisdictions were as accommodating.

The 1953 Indian Health Regulations filled the void by providing the necessary authority for detention "when a province is unable or unwilling to take the appropriate action in connection with some communicable disease among Indians."[98] On director Moore's recommendation, the 1951 amendments to the Indian Act (section 72) included the authority to make regulations to provide "compulsory hospitalization and treatment for infectious diseases among Indians."[99] The Indian Health Regulations that soon followed made possible the detention and incarceration of the dangerous. Exposing the limits of Canada's liberalism, the Regulations' expressed intent was to "eliminat[e] any discrimination between those Canadian citizens of Indian status and other citizens of Canada" by applying all provincial public health laws to status Indians. But in order "to protect and promote the health of the Indians" the regulations contained compulsory provisions.[100] The Regulations applied to all Indians who lived on reserve and "every Indian who follows the Indian mode of life" (to cover those in the north where reserves were not set aside), as well as those who lived in non-Aboriginal communities. Thus, "an Indian who suspects himself to be infected with an infectious disease" must be treated by a doctor. Violators faced a $100 fine, or three months' imprisonment, or both. Patients could appeal their detention by petition served on the superintendent (Indian agent) before a magistrate or two justices of the peace, with the physician present, though one wonders if patients were informed of their rights, or indeed of the Regulations themselves. Included in the Regulations were IHS Forms 7018 parts a, b, and c authorizing (respectively) compulsory medical examination and treatment; apprehension and detention; and the forced return of patients to hospital. The new Regulations recognized that "some Indians object strongly to having the police called in to force them to undergo examination and treatment ... [but] it is necessary to take compulsory action."[101] Not unlike the efforts to identify Inuit patients through fingerprinting by the RCMP in the 1930s, the Indian Health Regulations made clear the association of Aboriginal illness with criminality and subsequent incarceration.[102]

Dave Melting Tallow recalled how he left Camsell Indian Hospital against medical advice to attend the Calgary Stampede. His cousin brought him clothes and he climbed out a window, though the police eventually caught up with him. On another occasion he did not get as far:

> See what they used to do was they could put you in jail. They'd put you in jail in a cell. You had to go to court. I did one time. I had to go to court. I was running away from the hospital, they took me up there. I don't know what I was charged with, but they charged me with something. I just had pajamas on – in jail with pajamas on. The judge said that I had a choice – if I didn't want to go back to the hospital, he'd put me in jail and I'd have to stay there in jail until I was cured or something. Or I could go back to the hospital. Naturally I chose to go back to the hospital. They told me that I was giving TB to everybody.[103]

After three years in hospital Melting Tallow was finally released after undergoing a lobectomy and the removal of several ribs (see chapter 3). Not surprisingly, Indian hospitals maintained locked detention wards, usually constructed during renovations before the hospitals opened, and well before the Indian Health Regulations were enacted.[104]

A former nurse recalled hearing about, though never seeing, the "jail," a small room on the roof of the Charles Camsell Hospital where patients were kept under guard.[105] The RCMP delivered a man in leg irons to the ward in 1958. The superintendent warned, "Any patient who has tuberculosis and who runs away from the hospital will be locked in a private room when brought back to the hospital and all privileges suspended for one week, e.g. radio, visitors, etc."[106] Most provincial jurisdictions did not infringe on civil liberties of the tuberculous through compulsory detention, but the sweeping powers of the Indian Health Regulations were another reminder that Aboriginal people remained wards of the state without the liberties of citizens.[107]

Indian Health Service, a centralized bureaucracy with a network of interrelated institutions and a wide legal mandate, used its authority to move patients into and within its system, and, later, to provincial sanatoria. By the mid- to late-1950s the trends in tuberculosis treatment were mirrored in Indian hospitals: the success of antibiotic treatment further slashed already falling tuberculosis rates. But, Indian hospitals, unlike sanatoria, did not quickly empty because the institutions admitted patients with all medical conditions, determined by race not disease. What were once "tuberculosis" beds became general treatment beds since only a full hospital kept per diem rates from rising. Perhaps not surprisingly then, Indian hospitals continued to rely on compulsion. For example, asked to explain the cause for vacant beds at Miller Bay Indian Hospital in 1956, medical superintendent G.R. Howell suggested that tuberculosis in the region was coming under control. To fill the beds in his hospital would involve "scraping the bottom of the tuberculosis barrel" through more intensive surveillance and "the persistent use of persuasion and I.H.S. 7018a [Indian Health Regulations] to bring unwilling patients to hospital."[108] In 1957 Alberta's zone superintendent, Dr Falconer, informed Moore: "practically all the T.B. patients found in the province are under treatment and there is no waiting list. All the patients in the N.W.T. recommended for surgery have been admitted."[109] Saskatchewan, with its three provincial sanatoria, began accepting more Aboriginal patients in the 1950s, but patients who left against medical advice often found themselves admitted to the more "secure" Fort Qu'Appelle Indian Hospital.[110] Nevertheless, some patients chose to resist by isolating themselves from family and community in the bush rather than in hospital. Nevertheless, arrest warrants were issued. In Saskatchewan in 1961, IHS bureaucrats complained that patients who should be institutionalized "are hiding in the bush, even though a warrant has been issued for their apprehension ... Right now there is an old lady 77 years old who is hiding herself somewhere in the bush to avoid the RCMP."[111] As late as 1966 Dr Matas assured tuberculosis professionals that recalcitrant Aboriginal patients were not a problem. But, he continued, since provincial public health regulations "are much less severe than are the Indian Health Regulations," if the latter were ever abolished he hoped that "with patience and persistence" the provinces could be convinced to make full use of their regulations when required.[112]

Patients, first relocated to distant hospitals, were then shifted between institutions for medical reasons, to undergo surgery for example, or for bureaucratic convenience – to make use of bed space. Parallels can be drawn with the colonizing state's disturbingly frequent relocations of individuals and communities in the interests of resource development, bureaucratic convenience, and national security, while the "removed" were assured it was "for their own good."[113] Inuit, the most dramatic example, were transported thousands of kilometres to southern hospitals with minimal consultation and few opportunities to question their fate.[114] In October 1945 the Clearwater Lake Indian Hospital at The Pas in northern Manitoba received thirty-nine patients from Norway House Hospital without names, treaty numbers, histories, or records, including an infant of seven months – "nameless, numberless with no instructions for treatment. It has recovered at the Pas, on Penicillin, but no one knows who it is."[115] Children were especially vulnerable. Harry Kegiuna spent seven years in hospital as a child. Sent from the north by ship, where he sat in the corner by himself, then by airplane, he eventually reached Charles Camsell Indian Hospital. No one knew his name so he was simply called "Harry Hospital." After spending years in the hospital he was woken one night, told to put on some clothes, and sent across the country to Ottawa by train, with no chance to say goodbye to anyone: "They never told you what was going to happen."[116] Working as a government translator, Minnie Aodla Freeman visited Inuit patients at the St Boniface Hospital in Manitoba in 1957: "We saw a child there who had forgotten his language completely. This was as sad as any illness. How will he communicate with his parents when he goes home?"[117] Author Grygier notes that Inuit infants and children whose mothers were in treatment were fostered out on southern reserves, or more usually placed in Indian hospital wards, while others were informally adopted by white staff.[118] The medical superintendent at Dynevor Indian Hospital hoped to keep one of his "cute" Inuit patients. "In fact,

I told him [Louie] if he wanted to stay I would take him over myself for adoption. But he wanted to go back to his family and no doubt, it was the better plan."[119] Patients also found themselves moved about (and it is fair to assume they were never consulted) for reasons that had less to do with medical treatment.

The rapid change brought about by antimicrobial treatment for tuberculosis in the 1950s was celebrated as the "miracle" of the empty beds only in retrospect. At the time, sanatorium boards and their business managers faced rising per diem costs and growing deficits. In a particularly pathetic irony, not lost on IHS director Moore, sanatoria competed with each other and with Indian hospitals for Aboriginal bodies that had been for so long denied admission to their institutions.[120] In 1954, for instance, seven patients from Athabaska reserve in northern Alberta, and twelve from Yukon were taken south to the Charles Camsell Hospital and subsequently found themselves on the prairies in the Fort Qu'Appelle Sanatorium in southern Saskatchewan.[121] In 1955, C.B. Ross, superintendent of the venerable Muskoka Hospital in Ontario (established in 1896 as the first sanatorium in the country), thanked Moore for "another shipment of eleven Indians." With forty empty beds Ross wondered if Moore might direct more patients his way: "Anything which you might be able to do along this line would be greatly appreciated."[122] In an arrangement with IHS, Moose Factory Indian Hospital on James Bay sent Inuit patients to Mountain Sanatorium in Hamilton and Indian patients to Muskoka. But confusion set in when some Indians were sent to Hamilton; they were to be sent back to Moose Factory, like so much freight, as soon as beds were made available by shipping "new Indians" to Muskoka. The IHS regional superintendent reminded Moose Factory to advise the office when moving "Eskimos ... giving name, number, age and diagnosis and name of place he came from or to which he was sent."[123] Patients who did not understand English were at times "misplaced" in the system, and without communication with home, families were left to wonder what had become of their loved ones.

Clearwater Lake Indian Hospital in Manitoba, operated by the Manitoba Sanatorium Board on behalf of IHS, likewise felt the financial impact of increasingly effective treatments. In 1952, 195 patients were in residence; although this number eventually rose to 207, occupancy dropped sharply after 1959. By October 1961, the hospital reported a financial loss of $18,377, and the year was not yet over. But arrangements were soon made to improve the bottom line. As the hospital reported to the Sanatorium Board, "It was extremely difficult to see how these liabilities could be met, but as a result of discussions with Dr Moore, arrangements were made to transfer 58 tuberculosis patients to Clearwater Lake from Hamilton. As a result of this, and other increases in our tuberculosis occupancy, we are now in a satisfactory financial position."[124] The hospital committee minutes in October 1962, however, reported that the Inuit patients were transferred from Hamilton because of "disciplinary problems."[125] The trip from southern Ontario to northern Manitoba would have been particularly exhausting for the ill and increasingly perplexed patients. As noted in chapter 2, Aboriginal patients were kept in the institutions for one to two years in spite of the effectiveness of chemotherapy. Patients who survived were eventually relocated home (although some Inuit patients chose to remain in the south), but that process too was made more difficult by shoddy record keeping and at times callous disregard for patients' needs.[126] Many patients died at hospital and were never returned home, their families left to worry and wonder where they might be.

From the outset, IHS did its utmost to avoid responsibility for an issue it hoped to ignore: what to do with patients who died at its hospitals. Indian Affairs, for its part, was steadfast that it would pay no more than "absolutely necessary for the burial of indigent Indians." If the family wanted to transport and bury their loved one at home, it would be at their own expense.[127] When Dynevor Indian Hospital opened in 1939 the dead were buried across the Red River at the local parish, though the Sanatorium Board's George Northwood decried Indian Affairs' policy of limiting costs to $25 when the government allowed $100 for military burials.[128] At the Charles Camsell Hospital the issue emerged as soon as the institution opened. Regional superintendent E.L. Stone suggested that in the interests of good relations with local reserves IHS should show a "reasonable appearance of generosity" by notifying the undertaker and paying for embalming and a rough box to prepare the body for shipment to reserve, about $15.[129] But IHS refused to assume any responsibility for the burial of Aboriginal patients. Moore's assistant did acknowledge that families might be reluctant to send their sick to distant hospitals if they were not assured that in the event of death they would be buried at home.[130] Indian Affairs, rather unhelpfully, proposed that IHS develop a form to be completed by hospitalized patients outlining their financial resources and also indicating whether, in case of death, the patient's family wanted the body returned to the reserve. Failing that, Indian Affairs agreed to pay the costs of a burial in a cemetery closest to the Indian hospital if the family lacked the funds to return the body to their home community for burial.[131] By August 1947, with "considerable" mortality at the Camsell Hospital, Protestant patients were interred on the grounds of the Edmonton Residential School (where students were paid to dig the graves), and Catholics were buried at Enoch's on the Stony Plain reserve.[132] When they could, the hospital carpentry shop made small coffins for parents who wanted to take their deceased infants home with them.[133]

This policy, maintained across the country, was particularly harsh for northern communities, who could rarely afford the costly flights to return their family members. Yet into the 1960s Indian Affairs continued to refuse to provide transportation for deceased patients "if this will exceed the cost of burial at the place he died."[134] The policy also provided IHS with access to bodies for autopsy without having to secure the family's consent. In 1964, the IHS regional superintendent for Saskatchewan, Dr Orford, blithely stated: "Disposal of the body of an Indian after death is a matter which concerns Indian Affairs Branch. Indian Health Services is concerned only with the living."[135] Given the frequent and arbitrary shifting of patients throughout the IHS hospital system, the incomplete record keeping, and unmarked graves in back corners of cemeteries scattered across the country, it is little wonder that families lost forever their sons and daughters, mothers and fathers. It is only in the last decades that communities have begun to locate and honour some of the lost patients who lived and died in Indian hospitals.[136]

A far more pervasive and progressive narrative of life in Indian hospitals, constructed by and for IHS, demonstrated the state's noble intentions and its heroic efforts to cure the Aboriginal condition. From its founding the Charles Camsell Indian Hospital was to be the showcase of IHS efforts to provide care and, as importantly, to be seen to provide care. In February 1946 the hospital superintendent proposed having the National Film Board feature the hospital: "This film would be useful for showing to groups from various agencies and would be excellent propaganda."[137] It would be a decade before the film appeared, but in the meantime IHS and hospital staff went to considerable effort to educate and inform its Aboriginal constituency and the public generally about the hospital's good work. Staff produced the *Camsell Arrow*, an in-house newsletter, not uncommon in sanatoria, intended to help with patient morale and develop literacy skills (though it is unclear how much patients contributed). The *Arrow* featured short, gossipy "ward news" (including the apparently obligatory expressions of gratitude to nurses and doctors), and longer articles, such as travelogues submitted by vacationing staff. The *Arrow*, like newsletters in other large Indian hospitals (for example, the *Coqualeetza Courier* and Miller Bay's *Totem Tattler*) was also a convenient vehicle to discipline patients in correct attitudes and behaviour. However, the Miller Bay patients' committee had to ask when the *Totem Tattler* was produced and whether patients would be allowed to participate.[138] In the interests of public relations, the *Camsell Arrow* was combined with an annual *Pictorial Review* and distributed to Indian agencies and visiting dignitaries.[139] IHS and the National Film Board created hundreds of images of smiling and, oddly, healthy-looking patients (illustration 4.3). Indian hospitals also welcomed curious local citizens to tour their wards to view the curiosities. At the Camsell Hospital a heavily tattooed Inuit woman gave the gawking onlookers something to remember by lifting her top to show her tattooed chest. Dynevor Hospital invited visitors to see "our two very cute Eskimos."[140] In 1952 the gifted portrait photographer Yousuf Karsh, already famous for his 1941 portrait of a scowling Winston Churchill that graced the cover of *Time* magazine, visited Edmonton and the Charles Camsell Indian Hospital for *Maclean's* magazine. His compelling portraits of patients Mrs Susan Philippe, Daniel Makokis from Saddle Lake Cree Nation, Lucy Michel from Fort Nelson, BC, and young boys, Joe Koaha and Peter Naitit, from Cambridge Bay, and a "Metis lad" from Whitehorse, capture their loneliness and frustration (see illustrations 4.4 to 4.7).

In 1956 the National Film Board, with the cooperation of Indian Affairs, Indian Health Service, and the Camsell Hospital, produced the short film *The Longer Trail*.[141] Although the film is a fictionalized narrative ostensibly about "Joe Lonecloud" and his successful struggle with tuberculosis in the Camsell Indian Hospital, the film's real hero is Mr Mosley, the intrepid Indian Affairs rehabilitation officer who fights to win Joe's trust and battles the prejudices of Edmonton's employers and boarding-house owners. Like the National Film Board's other short film on the subject, *No Longer Vanishing* (1955), it is a narrative about Indian struggles with modernity. Protected and sheltered on reserves, they must inevitably relocate and integrate into Canadian society as useful manual labourers.[142] *The Longer Trail* opens with Joe happily riding his horse on the prairie when a nurse approaches with the unfortunate news that his chest X-ray is positive. He is delivered to Charles Camsell Hospital, where doctors give him a 95 per cent chance of recovery through "drugs and sometimes surgery." Joe, however, can never

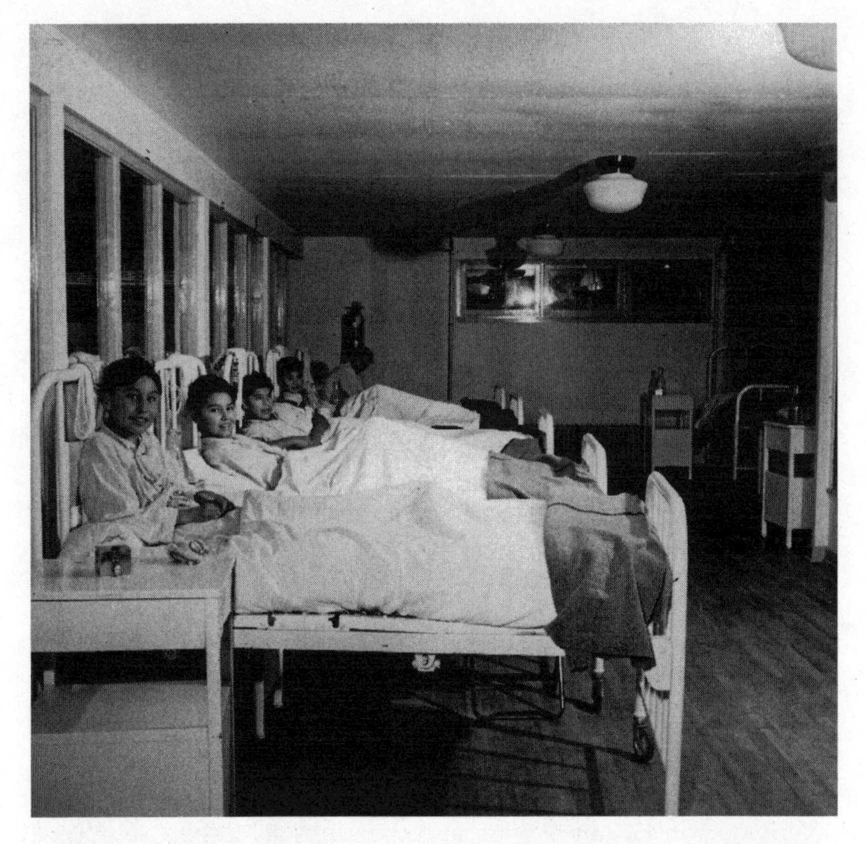

Illustration 4.3 Charles Camsell Indian Hospital. Indian Health Service enlisted the National Film Board to create hundreds of images of Aboriginal patients who are invariably portrayed as smiling and happy. The NFB also produced films depicting the hospitals as fundamental in the process of integration and assimilation.

Source: PA-139319, LAC.

return to his strenuous work on the "ranch." Joe, mute throughout the film except for his interior dialogue, admits to being afraid, misses his family and his horse, and muses, "I wonder if horses cry at night?" He escapes from hospital, but soon realizes his error and returns. Mr Mosley finally reaches Joe with an impassioned speech telling the young man that he is not the first to get TB. He can stay in hospital for five years, ten

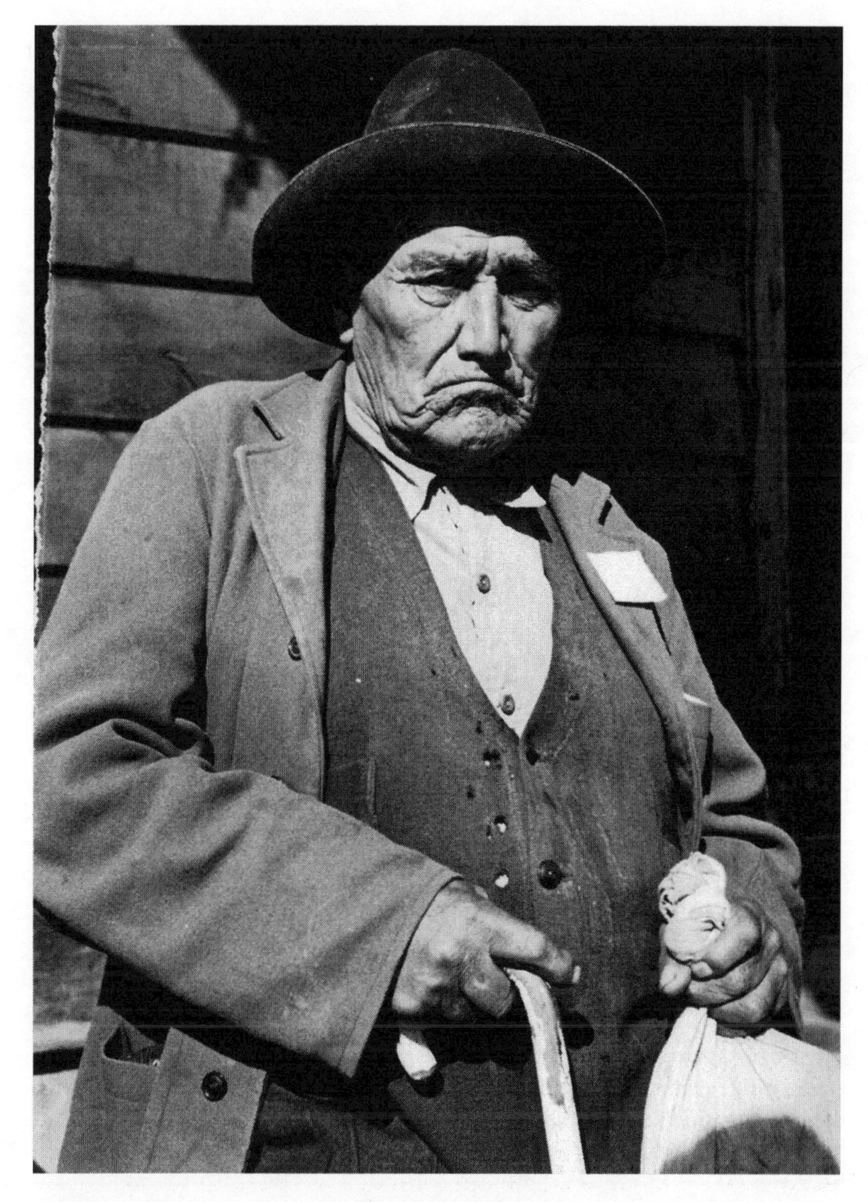

Illustration 4.4 Daniel Makokis, Saddle Lake, Alberta, at Charles Camsell Indian Hospital. Yousuf Karsh 1952.

Source: PA-165895, LAC.

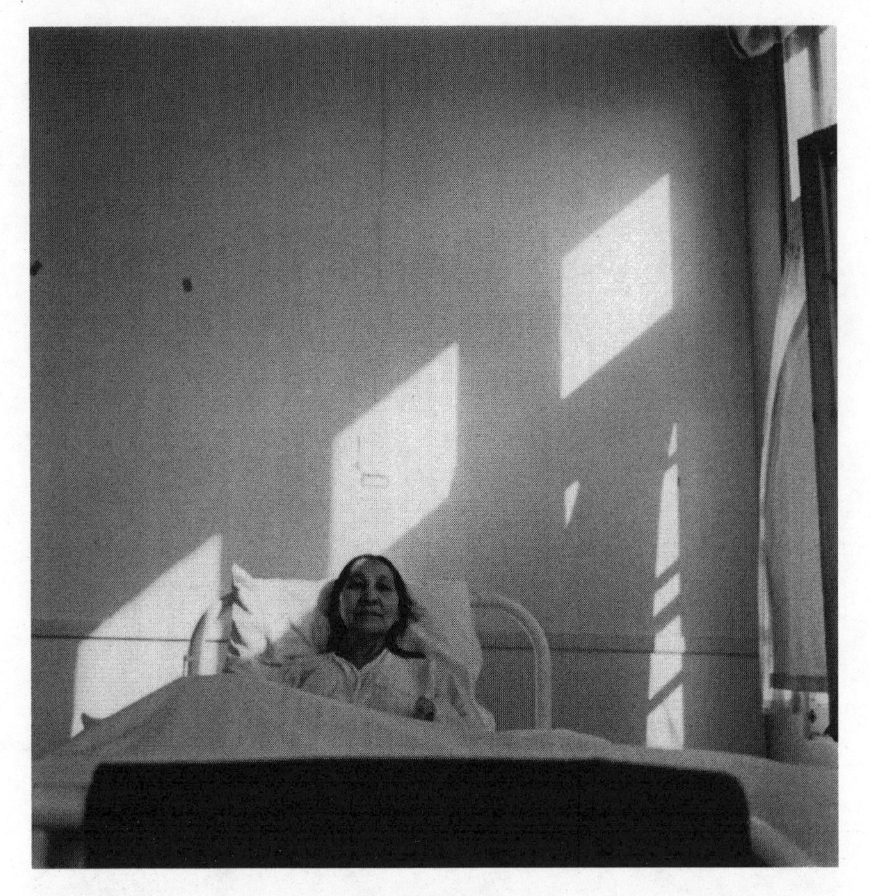

Illustration 4.5 Mrs Susan Philippe, Charles Camsell Indian Hospital. Yousuf Karsh 1952.

Source: e011083918, LAC.

years, or he may never leave, because with TB "you have to want to get well and right now you don't want to." Joe must change. Mosley promises to help him get an education in hospital and a job upon discharge. When Joe asks what job an Indian can get, Mosley has no answer, except to point out that there are no opportunities on the reserve. Joe subsequently embraces leatherwork, demonstrating that he is "good with his hands." And so, after two years, he is finally released. With a job in a carpentry shop and a quiet room, he does not think too much about his

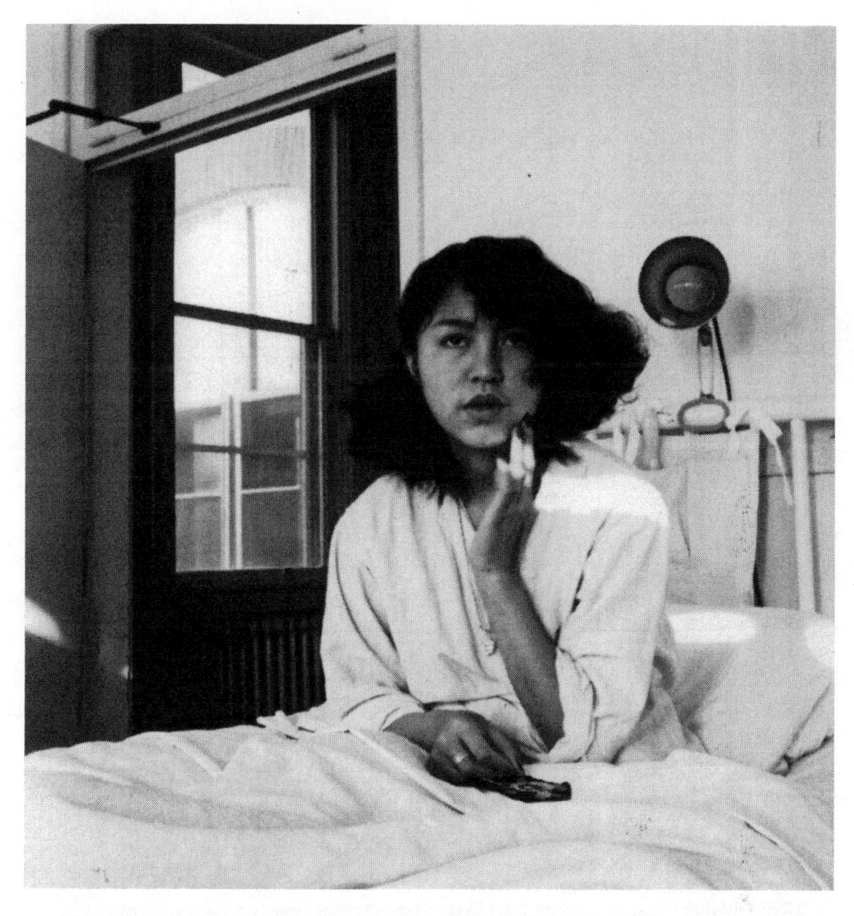

Illustration 4.6 Lucy Michel, Fort Nelson, BC, at Charles Camsell Indian Hospital. Yousuf Karsh 1952.

Source: e011083919 LAC.

horse or his home anymore. In the final scene Joe walks alone through a suburban Edmonton neighbourhood dreaming about someday fitting in on a quiet street with good neighbours, a wife, and kids. "I dream. I think, who knows?" *The Longer Trail* articulates a mid-century view that equates reserves with disease and dependency and professes faith in medicine and its institutions to solve the "Indian problem" through urban relocation and assimilation. Joe's trail to healthy citizenship,

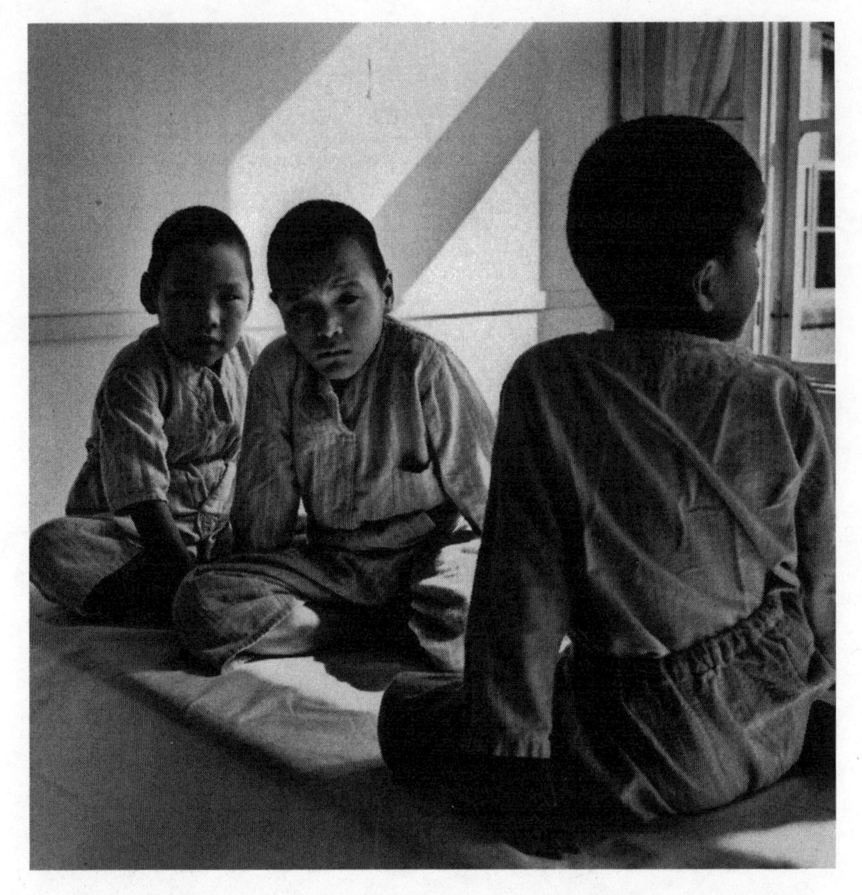

Illustration 4.7 Joe Koaha and Peter Naitit, Cambridge Bay; "Metis lad," Whitehorse at Charles Camsell Indian Hospital. Yousuf Karsh 1952.

Source: PA-165896, LAC.

made longer by his own ignorance and society's bigotry, was finally successful when he accepted his place in the economic order and left the reserve behind.

It is not clear what the Aboriginal participants in these carefully constructed narratives made of their experience, but Minnie Freeman, working in Ottawa was outraged and sickened to find herself being used as a token Inuk for state propaganda. Told to report to an unfamiliar bureaucracy, she was directed to smile and hold up a Canada Savings Bond while gazing at an Inuit carving; a photographer took her picture. Upset to find her image in the local newspaper the next day, she recalled: "The story read: 'Eskimos buying bonds, keeping up with progress,' some remark like that. I felt sick. I had no idea what bonds were … I felt sick because I was being used to show the *qallunaat* in the South how well the Inuit are treated in the North … I became very apprehensive after that when someone phoned, asking to interview me. I felt I could not be a part of something which was not really happening. Never were there photographs that showed the truth about my people's lives."[143]

Positive images of life and death in Indian hospitals, "excellent propaganda" in the construction of the welfare state, reassured Canadians that even the most recalcitrant and irresponsible received care, by force if necessary. In the hands of harried, if not unqualified staff, in crowded and dismal institutions, patients endured medicine's supposed great benefits. Their narratives of abuse, compulsion, and incarceration demonstrate a grim determination to survive at times despite, rather than because of, their institutionalization. Medicalizing inequality and pathologizing Aboriginality in the interests of the wider Canadian community, IHS carried out the colonizing state's contradictory policies: to segregate in order to assimilate and to isolate in order to integrate. But despite the Indian hospitals' obvious shortcomings, they remained a tangible state commitment to the people's health care, if not an acknowledgment of the treaty right to health care that communities would not easily forfeit.

Chapter Five

Getting Out of the Hospital Business

In early 1961 Indian Health Service bureaucrats mused that their objective should be to "get out of the hospital business wherever we can. The key word is *quiet*. There is no need to make a big to-do."[1] In particular, they had in mind the on-reserve hospitals in southern Alberta. That IHS policy makers presumed such a fundamental shift in health care delivery would escape notice highlights their continued insularity and paternalism, but it was also a tacit admission of the hospitals' serious deficiencies. By the 1960s there were more than enough empty sanatorium beds to meet the steadily declining need for in-patient tuberculosis treatment. Heavy investment in hospital and health care infrastructure under the continuing National Health Grants program meant that Canadians who could afford it had access to care in modern, well-staffed acute care hospitals. And by 1957, with the introduction of national hospital insurance, federal and provincial funds helped pay the spiralling hospitalization costs for all Canadians. New definitions of the "national health" meant that Indian hospitals would be quietly closed and community hospitals would be prevailed upon to expand (using IHS funds) to accept Aboriginal patients. Part of the broader postwar push for integration and "equality," Indians would disappear finally into the larger fabric of society and with them would go their "special status," treaties, and reserves.[2] Warning that the move to close hospitals would be "resisted by the Indians," bureaucrats assured their minister that they only needed to point out that community hospitals would provide better care.[3] Indeed, resistance emerged from all sides as the national projects of integration and Medicare became snarled in nasty federal–provincial jurisdictional disputes. Aboriginal communities argued that funds intended for their health care should be spent on much-needed improvements in Indian hospitals, and not invested in non-Aboriginal community institutions. For their part, some community hospital boards and provincial health departments also resisted Indian hospital closures, deeming Aboriginal patients a burden best cared for by the federal government. Aboriginal communities had good reason to fear a return to restricted access and basement wards in community hospitals. A focus on the experience in Alberta provides an opportunity to untangle the threads of these broad programs to assess their impact on Aboriginal health and health care. "Getting out of the hospital business" by starving the Blackfoot Indian Hospital while rebuilding the Charles Camsell Hospital suggests that integration in hospital care had as much to do with asserting medical authority and bureaucratic control as improving health. Likewise, the march to Medicare – hospital insurance and health care insurance – widely considered a great national success, was particularly damaging to Aboriginal people, who, caught between jurisdictions, came to be seen as unwanted patients in community hospitals and less deserving of care.

Particular targets for closure were the Blackfoot and Blood Indian hospitals in southern Alberta. Both hospitals, substantial three-storey brick structures built in the 1920s on their respective reserve lands, pre-dated IHS postwar expansion. Serving their reserve communities exclusively, the hospitals developed to meet local needs. The Blood Hospital, a Catholic missionary institution operated by the Sisters of Charity and built in 1928 on the southern edge of the reserve, sat on the main street of the Mormon settlement at Cardston, across from the community hospital. The Blackfoot Hospital further north replaced Anglican missionary care on the reserve in 1924. Owned by the Siksika (Blackfoot) and built with funds realized by the sale of nearly half their reserve lands, the hospital was unique as the only band-owned "Indian" hospital in the west and one of only two in the country.[4] The Siksika agreed to fund the hospital on the condition that their indigenous healers and midwives be allowed to continue their practice.[5] Over the next thirty years or so both reserve communities developed a medical syncretism or pluralism combining Western medicine with indigenous healers, a pragmatic accommodation to the changed circumstances of colonization.[6] With the independence that ownership conferred, the Siksika cultivated a measure of local control that became increasingly unpalatable to IHS. To understand why IHS planned to close the Blood and particularly the Blackfoot Hospital, it is necessary to examine the tensions between local pluralism in health care and the ascendant authority of medical bureaucrats to define and direct care in Indian hospitals.

While the Blood and Blackfoot hospitals replaced the rudimentary missionary hospitals that had been established in the nineteenth century in conjunction with denominational boarding schools, the majority of patients continued to be schoolchildren. As historian John Milloy notes, contagious disease spread easily among the weakened and poorly clothed children in badly constructed school buildings.[7] At the new Blackfoot Hospital, the resident Indian Agent George Gooderham reported in 1926 "children from the schools are admitted without asking the consent of the parents except when it is an operation case of a serious nature. It is among the children of 8 to 16 years of age that very good results have been obtained ... The doctor does minor operations when necessary; tonsils, adenoids, light tracoma cases and curettating tubercular affections [*sic*] make up the large proportion of these operations." Convalescing patients, especially older schoolgirls, were put to work washing and scrubbing at the hospital.[8] While children were forced into the hospital and kept there, their parents remained sceptical, preferring the services of their own healers and midwives.

Male physicians, in particular, had little to offer Siksika women. But the appointment in 1928 of Dr Frances Evelyn Windsor as medical superintendent of the Blackfoot Hospital may have attracted women to the hospital. Windsor, single and with a young child to care for, gladly accepted the appointment as medical superintendent, which came with regular rations and a house. Few other physicians wanted the small salary on an isolated reserve, though, as the 1920s slid into the Depression and private practices dried up, male physicians jealously eyed her appointment. As a friend of Calgary's member of parliament and prime minister, R.B. Bennett, Windsor was secure in her position.[9] She may have encouraged women into the hospital by acknowledging the Siksika's great reluctance to leave sick family members in the care of strangers. Though the Blackfoot Hospital's records are not extant, admissions at the Blood Hospital, especially among women, increased in the 1920s and 1930s. That hospital's records may point to a cultural explanation for increased use. Owned by the Department of Indian Affairs, but managed by the Catholic Sisters of Charity, the Blood Hospital allowed ill women to keep their young children with them in hospital, and permitted mothers to stay with their sick children, often bringing along healthy siblings as well. Moreover, government doctors did not attend the hospital unless called for. In October 1923, for example, the hospital admitted fourteen women, thirty-six children, and two men. Nine of the women were not ill, but accompanied their sick children; thirteen of the children were healthy and staying with sick mothers or siblings. Nearly half the hospital's residents (42 per cent) were not sick, which suggests the hospital was made to fit larger Kainai (Blood) cultural and social perceptions of health care.[10] However, the reserve's DIA physician Dr Alan Kennedy disapproved, urging "discipline" to make the institution a "true hospital ... not a comfortable place to stay, as some of the Indians seem to consider it now."[11] It seems likely that the Siksika made their hospital a "comfortable place" since they owned the institution.

Young women on the reserves, particularly residential school graduates who spent years under Christian influence, chose to attend the hospital's maternity ward, where they also learned to sew a complete layette for their newborns. In a 1926 photograph Siksika women proudly display their chubby infants at the hospital's baby clinic[12] (illustration 5.1). Certainly the Indian agent believed the maternity work would bring the "greatest beneficial results to the general health of these people."[13] But the hospital also had more practical advantages, namely running water and reliable heat in winter, services that reserve homes lacked. Gooderham advocated for an additional bathroom in the hospital "where Indians, not patients, could secure a bath. At present they flock to the Ward baths and although we want to encourage cleanliness, we wish to improve the situation."[14] Nurse Pesquot, a hospital employee in the late 1930s, suggested that women used the maternity ward in winter but preferred their own midwives in summer. As she told anthropologists Lucien and Jane Hanks, "Women seldom come in summer for childbirth ... In winter women come in with their children even though there is not much wrong with them. It is in order to get warm." Pesquot, who clearly resented the peoples' pragmatic hospital use, deemed them "hard to care for ... [T]hey always want something." She also supposed that the women did not feel pain. "At childbirth we never give any (analgesics). They may groan a little." When the anthropologists suggested that the women felt pain but did not express it, Pesquot replied, "they are just like animals." Her invective, prompted in part by her disapproval of the peoples' continued autonomy, was also a reaction to her perceived subordinate position in relation to the Siksika, whom she saw as inferiors.[15] Nevertheless, the Siksika used the hospital according to their social and cultural notions of care. But that autonomy would soon be undermined by rising costs and the continued poor health of the residential school students.

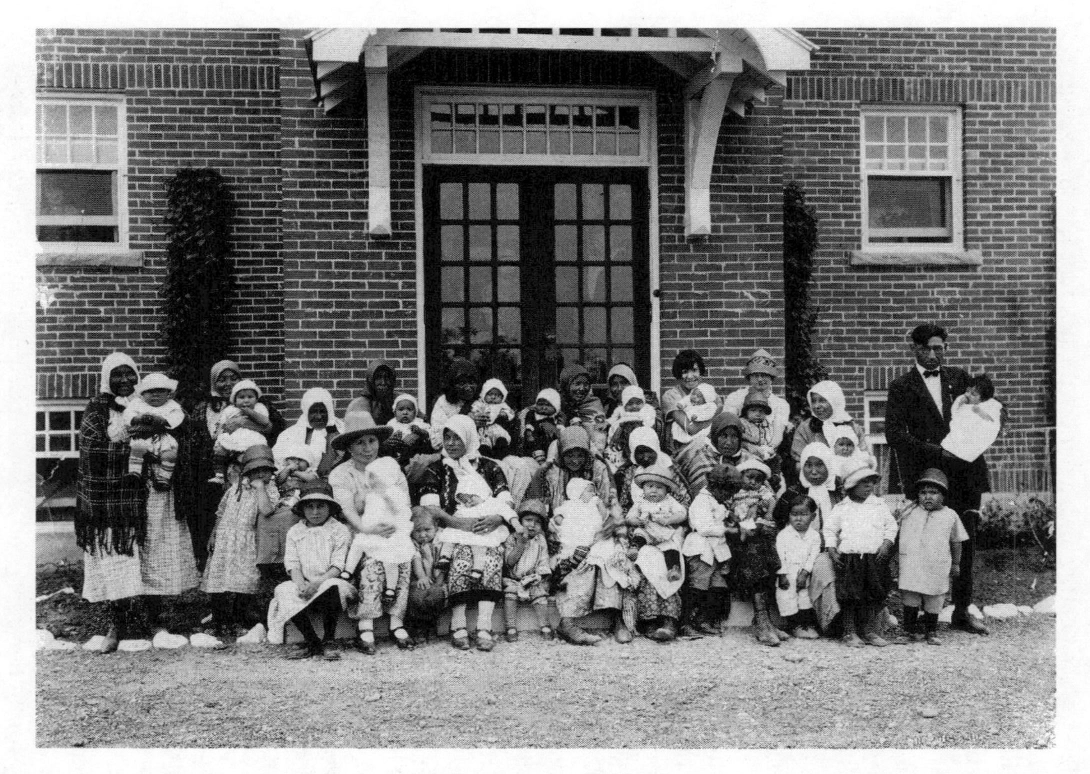

Illustration 5.1 Contestants in the first baby show held at the Blackfoot Hospital, 1926. Front row, L-R: Mrs Charles Joe Royal (1st prize winner); Mrs Harry Red Gun (2nd prize); Mrs A. Youngman (3rd prize). Mrs Jack McHugh is in the back row, right, in the cloche hat. Earl Calf Child, on the extreme right, the Indian agent's interpreter, is holding the baby of Mrs Spring Calf, who died in childbirth. The child was raised in the hospital.

Source: PA-32–1, Glenbow Archives.

A 1934 X-ray clinic at the Siksika's residential schools found a number of children requiring observation and eleven pupils who required immediate hospitalization. Students filled the enlarged forty-six-bed hospital, leaving little room for "ordinary cases."[16] It was clear to the agent that ill children could not be left in school under missionary care. While the Anglican Old Sun's School had plenty of dormitory space, it had no nurse, and the Catholic Crowfoot School had a nurse but was so overcrowded that staff slept in the infirmary. "Beds in the dormitories are so close together, one can barely move about. This school cannot keep a diseased child at present."[17] But despite children's poor health, missionaries resisted the loss of their students to the hospital, and the per capita grant that went with them. Crowfoot School's Father Jacques Riou insisted that the school, with its "home atmosphere," actually provided better care than the hospital.[18] Missionaries opposed what they considered unwarranted interference in their schools, while Gooderham pressed for hospital expansion.

Dr Windsor, in keeping with accepted tuberculosis treatment at the time, suggested a two-storey addition with balconies, where patients could enjoy complete bed rest with access to sunshine and the open air.[19] Instead, the agent thought it better to build a new residence for staff, while tuberculosis patients could be isolated in the old staff wing. While he was sure Siksika Council would approve the estimated $8,000 for a staff residence, he cautioned his superiors: "The Indians do not want to spend one more cent for medicalization than is necessary but they realize the need of more ward space and also the desirability of segregating the tbs [*sic*]. They will agree to this suggestion, I am sure."[20] The following day, in a more candid letter to the DIA's medical director, Dr EL Stone, the agent admitted they were spending Siksika funds like a "bloated Millionaire." As the Depression worsened the Siksika Council became increasingly concerned about DIA management of their funds. And while they paid for all medical services, Siksika Council worried that their hospital was no longer able to provide needed care for tuberculosis patients. As Gooderham put it, "Our young Indians know the situation in this regard and are, even now, complaining that the Department makes the Blackfoot pay the bill when other Bands receive equal or better hospitalization from Consolidated Revenue [DIA]."[21] Moreover, by 1940 the Siksika also paid for the treatment of up to six patients in the Central Alberta (Keith) Sanatorium. Aboriginal people were not usually admitted to provincial sanatoria because of community prejudice and the DIA's reluctance to pay for treatment, but the Siksika paid $5,875 annually to the sanatorium, even though other Albertans received free treatment under the 1936 Tuberculosis Act.[22]

The Siksika's large trust fund was an anomaly in Canada, and the DIA used it to pay for all its reserve operations, including items promised in the treaty such as aid for agriculture, equipment, and wages for white employees. By the terms of the original 1910 land surrender agreement the Siksika insisted that everyone receive annual cash payments, rations, and extra assistance for the elderly from the interest payments on invested capital, a reasonable reaction to years of poverty. As the Depression continued and interest rates fell, so too did their annual income. Agent Gooderham worried that they might cut funding for the DIA operations: "The minute the Interest Rate is reduced and the income lowered to a point when the major services such as Medicalization Staff salaries, take so much of the income that the Indian cannot get that direct assistance or payment which he had been receiving, there will be a wild cry to get rid of hospitals, Doctor [*sic*], farming Instructors, Stockmen etc. This time may not be far distant."[23] Nevertheless, by 1940 the Council's annual expenditure was $115,000, which included $30,000 for medical care, $10,000 for equipment, $7,000 for livestock, $6,000 for maintenance, and $9,000 for wages for white employees; the remainder went for the mandated distribution of cash, food, and clothing. As was the DIA design in 1910, all expenses besides wages for the agent and his clerk and the five-dollar annuity promised in the 1877 treaty were paid from Siksika funds, which meant a considerable saving for the DIA.[24]

When, in 1942, the Central Alberta (Keith) Sanatorium warned that the beds occupied by Siksika patients would be required by the military, the DIA's assistant medical superintendent, Dr W.L. Falconer, urged the Blackfoot Hospital to treat more tuberculosis patients. The Siksika were uncooperative, according to the doctor, with their "'millionaire' complex ... [they] do not object to being admitted to Keith Sanatorium [but] they are more difficult to handle in their own hospital. They consider this hospital as their own." The Siksika needed to be disciplined to use their hospital properly, as Falconer put it; with "control and supervision ... persuasion and instruction" the Blackfoot Hospital could be made to treat more patients. Moreover, he disapproved of Dr Windsor's management and urged her to show "more enthusiasm" for the work by undertaking surgery on her patients. Ultimately, he advocated complete bureaucratic control of the hospital in order to impose compulsory hospitalization.[25] As it happened, veterans did not need the sanatorium beds due to thorough X-ray screening of recruits and the steady decline of tuberculosis generally. Nevertheless, the tendency to compulsion, while a long-standing DIA policy, gained new vigour after 1945, when IHS was incorporated into the Department of National Health and Welfare.

The Blackfoot Hospital came under IHS management while the Siksika continued to finance its operation and maintenance. Immediately, Dr E.L. Stone, now the IHS regional supervisor in Alberta, advised complete bureaucratic control of the Blackfoot Hospital; the Siksika trust fund should be relieved of all operational costs. As he explained to IHS director Moore, "If they contribute to annual operations they will naturally want to exercise about as much control as they now do."[26] Stone, like Falconer, considered the Siksika's continued medical pluralism a direct challenge to their authority. Likewise, further north at Hobbema, where local reserves wished to help finance a new hospital, Stone actively prevented it: "A money interest implies a share of control. It does not work well."[27] Meantime, reacting to minister of national health Brooke Claxton's 1946 statement that IHS would pursue a hospitalization program, Siksika Council announced that it would no longer fund the hospital operations. Council reasoned that since it was "tacitly accepted throughout the Dominion that hospitalization of Indians is a Government obligation ... the Department [should] pay all costs of operation of the Blackfoot Hospital as they are doing in every other Indian hospital."[28] Stone, of course, fully supported their decision, explaining that as long as the Siksika paid the expenses, the department would have little control over the people or the hospital. While director Moore considered the issue a matter of "high policy" to be decided at the ministerial level, he dismissed Stone's concerns, arguing that the Siksika should be made to pay for their own health care. He heartily endorsed state policy that Aboriginal people, unless absolutely indigent, should pay for their own medical care, agreeing with many of his contemporaries that medicine was most effective when paid for. Moore considered Stone's suggestion to finance the Blackfoot Hospital a "retrograde step." Instead, he urged the Indian agent to exert "some persuasion" on the Siksika Council to reverse their decision.[29]

The new minister of national health in 1947, Paul Martin, agreed with Moore that the Siksika should be forced to pay for medical care by the terms of their 1910 land surrender agreement. Moreover, he warned, if the Council continued to object he would have the Indian Act amended to override its wishes.[30] Moore meanwhile assured his minister that the Siksika were indeed millionaires with $1,147,304.40 in their capital fund. But Moore failed to also note that the seemingly impressive fund amounted to slightly more than $1,000 per person; moreover, it could only be used for capital expenses and to generate interest, which, at 5 per cent, netted $57,365 annually, with hospital expenses taking 60 per cent. Just days later Siksika Council reversed its position and authorized an expenditure of $35,000 (a 28 per cent increase over the previous year) for the Blackfoot Hospital for 1947–8.[31] It is not clear what prompted Council to reconsider, but the influence of both the minister of health and the minister responsible for Indian Affairs Branch was not inconsiderable. For Moore and minister Martin, their policy to make the Siksika pay was doubly virtuous: it would teach them to value medical care while relieving the beleaguered white taxpayers of the cost. But, as the 28 per cent increase in the Blackfoot Hospital accounts revealed, the costs of hospital care in Canada soared in the postwar period, prompting the federal government to embark on its National Health Grants program of generous aid for health care.

By 1946 the federal Liberal government had retreated from its expansive and expensive postwar promises of social security including universal health insurance.[32] Canadians nevertheless continued to demand and were willing to pay for modern hospital care though fewer and fewer could afford the postwar ballooning costs.[33] Instead, in 1948 Mackenzie King's government established annual matching federal grants to provinces, targeting, among other things, public health, tuberculosis control, mental health, and $13 million annually for hospital construction. Minister Paul Martin publicly announced each of the thousands of hospital project grants, prompting journalists to dub the program "milking Martin's millions."[34] National Health Grants funded Canada's hospitals to expand and modernize, aiding their efforts to attract the paying patient, while the burgeoning system of IHS Indian hospitals relieved them from treating Aboriginal patients. But the Blackfoot Hospital, not considered a normal hospital, was deemed ineligible for any grants. By 1954 the hospital seriously depleted the Siksika trust fund, prompting the new agent, J.E. Pugh, to plead with the IHS to relieve some costs, if only staff salaries.[35] But Moore refused: "I do not believe that it would be in the public interest to relieve the Blackfoot Band from the costs they are carrying in connection with the hospital and the doctor providing medical care to the Band at present. It is our objective to make more and more Bands who are in a position to meet all, or a share of, their medical costs, assume this responsibility."[36] Neither minister

Martin nor Moore acknowledged the stark irony that the wealthiest provincial hospitals received considerable support from public funds through the National Health Grants, yet the Siksika were made to bear all hospital costs. Moore, characteristically overbearing, demanded that the Siksika "millionaires" pay. An unsigned note in his own office questioned Moore's policy: "We are rather hard on the Blackfoot. No one else can support a hospital these days."[37]

By July 1954 Moore relented. He subsequently retreated to a familiar discourse that characterized Aboriginal people as diseased and careless about their own health, and posing a threat to the nation; they required the control and regulation that only IHS could provide. He declared that Siksika control of the hospital was not in the best interests of the "Indians, the hospital, or the staff employed." In particular, he objected to the Siksika's continued autonomy in presuming to dictate hospital policy that threatened medical authority: visiting hours were too lax, patients left hospital when they felt better, and young children and the elderly were admitted to hospital when their caregivers needed to travel. Moreover, he noted, the building was deteriorating because the Siksika could no longer afford to replace equipment and furnishings. He proposed that the IHS assume responsibility for all operating costs, while the Siksika would still pay $6 per day for adults admitted to the hospital and $1.50 for newborns.[38] Council accepted the offer for a fifteen-month trial beginning January 1955, but argued that maternity care should be free, as was the accepted practice in all Alberta hospitals.[39] Sharing hospital costs might also address Council's anxiety for patient safety in the deteriorating building. Fire, caused by bare wiring and overloaded fuse boxes, was a constant concern, while the already inadequate water supply and leaking pipes would be completely overwhelmed in the event of a fire. The building needed paint, and a ruptured sewer line contaminated the soil and rotted the floor.[40]

When the cost-sharing agreement expired in April 1956, Siksika Council again refused to vote any more funds for hospitalization, arguing that hospital costs had nearly depleted their trust fund. Council was unmoved by rumours that Moore would shut down the hospital unless they paid.[41] Moore then threatened that necessary hospital renovations, especially rewiring, would not proceed, and he ordered individual Siksika patients to pay in advance for their care or they would not be admitted to the hospital. "I feel the Blackfoot have long abused their privileges in this institution and that it might be best for all concerned if we could abandon it." Moore was determined to refuse treatment rather than fund the hospital even while DIA officials assured him that Siksika finances could no longer meet essential community needs such as housing, water supplies, and roads. In late 1957, Moore, at his most autocratic, demanded complete control of the hospital buildings and all equipment. As he put it, he would accept nothing less than "unconditional surrender" from the Siksika.[42]

The shift in position, from insisting the Siksika pay all hospital costs to demanding they cede complete control, reflected increasingly coercive IHS policies. As more institutions came under its control IHS stepped up compulsion through, among other things, the 1953 Indian Health Regulations. Marking Aboriginal bodies as particularly dangerous justified legalized state coercion. Facing the intransigence of a coercive bureaucracy intent on regulating and disciplining bodies "for their own good" and in the interests of national health, the Siksika saw their trust fund diminish. Not coincidentally, in 1957 at the same time as Moore demanded unconditional surrender, the national health benefited by the federal Hospital Insurance and Diagnostic Services Act, which provided non-Aboriginal Canadians free care in the hospital of their choice.

In May 1958 Siksika Chief Clarence McHugh and councillor Matthew Melting Tallow travelled to Ottawa to meet with IHS officials and request a complete refund of all money expended on medical care and staff salaries. They also wanted the DIA to refund their expenditures on wages, vehicles, and housing provided for agency employees, $6 million by their count.[43] Moore, flanked by the department solicitor and four bureaucrats representing Indian Affairs and IHS, made it clear that he would not spend one cent on renovations until the hospital was turned over to IHS; moreover, the Siksika would continue to pay for hospital care. The chief countered, suggesting they would rent their hospital to IHS for $400 a month, since it was government policy to build and maintain hospitals for Aboriginal people. Moore acknowledged that the hospital building was increasingly dilapidated and threatened that Siksika patients would soon be hospitalized elsewhere. Nevertheless, for the previous year, the thirty-seven-bed hospital had only half the necessary staff with an average occupancy of only fifteen patients.[44] The IHS continued to refuse more than minimal care in a rapidly decaying building, forcing Siksika patients into state-run Indian hospitals. Patients, like Siksika Elder Roy Little Chief, were sent to the Charles Camsell Indian Hospital in Edmonton. Still resentful and suspicious fifty years later, he recalled the pain and loneliness of a year of bed rest and then chest surgery, and the anger and heartbreak upon his return to be told that his father had died.[45] The Siksika trust fund, created by the surrender of precious territory and intended to temper the impact of colonization for future generations, was all but gone by the late 1950s. When a reporter, in a 1958 interview about the Siksika's dire economic situation, asked Chief McHugh why they did not just sell the hospital to the government, he replied with not a little irony, "I suggested this to them and they told me we should give it to them as a grant!"[46] The Blackfoot Hospital – where resistance to assimilation emerged in the people's medical pluralism, and ownership created space for culturally appropriate care – was a direct challenge to medical authority. As a community the Siksika paid dearly for that autonomy as their trust fund dwindled and their health care deteriorated. But by the time of his retirement seven years later in 1965, Moore had yet to receive their "unconditional surrender."

In the meantime, in the late 1950s Moore was busy planning to rebuild the aging Charles Camsell Indian Hospital farther north in Edmonton. The hospital represented the best the IHS had to offer. With its close affiliation with the University of Alberta medical school's consulting faculty, its accreditation for postgraduate training that supplied much of its medical staff, and its urban location, it was quite unlike other Indian hospitals. It was the base for the IHS northern service in the western Arctic that sent often very enthusiastic physicians and nurses to northern nursing stations to remove patients to the hospital. Accounts of intrepid staff and pilots rescuing grateful "Eskimos" were a regular feature in the *Edmonton Journal*.[47] The Camsell Hospital was the public face of its bold humanitarian efforts, as well as the heart of the IHS system where medical bureaucrats got their training.[48] The hospital's senior nursing and administrative staff were remarkably loyal, most having worked at the hospital since it opened. Its on-campus residences for married and single employees created a healthy esprit de corps among non-Aboriginal staff that was maintained through regular rounds of parties and social activities. As one nurse recalled, "What impressed us the most at the Camsell was the friendly, 'happy family' atmosphere. Everyone, no matter what position, got along with everyone else."[49] In short, for IHS bureaucrats and staff, the Charles Camsell Indian Hospital was a source of both personal and professional pride. But physically, the institution showed its age. An ad hoc maze of wooden buildings connected by covered walkways, linked to a sagging fifty-year-old brick building, the hospital's dilapidated buildings caused great concern, not least for the Canadian Council on Hospital Accreditation. In

1957 the hospital received a three-year accreditation but was warned that it would not again receive accreditation (and access to trained postgraduate staff) unless it undertook radical renovations or rebuilt the hospital.[50] The hospital's tight-knit cadre of professional staff and IHS bureaucrats worked tirelessly to plan the new modern six-storey facility in which to continue their work.

But before construction of the new hospital could begin, the Diefenbaker Conservative government announced severe spending freezes and in September 1960 established a royal commission to rationalize its growing bureaucracy along a private-sector model in order to control government spending. Chaired by accountant and business executive Grant Glassco, the commission tabled its five voluminous reports in 1962. Its brief examination of the Indian Health Service, written by a group led by Dr John McCreary, dean of University of British Columbia's faculty of medicine, was highly critical of the Camsell Hospital facilities and staff.[51] It began by stating that the "extent and nature of the responsibility of the federal government to provide free health services for Indians in populated areas of the country is not clearly defined." It recommended scrapping entirely the planned $7 million Camsell Hospital construction project. Noting that tuberculosis patients constituted two-thirds of the patients in the Camsell Hospital, the commission recommended they be treated in empty provincial sanatorium beds, while the remaining 120 patients could be accommodated in local Edmonton hospitals. In general, the commission endorsed the larger program of integration actively pursued by the government. It therefore recommended the rapid transfer of Indian health care to "normal community facilities"; medical and dental care should be provided by privately practising physicians and dentists with the federal government covering prepaid medical plans where necessary.[52] The Glassco Commission's decision that a new Camsell Hospital was neither necessary nor desirable caused the bureaucracy to mount a vigorous defence of its plans, while the other recommendations aroused considerably less comment.

Before the commission's findings were made public, a draft report was forwarded to National Health and Welfare for comment. In marshaling arguments in defence of a rebuilt hospital, IHS director Moore provided the Treasury Board and his deputy minister, G.D.W. Cameron, with a list of "points to stress." It is hardly surprising that Moore would vigorously defend the institution that he viewed as his crowning professional achievement. He stressed the Camsell Hospital's efficient and economical operation, its importance as a base for its northern programs, and its role in medical education, with its "excellent teaching material," and as a training ground for new recruits, including a two-month appraisal program for "Indian girls" hoping to enrol in the provincial nurse's aide school.[53] Essentially, the Charles Camsell Indian Hospital was good for the IHS. Moore went on to argue that Aboriginal patients could not be treated successfully in provincial institutions such as the Aberhart Sanatorium in Edmonton. Geared to the "total needs of the patient," tuberculosis treatment at the Camsell Hospital recognized differences in social custom and language in a way that community institutions could not. Moreover, he argued, the "freedom and liberties provided [Aberhart] patients would be the ruin of a [IHS] treatment regime."[54] Moore refused to even consider admitting tuberculosis patients to the older Baker Sanatorium near Calgary because the buildings were in a worse state than the Camsell Hospital. He noted that, though there was a time when public opinion would tolerate care in ramshackle buildings, "that era is gone and conditions cannot excuse congregating Indians in a second-rate facility." It was also noted that Aboriginal people might also object to the hospital's closing, a "distinct shock ... and a thoroughly unpopular move." Though Moore did not mention that most patients had no choice of hospital, he claimed that many Aboriginal people "have shown a marked propensity for admission to this hospital. It enjoys a most favourable reputation despite a more disciplined regime than is imposed on natives in many other institutions."[55] As for the director's recent pronouncement that IHS wanted to "get out of the hospital business," Moore claimed that the policy "derived from my own personal conviction." As he continued, "There is ample evidence that we are pursuing it vigorously on many fronts and to an extent perhaps not generally known. I hope this will not now be pushed down our throats and our long-term objective thereby sacrificed or imperiled by what might seem expediency at the moment."[56] In other words, Moore wanted a new hospital at Edmonton while being free to close hospitals elsewhere. Nevertheless, while many of the rationales for rebuilding the Camsell Hospital served bureaucratic and professional needs, they also touched on the very arguments that Aboriginal leaders were urging on IHS to maintain hospitals close to their communities – without success. Though hardly sharing Moore's insistence on the need for rigid discipline, Aboriginal leaders did agree on the need for hospitals with Aboriginal employees who could mediate between medical staff and elders and children who did not speak

English. They also wanted their hospitals to stay open because of the continued discrimination Aboriginal patients faced in provincial institutions, and, Aboriginal communities argued, funds that were intended for their health care should be used to improve existing hospitals rather than being invested in non-Aboriginal institutions. Of course, they also argued that Indian hospitals represented the state's acknowledgment of their treaty right to health care, a position that would be emphatically denied by the government.

Whatever else the Glassco Commission meant for government organization, it had little impact on IHS operations; the defeat of the Conservative government in early 1963 allowed the Department of National Health and Welfare to ignore its recommendations. By December the minority Liberal government approved plans to replace the Charles Camsell Hospital (notably dropping "Indian" from the name), citing the ongoing need for a hospital to serve the Arctic and the provincial north, while blaming the Alberta government for rejecting further hospital integration.[57] Director Moore officiated at the formal sod-turning ceremony in October 1964, declaring it "one of the happiest days of my life."[58] The new Charles Camsell Hospital opened in 1967, dubbed a "centennial gift from southern Canada to our northern people."[59] At the official opening, Minister of Health Allan MacEachen's address praised the doctors and nurses for their "love of humanity ... courage, curiosity and spirit of adventure." The new hospital marked a milestone for his department, he noted, and "indicates the ever expanding services" provided for the north and the Indians of Alberta.[60] Of course, services were contracting, not expanding, as IHS actively worked to close other hospitals.[61]

While IHS bureaucrats defended their decision to rebuild the Camsell Hospital, they were continuing their efforts to quietly close the other Alberta institutions – the Blackfoot, Blood, and Hobbema Indian hospitals. Unlike the Charles Camsell, these were all small hospitals situated on reserves, and without influential supporters. Apparently aiding IHS efforts was Alberta's hospital insurance scheme, which refused to include the small, inefficient Indian hospitals in their plan, insisting that patients be directed to community hospitals. Provincial health minister Dr J. Donovan Ross, at least publicly, assured federal officials that his government was committed to integrating community hospitals by accepting Aboriginal Albertans. In June 1961 the Bassano Municipal Hospital complained to the minister that it was unfair that it should be required to treat Blackfoot patients once their hospital closed.

Dr Ross advised the hospital that such attitudes were contrary to the larger "desegregation" policy. The federal government would contribute financially to hospital expansion, but the province would not approve separate wings for Indian patients. In July he informed the forty-bed Cardston Municipal Hospital that it should prepare to accept patients once the thirty-nine-bed Blood Hospital (that sat across the street) closed. Further, he advised the Cardston Hospital that he approved plans to develop a basement ward, but that it must render "service to Indians on the same basis as other residents without attempting to designate certain areas of the hospital for use by the Indians."[62] However, despite forwarding these letters to IHS to demonstrate his commitment to integration, privately Ross informed IHS assistant director Dr Harry Proctor that "integration" was a poor term and unattainable in the foreseeable future, preferring the term "simultaneous development in association." Even with its planned basement ward expansion Cardston Municipal Hospital remained too small to accommodate patients from the Blood reserve. In any case it remained adamant about not accepting Aboriginal patients. Ross announced he was "not anxious or in a position to force them." Proctor informed his director Moore that Alberta would insist that all hospital construction costs be met by the federal government: "Dr. Ross has a very strong opinion of what the federal govt [*sic*] should pay for its *past* neglect of Indians."[63]

Alberta, increasingly at odds with the federal government over the national hospital insurance program's imposed conditions and annual audit, resented federal intrusions on provincial autonomy.[64] Therefore, health minister Ross did not look kindly on any IHS initiatives that required provincial cooperation. At the same time he was determined to control how hospitals in the province were used. When, in 1961, the city of Wetaskiwin in west-central Alberta proceeded to build a new sixty-bed hospital, provincial health officials suggested that a new federally funded "Indian wing" for patients from the Hobbema reserves might be added to the hospital. They wondered if the federal intention was to absorb the "Indian patients into the general services of a hospital" or if there would be a separate wing, which was the local wish.[65] The new hospital project was expanded to ninety beds to accommodate the two thousand people of the nearby Hobbema reserves.[66] According to IHS officials, the people of Wetaskiwin were not happy to "provide for Indians but have been prevailed upon." A handwritten note on the file added "And How!"[67] Ross issued a press release to announce a third-floor addition to the Wetaskiwin Municipal Hospital to include patients from the soon-to-be-shuttered Hobbema Indian Hospital, frustrating IHS plans for a "quiet" closing.[68] IHS bureaucrats understood that their integration policy would require negotiations with provincial and municipal officials, but they refused to acknowledge that Aboriginal communities had any interest or, indeed, should be allowed any input in negotiations. The Hobbema communities were therefore shocked to hear that their hospital that had opened only ten years earlier was to be closed.

The Treaty Six communities at Hobbema had advocated for a hospital in the late 1940s. While their leadership welcomed and supported tuberculosis treatment at the Charles Camsell Hospital in Edmonton, ninety kilometres to the north, there was a very real need for more accessible maternity and paediatric care for the then more than 1,500 residents. The local Wetaskiwin hospital twenty kilometres away admitted some Aboriginal patients, but as regional superintendent Dr E.L .Stone put it, the hospital situation was urgent: "Indian heads are sticking out of both ends of the cribs at the Wetaskiwin hospital."[69] When the Hobbema leadership offered to help finance a new hospital from their capital account, Stone actively discouraged them, fearing that, as at the Blackfoot Hospital, a financial interest might imply a voice in the hospital's management.[70] On the eve of its opening in early 1951, Stone, having in mind the Blackfoot Hospital's challenge to IHS authority, set out the conditions and rules by which the people could access the new twenty-three-bed Hobbema Indian Hospital. He began by noting that the hospital was the property of National Health and Welfare and that no band funds were used for the construction or operation. Only the doctor or, in his absence, the charge nurse could admit or discharge patients. There would be no ambulance and the people would be expected to bring their sick to the hospital and take them home. Visiting hours would be strictly enforced. Local people would be employed "for any work which they can do well," as ward aides or janitorial help. And finally, "No sick Indian will be required to pay for his care in the hospital unless his sickness or accident is the result of drinking alcoholic liquor."[71]

Nevertheless, five years later, in July 1956 (and two years before national hospital insurance), IHS approached the Hobbema area leadership to announce that according to new policies, they were to "stand on their own feet and to become independent in matters relating to medical and hospital costs."[72] Though regional bureaucrat Dr T.J. Orford explained that it was a general policy change and not directed at Hobbema specifically, it was clear that their oil and gas income attracted IHS attention. They were now to pay $6.00 per patient day at Hobbema, Charles Camsell, or any other hospital and $1.50 per day for newborns for ten days and $6.00 per day thereafter. Accordingly, the area chiefs were presented with the Hobbema Hospital accounts for April and May: $2,443.50 and $2,137.50 respectively. At the same time, Indian Affairs and IHS worked to interest Blue Cross in providing hospitalization insurance with the premiums automatically deducted from the reserves' oil revenues.[73] Two months later the chiefs rejected the IHS ultimatum, refusing the principle of payment for hospital or private insurance costs. Citing Treaty Six, the chiefs argued that they had surrendered all their lands for $5.00 per year and other treaty promises including medical care; their hospital was the belated fulfilment of that promise. They were especially disturbed at not being consulted or given a voice in the policy changes. Despite increased income in recent years, the standard of living remained far from adequate and their funds were required for housing and other essentials. The chiefs explained that they already contributed plenty since the hospital and all houses occupied by Indian Affairs and IHS employees were built on reserve lands and given free rental by Council. Moreover, the treaty promised one quarter section (160 acres or 65 hectares) of land for each family of five, but with an increasing population there was not enough land available and no way to access more. The chiefs saw clearly that the IHS demands were the thin edge of the wedge towards making them pay taxes, removing all their treaty rights, and "integrating" them into the general population. Dismissing their concerns, Orford viewed their treaty right argument as a "lack of desire to understand plus the ingrained acceptance of everything for nothing – the perpetual welfare attitude."[74]

So, in early 1962 local IHS officials finally met with the Hobbema leadership to announce that their hospital would become an outpatient clinic, and they would be hospitalized at Wetaskiwin. Bureaucrats explained that the change would mean improved medical services. The Cree chiefs wondered how people would get to Wetaskiwin for treatment since few owned cars and IHS would not provide transportation. They also wanted to know if any hospital staff could speak Cree since many of the elderly could not speak English. They were met with vague promises that the matter would be considered. Perhaps to make their point, Chief Sam Curry of the Montana Band and Chief Jim Bull of the Louis Bull Band spoke in Cree to IHS officials. The chiefs argued that the Hobbema Hospital represented the treaty right to health care, and that IHS had no authority to break the treaty: "When the Queen and the Indian Chiefs signed treaty, it was understood that hospital and medicines would be given and there would be freedom from taxes." IHS bureaucrats replied that they were just following orders from their superiors in government.[75] The Wetaskiwin Hospital Board, in receipt of a letter from the Indian Association of Alberta, fully supported a resolution protesting conversion of the Hobbema Hospital to an outpatient clinic. Local newspapers reported the board's resolution that "the Indians should use every effort to maintain their present hospital ... and the new Wetaskiwin hospital will be filled as soon as it is opened."[76] When Harry Moore, local Conservative member of Parliament, also protested his own government's plans to close Hobbema and integrate the community hospital, minister of health Monteith explained that it was a common misconception that Indians were entitled to any special benefits. "The other point sometimes raised by Indians is the mention in Treaty Six, one of the 12 treaties [*sic*] ... of the provision of a 'medical chest' [*sic*] at the home of the agent." Though the provision of simple medicines has been "scrupulously observed," the minister informed his backbencher that Parliament only acknowledged a moral obligation to assist Indians until they could be integrated into the community.[77] The deliberate plan to exclude the most affected Aboriginal communities from any negotiations – to "quietly" close Indian hospitals – stemmed from the state's contention that health care was a humanitarian, not statutory, commitment. IHS alone would determine the Aboriginal people's best interests while dismissing any claims to a treaty right to care.

While provincial and federal bureaucrats insisted that hospitalization at Wetaskiwin and the conversion of the Hobbema Hospital to a clinic would improve health care, the reality was far different. In early 1963 the Hobbema chiefs and councillors met with the provincial minister of health Dr Donovan Ross to plead for their hospital to be reopened. Many people had no means to travel twenty kilometres to Wetaskiwin, or ninety kilometres to Charles Camsell Hospital in Edmonton. In any case, the reserves only had wagon roads, all but impassable in winter. The people were required to first see an IHS physician at Hobbema before referral to the community hospital, which was a particular hardship for the seriously ill and maternity patients. People felt considerable discrimination in the Wetaskiwin Hospital. As the chiefs put it, "White people in Wetaskiwin feel that they are being displaced by the

Indians due to the tight bed situation in their hospital and therefore feel resentful towards the Indians."[78] Ross lectured the chiefs that though integration would take many years, the Indians should become more self-sufficient. He told the delegation that his department would not approve the Hobbema Hospital under the hospital insurance plan. If it were reopened Ottawa would need to pay the full costs. Community hospitals "with their excellent facilities and larger medical staffs, were to the advantage of the Indians." He said he looked forward to the day "when Indians in this Province would consider themselves as Albertans."[79]

But the now more than 2,500 Hobbema-area people were left with singularly poor care. The Hobbema clinic was without a physician after April 1963, yet IHS, always reluctant to pay non-departmental physicians on a fee-for-service basis, left it to clinic nurses to provide treatment or refer patients to community hospitals. At the same time, the staff was "quietly cut down" to four nurses, but only two worked full time. Rather than pay for prescriptions in town, IHS required non-departmental physicians to send them to Hobbema to be filled. Patients then had to travel back to Hobbema to collect their medications, but with minimal staff and restricted hours at the clinic, as well as an average of 600 patient visits per month, they were made to wait for care. Recommended renovations to the clinic included more than $2,000 for the installation of more benches![80] In an understatement, IHS director Moore remarked: "The Indians are up in arms about this and much resistance is being encountered in getting our patients admitted to the general hospital at Wetaskiwin."[81]

Jurisdictional disputes over cost sharing and administrative control that accompanied provincial insurance programs highlighted the increasing vulnerability of Aboriginal people as the policy of integration played out. In Alberta, ideological differences between the premier Ernest Manning and the Liberal government in Ottawa over national health insurance did nothing to improve health care for Aboriginal residents. By 1963 the province established its own health care insurance plan, the Alberta Medical Plan. Fully endorsed by the Canadian Medical Association and health insurance companies, it required residents to pay health care premiums and offered government subsidies for those who were too sick or too poor to purchase private insurance. Intended to influence the sitting Royal Commission on Health Services (Hall Commission 1961–4) with an alternative to the 1962 Saskatchewan health insurance model that was funded through taxation, "Manningcare" as journalists dubbed it, rejected what health minister Donovan Ross called Saskatchewan's "socialistic type of program."[82] But more than half of those who were eligible for subsidies under the Alberta plan were not protected because they could not afford to pay the high premiums ($140 per family, $69 for individuals).[83] Likewise, under the tax-funded Saskatchewan plan things were little better. Aboriginal people were excluded because the province deemed they were not taxpayers.[84] When IHS offered to pay the modest medical insurance plan premiums ($24 per family, $12 for individuals) on their behalf, Saskatchewan countered that it would pay all the bills for their care, with the federal government refunding the total costs involved, ignoring the fact that Aboriginal people paid provincial taxes.[85] In British Columbia, the province included Indian hospitals in its 1949 insurance plan but by 1960 insisted that its plan would only pay for hospitalization in federal hospitals after denial of treatment in a provincial hospital. So, for example, Aboriginal patients were forced to provide proof of denial of treatment at Prince Rupert Public Hospital before they could be admitted to Miller Bay Indian Hospital. Again, when British Columbia established its health insurance plan, Aboriginal people were excluded on the basis that the federal government was responsible for their care.[86] The policy of integration and the quiet closing of hospitals, measures intended to shift hospitalization and its costs to provincial plans, ran up against considerable opposition, not least from Aboriginal people, who found their health care compromised by jurisdictional squabbles.

With the provincial health insurance plans denying access to Aboriginal people, IHS continued its long-standing policy of contracting with particular local physicians, or physician groups, to provide care for all Aboriginal patients. Intended to keep costs predictable, and to direct patients to particular hospitals, the practice also compromised care. Aboriginal patients could expect not only long waits until the physician treated the full-fee patients, but also hurried consultations. As George Manuel recalled, "If you sat in most doctor's waiting rooms ... you did not need to look at the patient's faces to see who were the Indians. You just had to time the length of each patient's visit in the examining room. Half a fee, half a visit."[87] It was a practice also widely resented by the medical community, with the Alberta Medical Association condemning the prorated fee schedule as "penalizing" physicians who were unfortunate enough to practise near reserves.[88] Moreover, as physicians and provincial governments maintained, the federal government's responsibility for the abysmal housing conditions, lack of rudimentary sanitation, and widespread poverty on reserves in turn created a federal responsibility for much of the ill health that was the consequence. The attempted integration of health services under the various western provincial plans left Aboriginal people as pawns in the negotiations between jurisdictions, but they fared worse under national health insurance or "medicare."[89]

In Alberta, Premier Manning's overheated rhetoric only increased when the Pearson government announced in 1965 its decision to fashion its medical care plan after the Saskatchewan model.[90] Manning derided the comprehensive and universal features of the national program as state compulsion that violated the fundamental right of every citizen to exercise freedom of choice; a state-run monopoly on health insurance violated the principles of a free enterprise society.[91] Indeed, so ideologically opposed was he to the federal plan, health minister Donovan Ross resigned the position he held for twelve years after Alberta decided to participate.[92] Needless to say, as federal bureaucrats working in Alberta, IHS officials did not expect a lot of cooperation with their provincial counterparts, nor did they offer much. Aboriginal people generally, and the Hobbema Cree specifically, bore the brunt of this tension. While the provinces, municipalities, and Aboriginal people themselves viewed their hospital care as a federal responsibility, IHS insisted that all health care was a provincial responsibility. When the Wetaskiwin Hospital became crowded in the mid-1960s citizens resented Hobbema residents taking up beds they considered rightfully theirs. A 1966 petition from the Alberta Local Council of Women requested that the Hobbema Hospital be reopened because the community hospital was overcrowded: "Often a bed is unavailable because of the large number of patients from the Hobbema reservation. We feel that this matter requires urgent attention."[93] After a further expansion in the late 1960s the Wetaskiwin Hospital fell into serious deficit, which the Hospital Board blamed on Hobbema residents, who accounted for about 30 per cent of admissions. Why should local taxpayers be expected to fund a federal responsibility? they asked. Appeals by the board to both levels of government were met with denials of responsibility.

IHS argued that the Wetaskiwin Hospital was a creation of the Alberta Hospital Commission and if it wanted to receive a federal contribution beyond what was already paid under the Hospital Insurance and Diagnostic Services Act then the province had to pay the "so-called deficit" and recover half of it under the terms of the Act.[94] But the per diem rate the province's hospital commission paid the hospital was so low that it continued to incur operating deficits of $75,000 per year.[95] The Hospital Board declared that its only alternative was to refuse service to Hobbema residents. The dispute only soured relations between the two communities, with the Hobbema residents cast as intruders and a burden on local ratepayers. Locally the hospital and the chiefs attempted to ease tensions by appointing a Hobbema representative to the Hospital Board, albeit in an "advisory" or non-voting position, but the province rejected the proposal since it interfered in what it claimed was an exclusively federal jurisdiction.[96] The national minister of health, John Munro, explained to the Hospital Board that he could not interfere. His department, he argued, already shared with the province half of hospital costs for all residents – including Aboriginal people. Moreover, he explained, IHS paid the Alberta hospital insurance premiums on behalf of most Aboriginal people as well as the hospitalization plan's deterrent fees ($5 for the first day and $2.50 thereafter). In reply to a request for financial help from Chief Simon Threefingers of the Louis Bull Band at Hobbema, Munro noted that he could do nothing since deficits were a problem between the hospital and provincial authorities, saying, "this is a matter in which unilateral federal action would be most inappropriate."[97] As Canada achieved its long-awaited program of universal health care, the Hobbema Cree found themselves without their own hospital and increasingly resented as a financial burden on their neighbours. One can imagine that the ever more strained relationship in town caused Hobbema patients to think twice about travelling to Wetaskiwin only to be turned away. What kind of reception might children and elders expect? The local impact of hospital integration was largely damaging to those in most need of care, and caught between jurisdictions, the Hobbema Cree had no voice in the negotiations. What they understood to be a treaty right to health care was sacrificed to the imperatives of health insurance plans that entitled other Canadians greater access to care but left them begging. The sad irony of the Wetaskiwin situation was not lost on other communities that still had hospitals, particularly the Siksika and the Kainai in Alberta. It served as a vivid demonstration of what to expect if their care passed into municipal and provincial hands.

The Siksika refused to surrender their Blackfoot Hospital as director Moore had demanded in 1957, but as a result the building was allowed to continue to deteriorate. By the mid-1960s the hospital had been "obsolete for many years." Its fourteen beds, maternity, pediatrics, and medicine, were all on the same floor since there were not enough nurses to cover two floors. As a result, it could not accept adult men, who were sent to other hospitals for treatment. Physicians from a group medical practice at Bassano visited once or twice a week, an arrangement IHS officials agreed was unsatisfactory.[98] Further south at the Blood Indian Hospital, IHS bureaucrats agreed "nothing could make it into a good hospital." Though there was medical attendance available locally, physicians only reluctantly treated patients in the aging hospital.[99] Alberta's hospital commission refused to insure the small Indian hospitals, forcing IHS to continue funding operations, though it did so by restricting admissions. At the same time, as was made glaringly obvious at Wetaskiwin, municipal taxpayers were responsible for any hospital deficits. Unless Indian reserve lands were included (and taxed) as part of the municipal district, community hospital boards were not inclined to open their doors to reserve residents without firm assurances of support from the federal government. Other integration policies such as education, where Indian Affairs devolved its responsibility to the provinces through cost-sharing in lieu of property taxes on reserve lands, were effective with nearly 60 per cent of Aboriginal children attending provincial schools by 1969.[100] IHS likewise had a long-standing practice to make special grants to community hospital construction or expansion costs in proportion to the local Aboriginal population to be served, but under provincial hospital insurance plans, IHS refused to recognize any responsibility for operating deficits regardless of the cause.[101] Neither the community hospital at Bassano, near the Siksika reserve, nor the community hospital at Cardston had any plans to expand their institutions to accommodate reserve residents. As bureaucrats noted, there was "a certain amount of racial discrimination in Cardston against the Indians and 'incidents' occur from time to time in this connection."[102] By the same token, the Siksika and the Kainai viewed with growing suspicion federal plans to shut their hospitals, though the reality was such that care was deteriorating as quickly as the buildings themselves.

In early 1968, on the eve of Medicare, IHS announced its "Health Plan for Indians." An effort by National Health and Welfare to cut budgets in anticipation of the costly national health insurance to begin in mid-1968, it was couched in the same language of "equality" and "non-discrimination" for Aboriginal people that would inform the disastrous White Paper on Indian Policy the next year. Like the White Paper, it was a move to force Aboriginal people to receive services from provincial agencies, but unlike the White Paper, the Health Plan did not bother with even the pretence of consultation with Aboriginal communities. Letters were simply sent to band councils announcing that IHS would no longer subsidize their health care. It was a mean-spirited and draconian measure that required individuals to provide evidence to hospitals, doctors, druggists, transportation companies, and IHS that they were indigent and that they had applied and been refused assistance from their band funds. They had to prove that they could not obtain assistance from the provincial health or welfare departments, and only then would IHS provide assistance for any or part of their costs. IHS contemplated that a "health assistance card" as proof of indigency might ease the plan's administration but advised that "there should be nothing on the card to indicate Medical Service's Branch [IHS] responsibility, either directly or indirectly, now or in the future."[103] As provinces adopted Medicare plans Aboriginal people would be responsible for payment of all premiums and co-insurance charges, and if indigent they would need to apply to the province for assistance. Only after provincial assistance was denied would IHS "consider" making the payments, and only with proof of indigency. But access to all health services was also limited under the Health Plan, with IHS staff, dentists, and medical officers ordered to "give priority to diagnostic and preventive care." Where IHS did provide health care services or medications, patients were to be charged in the absence of proof of indigency. Admissions to hospitals were to be "controlled to prevent over-utilization" and outpatient care emphasized. Active case finding for mental illness would cease, and IHS would not be responsible for any hospitalization accounts. Limits were placed on all physicians', dentists', and optometrists' accounts, and available funds would be distributed on a proportionate basis. Health professionals were warned that current rates would not increase and would likely decrease. Dental care, glasses, and prosthetics would only be provided with proof of indigency, and IHS dental officers were only to provide "preventive dental care" for schoolchildren. Only "necessary" personal health care costs were to be paid by IHS and only with proof of indigency, though IHS would determine "necessity." Indian Affairs undertook a survey of all reserves to create an "indigent list," and band councils were told to determine who was eligible for care and who was not. Aboriginal people would become equal to other provincial citizens through a policy that severely limited access to medical services for all and in effect required the ill to exhaust all their resources before they would be helped, the very situation that Medicare presumably sought to remedy for other Canadians.

Not surprisingly, the Health Plan was met with considerable alarm in Aboriginal communities, and, coming in an election year, it received some comment in the press. In April 1968 IHS regional director O.J. Rath addressed the Alberta Chiefs' Conference with a brief statement explaining that there was really no change in policy after all. He quoted health minister Allan MacEachen's statement in the House of Commons that "Indians and Eskimos will receive the same consideration and treatment by this Department with regard to health as they received last year."[104] This was disingenuous, if not duplicitous, and referred to past unenforced IHS policy (more of a desideratum, in fact) that required payment for services by those who had the means, and by those who had not lived on their reserve for twelve months. Only the indigent were eligible for IHS medical services. It was not enforced because it was unenforceable without a means test, while the very aggressive protocols of the 1940s and 1950s, in the interests of protecting the national health, meant that IHS physicians, not patients, made decisions about hospitalization and treatment. As a result, it came as a distinct surprise to physicians, provincial officials, and Aboriginal people to learn that such a policy existed. Dr Rath reiterated the minister's claim that nothing had changed, and the only problem was a lack of communication of the true policy. He then told the increasingly hostile Chiefs' Conference that IHS wanted them to become involved in the "administration of health care programs"; essentially, band councils would be asked to decide which of their friends and relatives earned enough to pay for care so that assistance "may be directed to those of your people in greatest need." On larger policy direction, Rath quoted the minister directly:

> I believe it ought to be borne in mind that Indians are residents of the provinces. One of the objectives for progress of the Indian population is certainly to integrate them within the general population of a province. If they are to be regarded as separate citizens to be treated on a different basis in respect of education, health and welfare then the process of integration within the total community will be impeded and will never become equal citizens as we all want them to be.[105]

One had only to look to the experience of the Hobbema Cree to see how integration as "equal citizens" played itself out.

Cast in the language of equality and freedom, and part of the new Liberal Party leader Pierre Trudeau's broader liberal ideology that focused on political rights of the individual, the Health Plan would dispense with "special status" such as the treaty right to care.[106] The *Calgary Herald* reported that Dr Rath had a "rough afternoon" explaining the policy to an angry crowd. "Even when their protests came in Cree," the *Herald* reported, "the tones of bitterness and sense of betrayal needed no translation."[107] The chiefs wondered how this "middle-man" could simply announce their treaty rights no longer existed. Provincial governments were also alarmed. Alberta claimed that the plan to "slough off its responsibilities for the health care of Indians" made a mockery of the Constitution and the treaty agreements.[108] By the fall and with the election over, the new health minister John Munro repeated his predecessor's insincere claim that policies had not changed. Furthermore, he argued that IHS assistance for registered Indians who were living on reserves and were medically indigent was actually unfair: "While it appears to discriminate in their favour, it may not be to their ultimate advantage since it tends to differentiate Indians from other Canadians. Our hope is that Indians will become integrated in the main stream of Canadian life."[109] Nevertheless, bureaucrats continued to insist that limited medical assistance was provided because the people were poor, not because of any treaty right. Resistance to that claim emerged immediately.

Harold Cardinal, the youthful president of the Indian Association of Alberta, charged that the department's Health Plan was a clear abrogation of treaty rights. He advised that to pay health care premiums would be to lose the treaty right to health care; that once their care passed to provincial jurisdiction they would lose any claims to federal responsibility; and that to lose one treaty right would jeopardize them all.[110] In reply to Cardinal's concerns over the treaty right to health care, minister of health Munro informed him that Indian Affairs, not Health and Welfare, dealt with treaty rights. Moreover, he claimed that the provision of health care in the past, as in the present, was based solely on need, and stated: "Our efforts have never been related in any way to Indian treaties."[111] The following month, the government outlined its intentions and the logical conclusion to its integration policy in the *Statement of the Government of Canada on Indian Policy 1969*, or the "White Paper": to terminate completely the treaty relationship, dismantle the bureaucracy, repeal the Indian Act, and replace it with "Indian control" of reserve land that would eventually open them to provincial taxation. There can be little doubt that the Health Plan was developed to ease the process and prepare the ground for the White Paper. Aboriginal groups across the country responded with a clear rejection of the badly flawed policy that had been developed without consultation with the affected groups, articulating a defence of treaty and Aboriginal rights and demands for greater economic and educational development. The Alberta chiefs' response, its "Red Paper," or *Citizens Plus,* took its name from a phrase coined in the *Hawthorn Report* (1966), a survey of the conditions of Indians in Canada commissioned by the Indian Affairs branch itself. It recommended special status for Indian people as "citizens plus": "Indians can and should retain the special privileges of their status while enjoying full participation as provincial and federal citizens."[112] As *Citizens Plus* put it, the benefits outlined in treaty promises were not "handouts" as the White Paper implied, but the fair exchange for settler access to the Aboriginal peoples' lands and resources. One of those rights was health care: "the provision of health services to the Indian people on the reserve or off the reserve at the expense of the Federal government anywhere in Canada."[113] The widespread denunciation of the White Paper, supported by the press, led to its withdrawal by early 1971. But the White Paper's legacy, aside from being the impetus for regional groups to organize into a national Aboriginal voice, was the deepening distrust of government and a lingering suspicion that termination remained a "hidden agenda" in policy making.[114]

It was in this climate of cynicism arising from the Health Plan for Indians and the White Paper that greeted the continuing efforts to shut down southern Alberta Indian hospitals. Moreover, the Siksika and Kainai, closely watching the ongoing difficulties experienced by the Hobbema Cree, were increasingly wary of any further federal initiatives towards hospital integration. The White Paper may have been withdrawn, but the Health Plan remained the basis for National Health and Welfare's policy decisions. The Indian Association of Alberta advised its membership that they should present their treaty cards not Medicare numbers when receiving medical services, while IHS agreed to pay their premiums on a temporary basis.[115] Nevertheless, by 1972 IHS continued to insist that regardless of the legal responsibilities that Indian Affairs might have for education or social welfare, there was no legal responsibility for health services. The only guideline that IHS recognized was "those Indians who can pay for the health services, do pay."[116] As for reserve hospitals, IHS continued to negotiate with the provincial government for their closure, yet band councils saw their hospitals as the (now crumbling) bricks and mortar acknowledgment of their treaty right to health care. If there were funds for hospital construction, they argued, then it ought to be put towards improved Indian hospitals.[117]

Nevertheless, both the Blood and Blackfoot hospitals were closed by degrees. At the Blood Indian Hospital, serving nearly five thousand residents, IHS reduced the number of adult beds and limited the allocation of beds to physicians so that most adult patients were admitted elsewhere. The beds per room were gradually reduced and physically removed from the building so they could not be pressed into service.[118] The Siksika and the Kainai could keep their hospitals, but they certainly would not be good hospitals. Protracted and circular negotiations in an increasingly poisoned atmosphere continued throughout the decade. For example, the Blackfoot band council refused to sign any agreement to shut their hospital and open a health centre until the federal government agreed that this would not diminish their treaty rights, and until the Bassano Hospital began construction of an expansion to serve the Siksika; the provincial hospital commission refused to approve an expansion of the community hospital at Bassano to accommodate Blackfoot patients until IHS closed the Blackfoot Hospital; IHS maintained that treaty rights were an issue for Indian Affairs, not Health and Welfare.[119] At the local level, the impasse did nothing to improve relations between reserve and town. According to federal officials attending a Blood Band Council meeting to discuss the closure, "One of the main reasons the people of the Blood Band do not want to close the Blood Indian Hospital is the fact that they are afraid they will not get adequate services at the Cardston Municipal Hospital in view of the 'discrimination' against the Indian people by the people of Cardston."[120] Finally, with written assurance that treaty rights would not be affected, the aging hospitals were replaced by band-managed, but federally financed, reserve health centres, or outpatient clinics, though the Blood Indian Hospital, designated as a "Heritage Building" in 1991, continued as a seniors' long-term care facility until 1999.[121]

The Charles Camsell Hospital came to a more ignominious end. Shortly after the new hospital opened in 1967 it became something of a white elephant. With steadily falling tuberculosis rates, an increased emphasis on outpatient care, expansion of acute care facilities in the north, and its Aboriginal clientele directed by their physicians to other institutions, the hospital became seriously underused. To keep beds full, private local practitioners were accorded admitting privileges to the hospital, which subsequently developed into a community acute care hospital with only 23 per cent Aboriginal patients.[122] But, for its own reasons, the Alberta Hospital Services Commission would only approve a $78 per diem rate for the Camsell Hospital, compared to $125 for other city hospitals, forcing National Health and Welfare to subsidize what had become a general city hospital to the tune of $3 million annually.[123] No fewer than four different audits, reports, and studies between 1972 and 1976 attempted to find a future for the hospital, which senior IHS officials concluded was a "relic of an age that has already passed."[124] Yet in the hope of eventually transferring the hospital to the province, IHS sought to maintain it as a viable institution. However, in the politically turbulent post–White Paper years of unprecedented Aboriginal activism, the Alberta government wanted nothing to do with an "Indian" hospital. In 1972 IHS was prepared to transfer the hospital to Alberta for a nominal fee of $1, as well as a $3 million "transitional grant" (or the equivalent of one year's operating deficit) to the province to take it off their hands. The provincial hospital commission chair refused the offer, bluntly stating the provincial position: "We would prefer an empty hospital and no Indian involvement." Four years later and with negotiations ongoing, the hospital's annual operating deficit ballooned to $4 million.[125] Both levels of government agreed to leave the Indian Association of Alberta and other interested Aboriginal organizations out of the negotiations. Ultimately, the 1978 transfer agreement was reached only after the federal government agreed to two provincial demands: that it provide written assurances to "honour its existing obligations for the provision of health services" to the province's Treaty Indians; and that the federal government commit the substantial savings accrued from the transfer to enrich health services on reserves.[126] The formal transfer in 1980 was accompanied by national health minister Monique Bégin's announcement of a $2.5 million commitment to an Indian Health Care Commission to "promote and encourage native self determination" in the delivery of health services.[127] By 1996 the province closed and abandoned the Charles Camsell Hospital, in part due to asbestos contamination. The derelict building and its 4.7 hectare (11.5 acre) site, a frightening place patrolled by dogs, sits fenced, boarded, and scrawled with graffiti, "a nasty, nagging, neighbourhood eyesore."[128] It is a shameful and sorry end for a place that had such a profound impact, for good or ill, on so many lives.

Canadians are particularly pleased with Medicare, telling the latest Royal Commission that it defined their notions of citizenship.[129] Yet that healthy national citizenship excluded Aboriginal people, as the

"Health Plan for Indians" made clear. Limited health care would be withheld until and unless Aboriginal people remained destitute and on their reserves, while the "integration" policy constructed them as beggars at the doors of community hospitals. As Alfred Blood of the Blood Indian Hospital committee put it, "Since Medicare was introduced the Indian has been at a loss."[130] The slow demise of the Charles Camsell Hospital in the 1970s was only the most glaring example of how the integrationist agenda and the dark politics of Medicare came to damage those most in need of care. As the only new and modern Indian hospital, the Charles Camsell primarily benefited the non-Aboriginal population of Edmonton who made up the majority of its patients. The costs of that care, and especially the decade's operating deficits, conservatively estimated at $25 million ($3 million per year to 1975, and $4 million per year to 1980), funds earmarked for health care for Aboriginal people, instead went into the coffers of the nation's wealthiest province, while the small local institutions such as the Blood and Blackfoot hospitals were deemed too expensive to operate. One could be forgiven for viewing with cynicism the health minister's 1980 "gift" of $2.5 million for an Indian Health Care Commission to encourage "native self determination" in health care. Nevertheless, Aboriginal communities refused to accept a contingent citizenship and continued to press for better care based on their treaty rights.

"The Government's eyes were opened": The Treaty Right to Health Care

When the treaty was first made with the Queen the Indians were told the government that was to look after them was pretty nearly as strong as God. But the government was blind in both eyes, and the Indians suffered. As the years passed by, the government's eyes were opened, just enough to give us our own doctors and hospital.

– Sweetgrass Chief Sam Swimmer, North Battleford Indian Hospital, 1953

The treaty right to health care remains contested. The basis for the claim is the "medicine chest" clause in Treaty Six (1876) that included Cree communities in a wide swath of prairie and parkland in what became central Alberta and Saskatchewan. Over the course of the late nineteenth and twentieth centuries, the state's provision of medical care, at first sporadic and grudging, became increasingly comprehensive, including vaccinations, X-ray examinations, physician services, and Indian hospitals. As a result, Aboriginal communities, and Canadians generally, came to the not unreasonable understanding that health care was a federal responsibility, if not a treaty right. In government circles, however, the point was moot. Overwhelmingly paternalistic, IHS physician-bureaucrats dismissed treaties as dusty relics, and treaty claims as symptomatic of a stubborn backwardness that was surely as dangerous as disease itself. As tuberculosis receded as the primary threat to the national health, Indian hospitals came to be seen as costly obstacles to wider state efforts to "integrate" Aboriginal people to normal, healthy citizenship. Medicare, not medicine chests, would define access to hospital and health care. But, as we have seen, resistance to hospital closures emerged immediately. Though historians peg the resurgence of Aboriginal political organization to the White Paper and its aftermath, the process began earlier and emerged in many cases from grass-roots efforts that coalesced around issues of health care and Indian hospitals. For nearly two decades, Treaty Six community activists at the North Battleford Indian Hospital in central Saskatchewan struggled with countless bureaucrats and seven successive health ministers in an attempt to improve their health by holding government to its treaty promise of health care. A focus on one particular community's well-documented activism illustrates how bureaucratic surveillance and control maintained relations of power based on race that worked to undermine health.

The treaty right to health care emerged from the 1876 Treaty Six negotiations at Fort Carlton on the North Saskatchewan River between the Cree and the government's treaty commissioner Alexander Morris. While the nascent Canadian state understood the treaties as ultimately land cessions to facilitate agricultural settlement, Aboriginal negotiators saw the treaties as a mutually beneficial relationship whereby they agreed to share their land with newcomers in exchange for assurances of future livelihood secured by specific promises, such as aid to agriculture, schools, and annual cash payments.[1] Thus, at Fort Carlton senior chiefs Mistawasis and Ahtahkakoop, recalling the recent 1870 smallpox epidemic and alarmed by the rapidly dwindling bison herds, negotiated for, among other things, a promise of government assistance in the event of famine or pestilence, and a promise of a medicine chest. The written text of the treaty however does not reflect the actual treaty discussions, a point consistently made by Aboriginal people and only recently recognized by scholars and the courts.[2] During negotiations the Cree leaders presented treaty commissioner Morris with a request for additional terms. One witness to the proceedings, Metis trader Peter Erasmus engaged by the chiefs as their interpreter, noted that they asked for a medicine chest to be "placed in the house of every agent for the free use of the band." A.G. Jackes, secretary to the Treaty Commission, recorded the request slightly differently – "That we be supplied with medicines free of cost" – and the commissioner's reply – "A medicine chest will be kept at the house of each Indian agent in case of sickness amongst you."[3] The text of Treaty Six states "a medicine chest shall be kept at the house of each Indian Agent for the use and benefit of the Indians, at the direction of such Agent."[4] Slight differences perhaps, but the "direction" of the Indian agent was inserted in the treaty document. The "medicine chest clause" was exclusive to Treaty Six, though there is considerable evidence that requests and promises of medical care were negotiated at Treaties Seven (1877), Eight (1899), Ten (1906–7) and Eleven (1921), but no mention appears in those treaty documents.[5] For treaty Aboriginal groups across the west and north, the provision of medical care at subsequent annual treaty ceremonies no doubt confirmed the link between the two.

The first judicial test of the medicine chest clause came in 1935 when George Dreaver, chief of the Mistawasis Band in central Saskatchewan, sued the federal government to recover band funds that were spent on, among other things, drugs and medical supplies. The Exchequer Court found that from 1876 to 1919 the Department of Indian Affairs (DIA) provided medicine and supplies at Mistawasis, but after a land sale in 1919 medical supplies were charged to the band's funds. Chief Dreaver was witness to the Treaty Six negotiations and related for the court his recollection of the commissioner's promise. Justice Angers ruled that the medicine chest clause indeed meant that all medicines and medical supplies should be supplied free of charge: "I do not think that the Department [Indian Affairs] had, under the treaty, the privilege of deciding which medicines, drugs and medical supplies were to be furnished to the Indians gratuitously and which were to be a charge to the funds of the band." Angers continued: "The clause might unquestionably be more explicit but, as I have said, I take it to mean that all medicines, drugs or medical supplies which might be required by the Indians of the Mistawasis Band were to be supplied to them free of charge." He ordered the DIA to reimburse the Mistawasis Band $4,500.[6] Aside from supplies of medicines on reserves, often dispensed by the agent's wife or local schoolteacher, and occasional visits by government physicians, Aboriginal people were expected to pay for their medical care, while the state only sporadically and reluctantly provided care for the indigent. As part of a larger project of assimilation, the policy maintained the close collaboration between medicine and the colonizing state. To seek out Western medicine, and pay for its benefits, was long seen as a marker of progress towards "civilization," which necessarily trumped any quaint treaty promises.

Hospital care for Aboriginal people in the Treaty Six communities in central Saskatchewan's North Battleford area was severely limited.[7] An effort in the 1920s to build an "Indian annex" at the local Notre Dame Hospital was frustrated by denominational rivalry when the Anglican bishop objected to Catholic influence at the hospital (see chapter 1). By 1945 the Indian Affairs physician advocated for improved care for the area's 4,200 Aboriginal people, noting that beds were rarely available at the local Notre Dame Hospital, where "other patients rather object to Indians being placed in the same ward with them, and there are no wards that can be set aside for Indians only."[8] He had in mind the military's thirty-five-bed hospital in the redundant Commonwealth Air Training Camp at the airport. IHS director Percy Moore emphasized the economy in taking over the facility, including kitchen equipment, beds, and a complete supply of surgical instruments, that could be "turned over lock, stock and barrel" by the military. He also noted "hospital costs for the Battleford Agency for the past year were $38,662.50, of which $33,000.00 was for the care of sanatorium patients in the Prince Albert sanatorium."[9] The source of those funds (whether band funds or parliamentary appropriations) is not clear from Moore's statement, but it is clear that sanatorium treatment had become the overwhelming priority, highlighting the limited number of admissions to the local hospital.

In 1949 the IHS opened the North Battleford Indian Hospital with sixty beds under Dr P.W. Head, known locally as "Chief Medicine Knife," for the many surgeries he performed. Like other Indian hospitals opened in what were intended to be temporary military facilities, it was makeshift and drafty, pipes froze in winter and patients sweltered in summer, and fire was a constant threat. Cross-infection was a particular hazard in the military-style open dormitories. As noted previously, by the mid-1950s staff shortages had created a dangerous situation, especially in the two large wards for infants and children, where nursing staff moved from patient to patient without changing gowns or washing their hands. Children and infants were bathed in a common tub; infant formula was improperly prepared; bottles were propped for feeding and then left in cribs; soiled diapers were left in the ward and then laundered with other linens. The hospital's superintendent was advised to move adults into the large wards and keep children in smaller wards, and windows were to be opened whenever possible. Visiting hours were to be restricted to one hour a day and limited to close relatives.[10] But, despite its deficiencies, the hospital was much needed and became a valuable source of wage labour, as we have seen, though always in the least skilled positions. Nevertheless, patients felt comforted by Aboriginal staff who spoke their language and understood their culture, unlike many peoples' experiences in the community's Notre Dame Hospital.

The Treaty Six communities at North Battleford also viewed the Indian hospital as the government's acknowledgment of the treaty right to medical care. Sam Swimmer, the elderly chief of Sweetgrass, spent the last years of his life in the early 1950s in the hospital. He cultivated a close relationship with Dr Head and Mrs Wetton, a newspaper correspondent and local historian who referred to herself as an honorary member of the Sweetgrass band. Her columns focused on the hospital staff's quiet sacrifice and their life-saving efforts, while she characterized Chief Swimmer as enlightened by his hospital experience: "He cherishes no longings for the olden days of the medicine man and their crude tents and magic, but looks forward to the time when all his people will turn to real doctors to cure them of their ills." Chief Swimmer, for his part, used the media attention to praise the hospital as the state's commitment to the treaty right to health care. In his metaphorical style he stated: "When the treaty was first made with the Queen the Indians were told the government that was to look after them was pretty nearly as strong as God. But the government was blind in both eyes, and the Indians suffered. As the years passed by, the government's eyes were opened, just enough to give us our own doctors and hospital."[11]

The hospital was also a vast improvement over the public health facilities on the North Battleford area reserves, "fire traps" according to medical superintendent Cameron Corrigan, who visited them in 1956. At Onion Lake, 200 kilometres northeast of North Battleford, and at Mistawasis reserve, 130 kilometres west, the reserve nursing stations were fifty-year-old abandoned Indian agency houses taken over by IHS. Both were two-storey buildings with holes in the roof and cracked and leaking basements. At Mistawasis a woman with a cerebral haemorrhage was carried up the winding stairs on a blanket. She died immediately, as Corrigan noted: "I imagine the handling she got being taken up stairs would not have helped her cerebral haemorrhage."[12] No nurse had stayed in the house longer than six months. The water pump frequently quit, and in February when Corrigan visited, the attic was frozen. He sat with his feet on the table to keep warm, yet the kitchen wall was too hot to touch because of a cracked chimney. Corrigan suggested abandoning the cottages completely in favour of more beds at the North Battleford Indian Hospital. Instead, four years later IHS embarked on plans to "quietly" close the Indian hospital.

In early 1962 IHS actively negotiated with the province and the Notre Dame Hospital to close the Indian hospital, leaving the Cree communities out of the discussions. But in a small town nothing stays quiet for long. In March the chiefs and councillors from Sweetgrass, Poundmaker, Onion Lake, and Little Pine petitioned IHS to protest the hospital closure plans and the proposal for a new thirty-bed wing for Notre Dame Hospital. As the petition made clear, "If funds are available, we request that a new larger Indian hospital be erected." Besides, the petition asked, what would become of the Indian hospital's Aboriginal employees who cared for children and elders in their own language? Noting that the sixty-bed Indian hospital was overcrowded and the reserve populations increasing, how could a thirty-bed replacement suffice?[13] A week later regional bureaucrat and former hospital superintendent at both Hobbema and North Battleford, Dr Thomas Orford, surprised to be contacted at his Regina office by provincial media about the hospital's fate, told reporters that no decision had been made. Putting the best face on the government's self-serving policy, however, Orford told the press that closing the Indian hospital and adding beds to the general hospital would aid the "Indians towards becoming members of the community."[14]

IHS bureaucrats, facing similar resistance to their closures in Alberta and Saskatchewan, characterized Aboriginal opposition as illogical and disruptive, and as evidence of unredeemed backwardness of their leadership. According to Orford, Saskatchewan Indians were split into two factions, a "fairly large element who vaguely grasp at integration ... but who frighten easily when faced with reality" and a "more vociferous element who are not ready for anything different than reserve life and 'Treaty' agreements." The first group will "in time dig themselves out of apathy and indecision, while the other group will in ten, twenty, fifty years from now will [*sic*] still be clamouring for treaty rights." Orford maintained that the future of the hospital would rest on whether "we cater to the old guard or enhance the trend of swinging Indian thought towards full Canadian citizenship."[15] The dichotomy was seemingly evident and linked the hospital's closure and integration in the community hospital with progress and citizenship. However, IHS plans would have to wait as Saskatchewan's program for health insurance faced stiff opposition that summer with a bitter doctors' strike. Medical bureaucrats were advised to "temporise" in the meantime.[16] But the Indian hospital continued to deteriorate, requiring more than $50,000 in repairs to bring it to a "reasonable" standard according to the department's building inspector.[17] Instead, inpatient services would shrink, forcing admissions to the community hospital, if beds could be had, while maintaining a very limited outpatient service.

Complaints about the hospital increased as services deteriorated. Letters to the minister of health and to the local press charging discrimination, restricted access, and negligence causing death caught the attention of Ottawa bureaucrats. While Orford, as senior Saskatchewan bureaucrat, attempted to explain away the incidents as miscommunication between doctors and patients, it was clear that staff shortages and economizing had created a dangerous situation. But his reaction to charges of discrimination, calling them "unjust" and "unkind," was especially revealing of bureaucratic attitudes that stemmed from the state's insistence that its medical service was ultimately humanitarian. "I'm sure that if ... all the other Indians would reflect on the years of hard work and sacrifice undertaken by doctors and nurses in an effort to treat and improve health conditions for them, the suggestion of discrimination would be difficult to substantiate."[18] Orford's reaction was shared by many in the IHS who saw themselves as motivated by equal measures of service and science. Patient grumbling about treatment and conditions was further evidence of the ingratitude and fecklessness they were trying to uproot.

Nevertheless, the charges were serious enough for a delegation of senior administrators to visit the hospital in the spring of 1965. They found considerable cause for concern. Topping the list of their recommendations was a directive to stop talking about closing the hospital since staff were becoming demoralized; other problems stemmed from serious understaffing, resentment against senior staff, and an absence of privacy and security. They found that medical staff showed little respect for patients, in particular, refusing to discuss with patients their medical diagnosis or their course of treatment. For their part medical staff complained about the "rebellion of the Indian patients."[19] As a result of the visit by the Ottawa inspectors, the hospital's senior staff – medical superintendent, matron, and administrator – was all transferred elsewhere.[20] Moreover, as suggested by the community, an advisory board was established to deal with complaints.

Bureaucratic hopes that the "Lay Advisory Board" would smooth the choppy waters were quickly dashed. Chaired by Sidney Fineday from Sweetgrass, the Advisory Board saw itself as a liaison between the community, government, and hospital staff to protect patient interests while participating in major administrative decisions.[21] The election of two non-Aboriginal members, Zenon Pohorecky, newly appointed professor of anthropology at the University of Saskatchewan, and Reverend James Williams, minister of the Pentecostal Church of Christ, both outspoken critics of the hospital, worried medical bureaucrats. Dr Orford, in particular, suspected that the non-Aboriginal members had hijacked the Board. Displaying a newfound appreciation for the people's judgment, he recommended an all-Aboriginal Board: "I am confident that left to themselves, the Indians will amicably and satisfactorily resolve past difficulties and carry on a good partnership with hospital personnel."[22]

In August Orford and the new hospital superintendent, Dr M.L. Webb, attended the Advisory Board's first meeting and were dismayed to find Metis political activist Malcolm Norris speaking out against the "mediocrity of civil servants." Orford objected to the presence of non-Aboriginal people who "disrupted" the proceedings and a newspaper reporter who stirred up mistrust, undercutting the purpose of the board, which according to Orford was to "restore good will and respect between the Indians and the hospital." Speaking for Aboriginal communities, Orford contended they were "extremely capable of speaking for themselves when given the opportunity and I believe this is the way they would prefer."[23] The Advisory Board meeting revisited the previous year's incidents of discrimination and negligence at the hospital and the refusal of local Notre Dame Hospital to accept Aboriginal patients, which made front-page headlines in the *Saskatoon Star Phoenix* and the *Toronto Telegram*.[24] Worse yet, a CBC television program aired in October further publicizing for a national audience the problems at North Battleford Indian Hospital, and bringing the issue into the living rooms of Ottawa bureaucrats. Sidney Fineday told the CBC about charges of malpractice at the hospital, which the IHS director saw as "vague complaints which would not much impress any reasonably intelligent viewer." Anthropologist Pohorecky also appeared on screen, recounting charges of neglect that prompted the headquarters visit in April, while Dr Webb countered that major changes in the hospital's administration had resolved the problems. New IHS director Dr H.A. Proctor reassured himself that Webb's explanation left viewers with the impression that whatever grounds for complaint had existed, they were resolved.[25]

Back of the tensions and hostility at the Indian hospital were the ongoing negotiations with provincial authorities and Notre Dame Hospital for an expansion for which IHS offered $325,000 to accommodate Aboriginal patients. But in the middle of negotiations in April 1965 the hospital's owners, the Sisters of Providence, retired from the hospital field, forcing the city and surrounding municipalities to scramble to form a Union Hospital district to take over the hospital. With no hospital construction in the near future, IHS was forced to maintain and perhaps expand the Indian hospital to service the more than 8,000 people on twenty-one reserves in the Battleford and Meadow Lake agencies, especially since the surrounding small-town hospitals showed a marked preference for non-Aboriginal patients.[26] With the realization that the Indian hospital would not be closing for at least another five years, IHS took the Advisory Board's concerns more seriously, if only to avoid more damaging publicity.

Medical bureaucrats saw the Advisory Board as an exercise in educating and disciplining Aboriginal people to accept "integration" into the Union Hospital, and provincial society generally. Proctor and Orford, from their offices in Ottawa and Regina respectively, believed that much of the opposition to integration by the area chiefs was a gesture to "their so-called [treaty] rights," not sincerely held. But the chiefs, concerned especially about the treatment that elders would receive if none of the staff spoke their language, also asked the pressing question: was the Union Hospital prepared to receive Aboriginal patients? Dr Webb admitted that while the hospital management was ready to accept patients, it might take some time to convince other hospital patrons.[27] Burton Baptiste, councillor from Little Pine, raised the critical question at the Advisory Board meeting in early 1967: what would IHS do if the Aboriginal communities refused to accept an integrated hospital? Webb's reply was "rather unspecific." IHS would take this into consideration, but, as he put it, "I did not intimate ... that we would comply with such a request."[28] Despite medical bureaucrats' dismissal of treaty rights, the issue was especially pressing in the mid-1960s.

In 1965 provincial authorities charged North Battleford Indian Hospital employees Walter Johnston, Harry Wuttunee, and Andrew Swimmer with failure to pay the 1963 hospital insurance premiums under the Saskatchewan Hospitalization Act, a move apparently instigated by the hospital's administrator.[29] The charges stemmed from the IHS policy that it would only pay the provincial hospitalization insurance premiums, or tax, for indigent Aboriginal people living on reserves, and those who had lived off the reserve for less than a year. As hospital employees, none of the charged were indigent. Since all defendants intended to raise the same defence – that the treaty right to health care exempted them from the tax – Saskatchewan's attorney general proceeded against Johnston alone. At the time, IHS director claimed "it is not considered that Indian Canadians have any special entitlement to free medical care, hospitalization and similar services ... None of the various Treaties between the Crown and the Indians has been judicially interpreted as conferring this right."[30] This was narrowly correct, since the 1935 *Dreaver v The King* judgment dealt only with medicines, not medical care. Just days before Johnston went to trial, deputy minister of health Donald Cameron provided a strange, and vaguely threatening, interpretation that the medicine chest clause might well limit medical care to nineteenth-century standards. In response to an inquiry about the treaty right, Cameron said that when Treaty Six was drawn up in 1876 the contents of a medicine chest would have been rudimentary "since most of the medicines of greatest use today have been developed in the past few years. This development of new and presumably better medicines is going on all the time. If we were to interpret what is to be meant by a 'Medicine Chest' it might restrict the use of some of the latest proven materials as they become available. I believe that Indian Health Services tries to use good up-to-date medicines and other medical materials."[31] The government did not pursue this bizarre line of reasoning, but it reflects IHS thinking that, whatever else the treaty might mean, the benefits of modern medicine had long ago surpassed its outdated promises.

In March 1965 Walter Johnston alone went to trial and pleaded not guilty, arguing that the medicine chest provision of Treaty Six conferred a right to free health care and hospitalization. Interestingly, Johnston provided the court with the original Treaty Six document that had been carefully preserved in the community for nearly a century. The government's copy was compared closely for accuracy. Judge J.M. Policha, referring to the 1876 treaty negotiations in his ruling, said he was "greatly impressed by the representations and submissions made by various Indian Chiefs and the concern they felt with the welfare of their people." In acquitting Johnston, he ruled that the medicine chest clause of the treaty should be interpreted to mean that Johnston was entitled to receive all medical services and hospital care free of charge. Further, he stated, the "entitlement would embrace all Indians within the meaning of the Indian Act, without exception."[32] Shocked at this unexpected outcome, IHS director Proctor immediately advised that it would be "judicious" to suspend any further "Loss of Benefit" notices while the courts studied the Johnston ruling, and most especially since they were still in "negotiations to placate the Indians in the North Battleford area." He further directed IHS bureaucrats to say the "least possible" about the Johnston case. As far as IHS was concerned, treaty interpretation was an issue for Indian Affairs and the Department of Justice: "We will keep out as far as possible until the smoke clears."[33] An appeal of the ruling seemed inevitable, but only Saskatchewan's attorney general could launch it.

Though the ruling's impact would be more keenly felt in Ottawa than in Saskatchewan, both bureaucracies recognized that the Johnston ruling represented a major shift in how Aboriginal people and their rights would be understood. Orford summed it up succinctly, descending to a tactless stereotype to make his point: "He [Judge Policha] seems to think that in perpetuity the Federal government is stuck with supply [*sic*] of full and total medical care for Indians regardless of their place of residence or financial status. I imagine the Indians in Battleford and other areas of Treaty 6 are jumping with joy right now. Fortunately, I'm nearly bald so my scalp would be of little value."[34] His statement highlighted an increasingly acrimonious relationship with the local community, while betraying considerable anxiety that medical and bureaucratic control might be eroded. With Liberal administrations in both jurisdictions, the provincial health department's solicitor informally advised Orford in Regina that there were just ten days in which to launch an appeal, and that the federal government should make representations to the province's attorney general to do so. But neither Health and Welfare's IHS nor the Indian Affairs branch, both putatively representing Aboriginal interests, wanted to be seen to be supporting the appeal. Minister of health Judy LaMarsh, advised by her deputy Donald Cameron, declined to take any action "that could easily be interpreted by the Indians as opposition to their interests and legal rights."[35] She promptly advised her cabinet colleague John Nicholson at Citizenship and Immigration, the bureaucratic home of Indian Affairs, to contact the provincial attorney general regarding an appeal.[36] But Indian Affairs returned the volley, arguing that Health and Welfare should ask for an appeal since the matter concerned medical insurance paid from that bureaucracy's parliamentary appropriation. Advising his minister, assistant deputy R.F. Battle stated the obvious: "At the moment, the decision is in favour of the Indians. If the Department of Citizenship and Immigration takes action to appeal, then it will appear in the eyes of the Indians that we are not favourably disposed towards the decision." In case the minister had forgotten, Battle continued, "our role should be to defend the Indians' interests. If we initiate action to appeal then I am afraid it will have a damaging effect on our position with the Indians concerned." To be clear, Battle pointed out, "our relationship, which might be stated publicly, is to provide assistance to insure that in the event of an appeal the Indians' case is properly presented."[37] Bureaucratic manoeuvring aside, claims that either ministry was working in the "Indians'" interest were strictly for public consumption. For Aboriginal people, that mask had slipped years ago as the government continued its policy of restricting their economic, social, and political self-determination in the interests of assimilation to a Euro-Canadian norm. Indeed, in the wake of his apparent victory, Walter Johnston and his original co-accused, Andrew Swimmer, applied for necessary glasses and dentures at the North Battleford Indian Hospital. They were promptly denied. Orford advised IHS employees in Saskatchewan that policies had not changed, warning them not to speak to the press or to otherwise embarrass the government.[38]

Saskatchewan's minister of public health, Davey Steuart, pressed both ministers for an answer: "If you would like our Government to proceed with an appeal ... it would be appreciated if you would advise me in this regard at an early date."[39] The province subsequently launched its appeal in late October 1965 with covert support from Justice Department's lawyer R.E. Williams. Meeting with R.L. Barclay of Saskatchewan's attorney general's office, Williams proposed an argument: the medicine chest provision in the treaty was an ad hoc attempt to meet a specific problem before there was a provincial government, but with the advent of modern provincial medical services, the provision had become a "historical appendage." The costs for care, the argument went, were borne by Canada for some Aboriginal people, but Walter Johnston, integrated into the white community and a "normal citizen" of the province, was required to bear the same responsibilities as other citizens, including paying the hospitalization tax.[40] This argument, neatly reinforcing government policy, was particularly appealing to Indian Affairs, and, it was hoped, it might also appeal to the good sense of the Appeals Court justices. Williams also provided Barclay with copies of Treaty Six and other documents from Indian Affairs archives.[41]

In March 1966 Saskatchewan's chief justice, E.M. (Ted) Culliton, a faithful Liberal, delivered the court's judgment.[42] He began with the question of historical evidence, arguing that the words in the treaty should be interpreted literally. He referred to treaty commissioner Alexander Morris's 1880 account of the treaty negotiations as "authoritative."[43] But, as noted, in Morris's account the people asked for a "a free supply of medicines," and later, that they be "supplied with medicines free of cost," though the written treaty states that the medicine chest will be kept at the agent's house and used at his direction.[44] There is no evidence that Culliton looked further than Morris, but if he had, he might have consulted the acknowledged expert and government anthropologist Diamond Jenness's *The Indians of Canada*, first published in 1932 and in its sixth edition by the 1960s.[45] A durable anthropological survey of Aboriginal contributions to Canada's evolution, *Indians of Canada* placed their usefulness in the far distant past: "Doubtless all the tribes will disappear ... Some will merge steadily with the white race, others will bequeath to future generations only an infinitesimal fraction of their blood. Culturally they have already contributed everything that was valuable for our own civilization."[46] The discourse was pervasive in postwar Canada. Aboriginal people needed to be "Canadianized"; to that end Indian Affairs was made a branch of the Department of Citizenship and Immigration where, like European immigrants, they might take their place on the bottom rungs of Canadian society as reformed citizens.[47] In government policy and expert opinion, modernity demanded that Aboriginal people forget their past, shed their "Indianness," in order to become Canadians. Clinging to the "historical appendages" of treaties was symptomatic of their refusal to become normal citizens. Culliton's ruling, referring to the *Dreaver* case, found no reason to support a wider interpretation than had Justice Angers in 1935. Yet Angers's ruling did not consider medical services or hospitalization since only medicines were under consideration. Furthermore, in 1935 Angers had interpreted the "medicine chest" in a contemporary manner to mean all "medicines, drugs and medical supplies," as had the magistrate in Johnston's lower-court ruling. Culliton, however, ruled on the "plain reading" of the clause to mean "no more than the words clearly convey" – a first-aid kit.[48] Walter Johnston was ordered to pay the $72.00 hospital insurance tax.

The Johnston ruling did nothing to ease tensions at the North Battleford Indian Hospital. IHS bureaucrats naturally saw the decision as a vindication of their authority to make and change policy. Negotiations with the province and the Battlefords Union Hospital (the new entity operating the former Notre Dame Hospital) for a funding agreement continued, while local IHS employees were directed to "discreetly elicit" community and "Saskatchewan Indian Federation [*sic*]" support for their plan to withdraw from the hospital field.[49] The new IHS regional director felt sure that "deep down they appear to accept this closure as inevitable and will, I'm sure, agree with time and further discussion."[50] This was an increasingly common response from IHS officials in their correspondence with headquarters in Ottawa. As local bureaucrats, their role was to implement policy, and despite strong indications to the contrary, they assured their superiors that community opinion was swinging their way. But the 1968 "Health Plan for Indians" that required proof of indigency in order to access medical care from IHS, and the 1969 White Paper alarmed the Advisory Board. It refused to enter into any agreements. Besides, the treaty right to health care was again before the courts.[51]

In 1968 Andrew Swimmer, Chief Sam Swimmer's son, continued his father's struggle to protect treaty rights. He was charged with failing to pay the joint Saskatchewan hospitalization and medical care insurance tax. As in the Johnston case, the lower court ruled that the medicine chest clause in Treaty Six entitled Swimmer to free medical and hospital care, and thus he was exempt from paying the tax. The province was again preparing an appeal. Of more immediate concern to the Advisory Board were the deteriorating living conditions on the reserves, particularly the overcrowded and dilapidated housing that contributed to the high rates of hospitalization, especially among children. But IHS continued to deflect responsibility, directing the Advisory Board to take their concerns about housing, water, and sanitation to Indian Affairs bureaucrats. But by mid-1970 the climate had changed. In June, after a year of concerted and scathing criticism of government policy by an increasingly politicized national and local Aboriginal leadership, the Trudeau Liberals backed away from the disastrous White Paper proposals.[52] Echoing Trudeau's 1970 comments to the National Indian Brotherhood that the government "won't force any solution on you," a slightly chastised bureaucracy at Battleford promised that unless the community desired integration with the Union Hospital no one on the federal side would try to pressure them.[53]

Health minister John Munro assured the Advisory Board that he would make a substantial construction contribution to the Union Hospital on behalf of Aboriginal people, the generosity of which depended on the willingness of the hospital and the province to allow Aboriginal representatives on the Union Hospital board, and the assurance of Aboriginal employment in the new hospital. The total cost for the proposed 160-bed hospital was now estimated at $3.5 million. The province would pay half, the federal contribution on behalf of Aboriginal people would be $1.2 million, leaving $500,000 to be raised by the community. Regardless, over the previous decade the Indian hospital had been closing by inches. The maternity ward was closed in the mid-1960s and the outpatient clinic closed in early 1970. Aboriginal patients, mostly children, admitted to the Union Hospital increased from 8 in 1968 to 260 the following year.[54] Hospital integration, an increasingly difficult political position, was accomplished by other means.

Despite the government's more conciliatory tone, a pall of suspicion hung over discussions. The Advisory Board's chairman, Ernie Tootoosis, insisted that "integration" was an unacceptable term; amalgamation might be more suitable. They would not negotiate with provincial officials, since they had no treaty with the province. Furthermore, the Advisory Board could do nothing until all the band councils had consulted with their people about amalgamation. They invited the ministers of Indian Affairs, Jean Chrétien, and Health and Welfare, John Munro, to visit North Battleford to discuss how the proposed amalgamation would affect treaty rights.[55] Six months later band resolutions from five reserves rejected amalgamation. The leading negotiators on the Advisory Board, George Nicotine, Burton Baptiste, and the new chairman Joseph Weenie, argued that since the federal government was willing to spend $1.2 million for their health care, those funds should be used to build a new Indian hospital instead of investing in the community hospital. They also wanted all other hospitals to open their doors to Aboriginal people.[56] But an increasingly frustrated Advisory Board could only watch as IHS effectively abandoned the Indian hospital. The medical superintendent position remained vacant, and the steady succession of bureaucrats at the local and regional level did little to maintain a level of understanding of the Aboriginal position. Dr Hicks, the acting regional director at Regina, assured his superiors that the Advisory Board's concerns that their treaty rights be addressed before the hospital closed were not sincere: "finally they will allow themselves to be 'conned' into it, after making sure that still 'the rivers flow, the grass grows and the sun shines.'"[57] Besides, as the bureaucrats repeatedly intoned, only Indian Affairs, not IHS, could discuss treaty rights.

The increasingly acrimonious atmosphere did nothing to improve the racial discord in the town and at the Union Hospital. Some Aboriginal people were turned away without treatment, while other patients were left in the hallway. Union Hospital administrators cited overcrowding as the problem and stated that an expanded hospital would resolve the issue. But hospital patients, the community's most vulnerable elders and children, would also have been subject to the more fleeting and subtle sneers from admitting clerks and scowls from hospital personnel, subjectively felt and impossible to quantify. A bureaucrat familiar with the town later admitted that "there is indeed a great deal of discrimination in North Battleford," though he felt sure it did not affect hospital patients.[58] Furthermore, integration with community schools was proving disastrous for many Aboriginal children, especially since their parents had no representation on local school boards. Dr Webb, once the hospital's superintendent and now at headquarters, led a delegation from Ottawa to convince the Advisory Board to approve their integration plans. He suggested the only way to overcome discrimination in the community was to amalgamate. Sharing a hospital would be a great opportunity for Native and white people to get to know each other.[59] An exasperated Joseph Weenie insisted that the discrimination began in the hospital! But the colour line in North Battleford was clearly drawn. Police regularly rounded up Aboriginal patrons in public spaces and beer parlours and sent them on their way back to the reserve. The newspaper *Saskatchewan Indian* noted in 1972 that North Battleford "remains one of the most racist and anti-Indian towns in Saskatchewan."[60]

Impatient with the seemingly endless discussions, the Union Hospital threatened that it would proceed with a smaller expansion that excluded Aboriginal people unless it had a decision on the government's $1.2 million contribution by the end of November 1971. Adding urgency was the realization that, regardless of Aboriginal support, IHS would be forced to make a substantial contribution since every year more Aboriginal patients were treated in the Union Hospital. Health minister John Munro, in order to "sell" integration, invited Advisory Board chairman Joseph Weenie and six area chiefs to meet him in Ottawa on 22 November 1971. He promised to "sweeten" his offer with expanded public health facilities on reserves and improved transportation, which he calculated would cost less than $200,000 per year – the equivalent of the current deficit at the Indian hospital. Further, Munro attempted to convince the delegation that IHS was sincere in wanting to improve health services without compromising the long-term solution of the treaty rights question.[61] The minister's offer: to contribute $1.2 million towards expansion of the Union Hospital and the Indian hospital would close. He made a vague promise to convert the old hospital into a senior's home, and IHS would station a physician at the new hospital. The minister also promised to ensure adequate Aboriginal representation on the Union Hospital board, though provincial legislation made this impossible. Finally, Munro assured the delegation that discrimination would not be tolerated. The North Battleford delegation, for their part, explained that amalgamation would jeopardize their treaty rights, and they wanted to discuss Andrew Swimmer's case and the treaty right to health care. They explained that through the treaties Aboriginal people had already contributed plenty, in return for promises such as health care. The amalgamation of the schools was not working, and they wanted a new Indian hospital.[62] But Munro deflected the treaty issue since the Swimmer appeal was before the courts. The province had appealed Swimmer's acquittal and in December 1970 Chief Justice Culliton, referring to his judgment in the *Johnston* appeal ruled "the terms of Treaty No. 6 do not impose upon the Government of Canada the obligation of providing, without cost, medical and hospital services to all Indians."[63] Swimmer was ordered to pay the hospitalization and Medicare Insurance taxes. An appeal to the Supreme Court was filed, but it remained dormant.[64] In the meantime the Federation of Saskatchewan Indians negotiated a compromise with the provincial government to cease requiring individuals to pay insurance premiums, forcing the federal government to do so.[65] In short, since Munro would not discuss the treaty issue, positions became hardened with Poundmaker's David Tootoosis declaring at one point that they were in deadlock. The delegation left Ottawa, agreeing only to take the minister's proposal to their people. But, well before the meeting had begun, the minister had already determined that regardless of an agreement, the government would contribute the promised $1.2 million to the Union Hospital, and the Indian hospital would finally close.[66]

In anticipation of the minister's announcement to that effect, IHS bureaucrats attempted to reassure the Advisory Board that amalgamation was in the best interests of the whole community. At increasingly stormy joint Union Hospital–Advisory Board meetings, it became clear that amalgamation would proceed regardless of Aboriginal opposition. IHS officials and Union board members were particularly insulted when the discussion was held in Cree.[67] A frustrated George Nicotine feared that Aboriginal representation on the Union Hospital board could not counter the everyday discrimination felt in the community. "In North Battleford" he said, "there is so much discrimination … Let's trade hospitals."[68] Dr Webb assured his deputy minister that with the decision made, "the Indians will probably cooperate in arranging and effecting an orderly transition."[69] But beyond the concerns about discrimination in the community and at the Union Hospital, the Cree leadership remained adamant that until the minister assured them in writing that their treaty rights would not be affected, they would not consent to their hospital's closure. Despite the Indian hospital's many shortcomings, and the fact that IHS effectively abandoned it by admitting most patients elsewhere, it remained the community's touchstone in the continuing effort to assert the treaty right to health care. Like the efforts by the Kainai and Siksika in the 1970s, the leadership had little recourse but to defend what their hospitals represented. With the *Swimmer* appeal to the Supreme Court in abeyance, the issue also remained very much alive for IHS.

In early 1973 IHS asked its legal services for an interpretation of the medicine chest clause. Dr Webb, now assistant deputy minister, wished to know if there were any federal legal obligations to provide health care to Indians, especially in relation to Treaty Six. Regardless of the court rulings in *Johnston* and *Swimmer*, and despite bureaucratic efforts to deride, dismiss, and ignore the treaty right to health care as a fantasy not sincerely held, significant concerns remained. The arrival in late 1972 of the new minister of Health and Welfare, Marc Lalonde, likely prompted Webb's inquiry. In reply, legal services outlined that for many years Parliament had voted funds to provide health care services, including paying health care premiums for the indigent to provincial hospital and medical care plans, but that such voluntary payments did not endow Indians with an enforceable right to demand payment. However, the brief continued, "tradition, custom and usage (and dependency) may ultimately produce a strong moral right." After describing the case law including the judgments in *Dreaver*, *Johnston*, and *Swimmer* regarding the treaty right to health care, the legal brief noted that the provision of such medical care services over the years "will undoubtedly have made the Indians believe that they are entitled, as of right, to such services. It is a truism to state that, for governments, a benefit once given is very difficult to take away. There are undoubtedly many Indians today – particularly those who are politically active – who believe that the Federal Government has a legal obligation to provide such care." Legal services then cited a 1950 Supreme Court decision, *St Ann's Island Shooting and Fishing Club Ltd. v the King* (dealing with Crown leasing of Indian reserve lands, not health care), which nevertheless stated that Aboriginal people were in effect wards of the state "whose care and welfare are a political trust of the highest obligation." This Supreme Court statement, warned the legal services' brief, conveyed a "judicial attitude which cannot be ignored." Legal services advised that, in transferring health services to territorial and provincial jurisdictions, IHS should negotiate with affected Aboriginal groups to solicit their agreement.[70] Thus, despite the Saskatchewan appeal court's ruling, the federal state acknowledged a political imperative to consult, if only to avoid controversy.

The following July 1973 the Indian hospital's Advisory Board met with health minister Lalonde in Ottawa, where they pressed him to reconsider his predecessor's decision to contribute funds to the Union Hospital and close the Indian hospital. Unsuccessful on that front, the Advisory Board did persuade the minister to provide assurances, in writing, that membership on the Union Hospital board (made possible by amended provincial legislation) and cooperation in "amalgamation" of hospital services in the Union Hospital "will not in any way prejudice your legal rights under Treaty Six."[71] Wording his statement carefully so as to neither admit nor deny a treaty right to health care, the minister pledged to continue to pay health care premiums and other health services costs as a matter of government policy. Lalonde also made a vague promise to endeavour to have Aboriginal employees at the Indian hospital transferred to the Union Hospital or otherwise deployed in departmental activities in the area. But North Battleford ratepayers took some time to approve the hospital expansion plan, and coupled with construction delays, by late 1973 the original federal contribution would need to double to $2.2 million. The Indian hospital continued its limited operations, but was slated to close in April 1977.

As the 1977 deadline approached, Sweetgrass Chief Steve Pooyak and Gordon Albert, representing the Federation of Saskatchewan Indians, met with the deputy minister in late November 1976 to postpone closure of the Indian hospital until the situation could be studied. They argued that for the previous fourteen years since 1962 when the hospital's closure was first considered, there had never been meaningful input by the Aboriginal people; meetings with the Advisory Board were little more than gestures on the part of IHS and the white community. In particular, they argued that the hospital expansion plan was unworkable. It called for the closure of the Indian hospital's 39 beds and the Union Hospital's expansion from 167 beds to 168, or a net increase of just one bed. Though forty of the Union Hospital's chronic care beds were to be converted to acute care, there was no facility that could accommodate those patients. More pressing was the perennial concern about discrimination in North Battleford. The delegates termed it "rampant," and said that white people were "proud" of their low regard for Native people. Though the deputy minister dismissed their concerns, he told the delegation that if they had a counter-proposal he would convey it to minister.[72] They then produced a proposal by the North Battleford District Chiefs to study their concerns about hospital care.

The chiefs' proposal began with an articulation of the Treaty's promised right to health care and how their people's social and economic position had since deteriorated, creating many of the existing health problems. They claimed the right to "regulate and control" the treaty right to adequate medical services in the people's interests. Their concerns echoed those voiced since the Indian hospital's closure was first proposed. The elderly would be disadvantaged, and "non-Indian patients have in certain instances refused to share hospital rooms with Indians."[73] The proposal asked for one year and $60,000 to study the Aboriginal and white communities' attitudes to the Indian hospital's closure, and the experience in other integrated hospitals. Not surprisingly, deputy minister Bruce Rawson refused to consider the proposal, maintaining that there had been adequate consultation, though he recognized that there was no agreement between Aboriginal people and IHS on the right to care under Treaty Six.[74]

The Battleford chiefs took it upon themselves to study hospital services and the impact of the Indian hospital's closure on local health and health care. In March 1977, with the Indian hospital's closure imminent, they presented ministers Marc Lalonde of Health and Welfare, and Warren Allmand of Indian Affairs with evidence that the $2.2 million investment in the Union Hospital "will be of far greater benefit to non-Indians than it will be to Indians." They charged that negotiations with the Advisory Board over the years were "simply a public relations effort to convince the Indians this would be good for them." Their position – except for minor concessions such as a minority position on the Union Hospital board and vague promises to reduce discrimination – "has never seriously been considered."[75] These claims, as we have seen, are borne out by the documentary record, where a succession of bureaucrats consistently dismissed the Advisory Board's concerns. The direction of government policy, the chiefs contended, remained to unload its constitutional and treaty responsibilities. It continued to upgrade non-Aboriginal schools and hospitals, while facilities serving Aboriginal people deteriorated. The chiefs also charged that when they requested documents in 1976 relating to the ongoing negotiations, Health and Welfare claimed they only retained files for five years before being destroyed. Again, as we have seen, the documentary record still exists.

The chiefs' brief used hospital utilization rates and a 1975 Indian Affairs housing survey to calculate that the planned Union Hospital expansion would provide forty-nine fewer beds than required; moreover, the area reserves' appalling housing and infrastructure contributed to their misery.[76] They determined that from 1971 through 1975 infant mortality was ten times the national rate, and the average age at death was just forty-one years. Moreover, 37 per cent, or 422 families, had no home; 98 per cent of houses had no sewer or water, and no telephone to summon help in emergencies. There were just nine wells for 5,480 people. "This is the heritage," the chiefs stated, "of a people whose ancestors surrendered the land and resources, which produces all the wealth of Canada, in exchange for a guarantee of certain rights and services for as long as the sun shines, the grass grows, and the rivers flow. One of those services promised was health care."[77] The brief recommended that the on-reserve nursing stations "should be condemned," and that government fund training for personnel to operate proper clinics. They urged the government to undertake an extensive housing and infrastructure construction program. Finally, they recommended that the Indian hospital remain open until a task force of representatives from government and the community could investigate hospital care facilities.

The chiefs' brief was sufficiently alarming, and potentially damaging, for the ministers to agree to establish a task force inquiry. It was also the least costly of the chiefs' recommendations. The five-member task force – David Ahenakew, president of the Federation of Saskatchewan Indians; Steve Pooyak representing the Battleford area Chiefs; Alex Taylor, for the Saskatchewan government; Alex Pinter from Indian Affairs; with Luc Laroche, from University of Ottawa as chairman and representing Health and Welfare – was formed in mid-May 1977 and directed to report in just six weeks. It would receive no funding, the members were to pay their own way, and there would be no new research. Essentially, the task force was to investigate the chiefs' brief and to review existing health programs, hospital utilization, and problems relating to housing and sanitation. The task force operated under one further constraint: "In any event, it is important that the task force come up with a recommendation relating to a unified, integrated system. The minister is not prepared to consider any dichotomy in the health service, eg a special service for Indian people outside the existing health services."[78] But it was also made clear to all that the task force was to be the "court of last appeal." The minister would use its recommendations to finally decide on the dilemma of the Indian hospital.[79]

To appear impartial, Health and Welfare appointed an outsider, Luc Laroche from University of Ottawa's medical school, to chair the task force and represent the department. Alas, the appearance of impartiality was deceiving. After a hurried investigation, the task force chair submitted his report on 30 June 1977, and immediately health minister Lalonde announced the Indian hospital's closure. Of particular significance to the minister was the report's Recommendation #1: "The present physical entity known as the Indian hospital to cease existing as an active treatment facility and that the Minister consider the feasibility of replacing it with an Indian Health Centre."[80] This was precisely what the minister and his bureaucrats wanted to hear and the policy his predecessors had pursued for fifteen years. Unfortunately for the department, the task force had made no such recommendation. In fact, chairman Laroche, in his report, had unilaterally altered many of the task force's recommendations. The original task force recommendation read: "The present physical entity known as the Indian hospital to cease existing as an active treatment facility *and to be converted into an Indian Health Centre.*"[81] The change in wording, seemingly subtle, subverted the task force's authority by giving the minister the power to decide. More importantly for the community, the task force report's change from *converting* to *replacing*, meant that the Indian hospital, at once a tangible recognition of the treaty right to health care and a powerful symbol of their enduring struggle to have that right recognized, would be lost. Recommendation #2 was also changed. In the original task force report, the Indian Health Centre was to be under the direction and control of a board consisting of the North Battleford District Chiefs; the board would have responsibility for all aspects of management, from policy, to budget approval, to administration. However, in Laroche's report submitted to Health and Welfare, the board's responsibility would be "subject to the overall authority of the Government of Canada."[82] The change in wording also affected the task force's further Recommendation #11, that the proposed Health Centre lands, presently hospital lands, be declared a special reserve under the Indian Act and therefore under the control of area chiefs.

Laroche's other changes were not so subtle. Some recommendations were removed entirely, while other revisions completely altered the tenor and substance of the task force's most important conclusions. For instance, the original statement on the treaty right to health is as follows (with Laroche's deletions underlined and his altered wording in italics):

> The Task Force believes that the Indian people, [*The Indian representatives on the Task Force have expressed the view that the Indian people*] under the

Royal Proclamation of 1763, under Treaty #6 and the BNA Act, have a unique relationship to the federal government. This relationship requires the Government of Canada to accept and exercise the responsibility for the health and medical care of Indian people

There are indications that the health conditions of the Indian people have been deteriorating in recent years [*not improved as much as expected in recent years*] in spite of the present services being provided by Health and Welfare Canada.

Under the terms of Treaty #6, the federal government [*the Indian representatives strongly believe that the federal government*] is obligated to provide comprehensive health care services to Indians in the North Battleford District.[83]

In submitting his report to the minister, and before it became widely known he had substantially altered the original task force recommendations, chairman Laroche warned, "I know that the report will be controversial. It nevertheless expresses the mood of the Indians in North Battleford."[84] Even Laroche's significantly revised report was unacceptable to the bureaucrats. Preparing a counter-proposal despite the promise that the task force would be the "court of last appeal," deputy minister Bruce Rawson restated the government position: "We do not agree with the essence of the key recommendation to convert the hospital into a health centre and to grant Indians the authority to fully manage their own health services."[85]

Predictably, the four task force members (of whom only David Ahenakew and Steve Pooyak were Aboriginal) were outraged at the altered report. Minister Lalonde was at pains to explain away the fiasco. He explained that Chairman Laroche indicated some concern about the wording of the task force report and proposed changing it to make it more "palatable" to the government. Though Lalonde maintained that his officials advised Laroche to write the report as directed by the task force, Laroche himself claimed that senior bureaucrats recommended the changes.[86] Writing to task force member David Ahenakew, Lalonde apologized for the "confusion," which he claimed was the "result of good intentions and certainly not the result of a deliberate attempt to mislead."[87] Nevertheless, a telex from Lalonde's deputy minister, Rawson, to fellow bureaucrat Charles-E. Caron suggests duplicity, at best: "Personally I hope the confusion continues to mount around recommendation number one. I am sure that if the truth was known it would be quite clear and we would be in the soup."[88]

Recall, it was the Battleford chiefs' 1977 brief charting reserve conditions – homelessness, overcrowding, a lack of even rudimentary infrastructure, and the subsequent destruction of health – that prompted the task force inquiry. Although hampered by an arbitrary six-week deadline, it did not take the task force long to target a century of unfulfilled treaty promises as the fundamental problem. Recommending a renewed treaty relationship in which the Aboriginal people most affected would manage their own programs, the task force saw their work sabotaged. While bureaucratic obstruction and government intransigence marked the past fifteen years of struggle for the hospital, this was a grotesque perversion of sincere efforts to improve living conditions and health. The task force debacle was, moreover, the disturbingly logical consequence of the state's enduring assimilation project. At its core was the self-serving view that medical bureaucrats alone knew what was best for the people's health. In July, Marc Lalonde engaged independent consultant Graham Clarkson to formulate a health service plan for North Battleford. The minister promised, "I am prepared to accept any recommendations that Dr Clarkson may make after thoroughly studying this situation."[89]

Clarkson, the former executive director of the Saskatchewan Medical Care Insurance Commission and a respected health care consultant, began by interviewing all the task force members. Noting that they were "disturbed" by Laroche's report, calling his actions "inept at the best," Clarkson told Minister Lalonde, "I have no doubt that Dr Laroche is of the opinion that he acted with the interests of the Indians at heart. I also have no doubt that the Indians find it next to impossible to understand this."[90] Not surprisingly, Clarkson met considerable suspicion in North Battleford. As he put it, "Tension was high – and for good reason," not only because of Laroche's actions, but also because the government had already shut the hospital. He could not blame the people for their distrust. To demonstrate his independence to all concerned, Clarkson demanded the removal of the local IHS bureaucrat, Mr Burrows, who was increasingly distraught and unable to re-establish "sound relationships with the Indians."[91] Burrows was gone within the month.

In his recommendations, Clarkson followed closely the (original) task force report. Fundamental to his plan was Aboriginal administration of all health programs. While he agreed that the Indian hospital should remain closed, Clarkson proposed an Indian Health Centre under the authority of an executive board with representatives from each of the area reserves, a representative from each of Indian Affairs and Health and Welfare, and two non-Aboriginal community members. The centre's executive director would be appointed from among the Aboriginal members. Moreover, referring to "difficulties at the [IHS] Regional Office," Clarkson recommended that the Indian Health Centre report directly to Ottawa.[92] As Clarkson made clear, progress towards a solution of the health crisis required new, or perhaps fewer, bureaucrats at both the local and regional offices. His plan also called for a clearer focus on preventive and protective health services on the reserves, again administered by the bands and employing Aboriginal health workers.

Clarkson's study found that the long-standing local practice of contracting out medical services to a physicians' group had created unnecessary, excessive, and inappropriate hospitalization, especially of children. He noted that the volume of hospital care received by the Aboriginal community was more than three and a half times that of the non-Aboriginal community. The largest difference was for infants under one year, who were hospitalized five times more often than non-Aboriginal infants. Further, Clarkson compared just the Aboriginal population of the province, and found that the North Battleford area people were hospitalized one and a half times more often.[93] Much of the excess children's hospitalization was the consequence of poor housing and sanitation on the reserves. But calling some hospitalization "admissions of convenience," Clarkson thought it a "sad reflection on the Federal Government agency who operated the North Battleford Indian Hospital."[94] He examined the physicians' volume of practice and found that of the twenty doctors who admitted patients to either or both the Indian hospital and the Union Hospital in 1976, four had an average of 629 patients, while the other sixteen doctors collectively had 189. Clarkson could not imagine how these four doctors could spend adequate time with their patients. "Some of the doctors seemed to have little or no interest in providing medical services to the Indian community while one or two appeared to supply a remarkable volume which, to my way of thinking, would have to have been carried out all too quickly." Clarkson's plan called for the Indian Health Centre to retain two physicians on staff, under the supervision of the executive director. He quickly explained that this would not be a reversion to the designated doctor system of the past where IHS compelled patients to go to particular physicians, but rather Indian Health Centre physicians would form a nucleus whose "concern and involvement" would be working with the Aboriginal community.[95]

Organized medicine, locally and provincially, reacted negatively to Clarkson's plan and his criticisms of their work.[96] Clarkson understood the North Battleford district medical society's objections to the planned Indian Health Centre to be motivated by self-interest, specifically its impact on their incomes.[97] At a meeting with the Battlefords Union Hospital staff, IHS (properly Medical Services) director Lyall Black attempted to explain Clarkson's recommendations to a very hostile audience. He witnessed first-hand the bigotry and prejudice that Aboriginal people had long endured; as he reported, there was "little sympathy evident amongst the staff for Indian people." On the clear need for cultural orientation, Black noted the staff's confusion and surprise when he clarified that the orientation program would be necessary "for the doctors and hospital staff rather than for the Indians."[98] The Saskatchewan Medical Association's E.H. Baergen continued to oppose the Indian Health Centre in a letter to the *Canadian Medical Association Journal*. By way of "advising" any potential candidates for the staff positions at the Indian Health Centre, Baergen noted that since there was currently an adequate number of physicians practising in North Battleford, any increase would lead to friction among the medical staff of the Union Hospital, warning that "this will inevitably give rise to hard feelings against any newcomer to the centre."[99] This thinly veiled threat exposed the challenges that the Indian Health Centre posed to the medical status quo in North Battleford. Nevertheless, Clarkson's plan, accepted by the new minister of Health and Welfare, Monique Bégin, in December 1977, formed the basis for the Battlefords Indian Health Centre Inc., which opened less than two years later, while the new Battlefords Union Hospital celebrated its grand opening in June 1978.

The Indian Health Centre's board of directors stated its objectives: first "to ensure that comprehensive health services are delivered to the Indian Bands … as a matter of Indian right under the British North America Act, Treaty Number 6 between her Majesty and the Cree Nation and the Indian Act"; and second, "to provide direction to Her Majesty in the operation of the Battlefords Indian Health Centre Inc."[100] At the Indian Health Centre's grand opening in July 1979, National Indian Brotherhood President Noel Starblanket celebrated the achievement as an example of community-based and community-controlled health care. But he also used the occasion to elaborate on the political and economic roots of ill health, in particular "coerced dependence upon paternalistic and ever-shifting federal policies … [that] contributed to a great extent to the manifestations of social ill health now seen among us, including alcohol and drug abuse, family breakdown, suicides, accidents, and violent deaths."[101] Starblanket's remarks were especially poignant in light of the recently withdrawn federal guidelines for access to non-insured health benefits (dental care, drugs, glasses, and medical transportation). Hoping to trim budgets and stem a perceived abuse of benefits by the non-indigent, the Liberal government imposed a means test that hearkened back to the 1968 "Health Plan for Indians" a decade earlier. Protests emerged immediately with an angry march on Parliament Hill, while the St Regis Mohawk set up a $1 toll at the American border at Cornwall, Ontario, for a health fund to pay for needed medical care.[102] Experiencing its own "White Paper moment," the Department of Health and Welfare suspended the guidelines in January 1979. The government fell in June and the newly elected (albeit short-lived) Progressive Conservative government withdrew the guidelines, opting to rely on professional medical and dental judgment to determine eligibility for non-insured benefits. Starblanket praised the decision of the new health minister (and fellow platform dignitary) David Crombie. But, in language that would make any federal politician squirm, Starblanket framed the Indian Health Centre as a concrete example of self-government: "We can march with the sun to the brightness of a new and better day – through the total control of our lives and destinies – or we can retreat to the false security and darkness of government colonialist control."[103] Neither Starblanket nor the minister, in his remarks, mentioned the treaty right to health care. According to Crombie, the Health Centre was a landmark that demonstrated the government's determination "to *give* the Indian people" responsibility for their health, while confirming the willingness of the District Chiefs to "*accept* greater responsibility" for the delivery of health programs.[104] Nevertheless, the Indian Health Centre continues to stand as testament to the Aboriginal community's insistence that health services and the treaty relationship would not be severed.

Certainly, the North Battleford communities were not the only voices for change in health care delivery in the 1970s. The National Indian Brotherhood (NIB) in 1978 established a National Commission of Inquiry on Indian Health bringing together health representatives from provincial and territorial Aboriginal organizations. Taking direction from its members, not IHS or health professionals, the National Commission provided a distinctly Aboriginal perspective on health issues affecting its constituents.[105] Its 1978 brief, *Indian Control of Indian Health,* highlighted how federal policy, often formulated for political purposes and without input from Aboriginal people, lurched from crisis to crisis to the detriment of the very people it was to serve. The Indian Association of Alberta likewise characterized the federal government's approach to health care as unilateral, arbitrary, and piecemeal, while calling on the state to honour its treaty responsibilities.[106] By late 1979, taking some direction from national and provincial Aboriginal representatives, IHS developed yet another Indian Health Policy that, for the first time, acknowledged that health policy flowed from "constitutional and statutory provisions, treaties, and customary practice ... and from the commitment of Indian people to preserve and enhance their culture and traditions." Not quite an affirmation of the treaty right to health, but it did move beyond the long-held claim that IHS policies stemmed from little more than a moral obligation. As a Health and Welfare bureaucrat put it, "We always thought that, as health professionals, we knew what Indians needed with respect to health care ... [h]owever, not only is health status unimproved by today's standards, the situation is incompatible with both the aspirations of the Indian people and the tenets of self-determination and human rights."[107] Recognizing also the "intolerably low level of health of many Indian people, who exist under conditions rooted in poverty and community decline," the new health policy rested on three pillars: community development (socio-economic, cultural, and spiritual); the traditional relationship with the federal government to serve as an advocate and to promote local capacity; and an active federal role in the interrelated health system.[108] An unprecedented policy direction perhaps, but old habits die hard: six months *after* announcing its policy, the government appointed a commission of inquiry to determine how Aboriginal groups should be consulted in decisions affecting health care policies and services.

The Advisory Commission, led by prominent jurist Thomas Berger, who had recently completed the Mackenzie Valley Pipeline Inquiry, advised that consultation about communities' participation in the planning, budgeting, and delivery of health programs should be the first step in their actual planning and delivery of those services. His report celebrated the achievements of the North Battleford Health Centre as a model of self-determination in health care, while also pointing to programs already developed by Aboriginal communities across the country. There were health centres, health councils, health liaison programs, initiatives in environmental health, nutrition, breast-feeding, homecare, mental and spiritual health, and midwifery programs.

All were community-based and all were chronically underfunded or funded on a piecemeal basis.[109] These initiatives, he stressed, emerged not from government policy, but often in spite of it. Berger therefore recommended that the $950,000 Cabinet had earmarked for consultation (less than 1 per cent of the IHS budget, he noted) be distributed among the provincial and territorial Indian organizations affiliated with the NIB to be used to develop the consultation process, with a separate appropriation to fund the process for the Inuit. His further recommendation – the establishment of a permanent national Indian Health Council – was not implemented.

The creation of the Battlefords Indian Health Centre to deliver health care "as a matter of Indian right," as it declared, offered a new model that reflected a changed political and medical landscape. Aboriginal self-determination in health would join similar programs to take back control of education and social services. Programs focused on preventative public health initiatives, delivered in the community, became more appropriate in the 1980s as many Aboriginal communities underwent an "epidemiological transition" with declining rates of communicable diseases and infant mortality, and an increasing incidence of chronic conditions such as diabetes and cardiovascular diseases.[110] Moreover, Canada endorsed the World Health Organization's optimistic goal of "health for all by the year 2000" and its 1978 Alma Ata declaration on primary health care as an essential first element that "requires and promotes maximum community and individual self-reliance and participation in the planning, organization, operation and control."[111] But clearly, Canada's support of primary health care in 1978 did not envision local Aboriginal control of health services. As noted, the IHS top bureaucrat had declared just the previous year "we do not agree ... to grant Indians the authority to fully manage their own health services."[112]

It was certainly no coincidence that North Battleford Indian Hospital employees, Walter Johnston and Andrew Swimmer, triggered the court challenges of the treaty right in the 1960s, much to the outrage of their employers. The court's rejection of those claims supported the state's contention that health care services are provided as a matter of policy, not legal obligation, leaving it free to change policy. Yet, the 1960s Saskatchewan Court of Appeal decisions very much reflected their times. Subsequent Supreme Court decisions, such as *Queen v Sparrow* (1990), held that the courts should interpret Aboriginal rights in a flexible manner to permit their evolution. As the Federal Court noted in reference to the medicine chest clause in 1999: "Mr Justice Angers took a proper approach in his 1935 decision in Dreaver (supra), reading the Treaty No. 6 medicine chest clause in a contemporary manner to mean a supply of all medicines, drugs and medical supplies. Certainly, it is clear that the Saskatchewan Court of Appeal took what is now a wrong approach in its literal and restrictive reading of the medicine chest clause in the 1966 decision in Johnston (supra)."[113]

It seems likely that a legal challenge today would have a different outcome. Nevertheless, the question of "insured health services" (hospital and physician services) seems resolved under the Canada Health Act (1984), in which provinces agreed to deliver care to all provincial residents, including Aboriginal people whether they lived on or off reserve, in return for federal funds, ending the often rancorous provincial-federal disputes over payment.[114] Access to non-insured health benefits remains subject to government policy, suggesting that the judgment in *Johnston*, not the 1935 *Dreaver* decision defining medicines and medical supplies as a treaty right, is the judicial last word.

The protracted struggle over the North Battleford Indian Hospital reveals the community's considerable resolve to define and defend its treaty relationship with the state. Resistance to arbitrary and shifting policies became a generation's work that ultimately contested the value of treating illness bred in poverty only to return the cured to the same conditions. The history of the North Battleford Health Centre's creation exposes an entrenched bureaucracy imbued with the increasing authority of medicine, actively working to undermine the community. State control and surveillance shifted only reluctantly and incrementally in the face of determined resistance by Aboriginal communities, and only after many years of suffering and despair. That communities might know their own health care needs came as an unwelcome challenge to a bureaucracy that consistently viewed Aboriginality as a condition to be treated and cured.

Conclusion

The history of "separate beds" for Aboriginal people complicates our understanding of twentieth-century health care in Canada. Indian hospitals stood alongside their more modern white counterparts, putting racial segregation at the core of the nascent welfare state. The Indian Health Service (IHS), removed from Indian Affairs and attached to the national health bureaucracy, acknowledged that Aboriginal people would be included in schemes for postwar health care, if only to keep them excluded. Underfunded, poorly staffed, and racially segregated institutions isolated the putative threat posed by Aboriginal people, while Canada consciously defined national health as liberal white citizenship. First Nations communities that saw hospitals as a first step towards better health found instead that the state's commitment ended with hospitalization while reserve poverty continued unabated. Separate bureaucratic silos of Indian Affairs, responsible for reserve sanitation and housing, and Indian Health Service, in charge of health care, encouraged this "vertical" or disease- or treatment-specific approach to health services and all but ensured continued poor health. Medicare only made matters worse. Accomplishing what the 1969 White Paper could not, national hospital and health insurance finally provided the federal government with a golden opportunity to jettison its legal responsibilities for Aboriginal people's health. For more than twenty years communities wrestled with an entrenched bureaucracy that sought to undermine their efforts to improve health through an integrated approach based on a measure of self-government. While most Canadians celebrated Medicare, Aboriginal communities faced arbitrary and often punitive health policies that exacerbated persistent socio-economic inequities to maintain health disparities based on race.

The meanings of Indian hospitals are inextricably linked to the larger story of health care in modern Canada. As tuberculosis retreated in the 1930s, the migration of First Nations to towns and cities reawakened fears of infection. The concerns of medical experts transformed the "Indian problem" into a threat to the public health. In urging the federal government to take responsibility, the Canadian Tuberculosis Association (CTA) encouraged the state to confine Aboriginal people in institutions well segregated from white patients. As the voice of sanatorium directors and provincial health bureaucrats, the CTA constructed the problem of "Indian tuberculosis" and devised its solution in racially segregated institutions financed by the federal state. While the first Indian Health Service hospital at Fort Qu'Appelle in 1936 was intended to provide a maternity ward to further the BCG vaccine trial on First Nations infants, the "remarkable economy" of the institution that operated at half the cost of sanatoria quickly recommended it as an ideal prototype. That model of maternity/general hospitals that also treated tuberculosis – an "unholy combination" according to one physician – underscores the baleful role of Indian hospitals as institutions of segregation and confinement.

First Nations communities initially greeted Indian hospitals as the harbinger of a brighter future where the state acknowledged its treaty obligations to better health care. But the promise rang increasingly hollow in the coercive and dangerously underfunded institutions. Shipped from their homes like spoiled cargo, patients often found themselves isolated by culture and language, unable to understand their situation, their treatments, or their prognosis. Those who challenged IHS control, like the Siksika at their Blackfoot Hospital, paid a heavy price. Overwhelmingly paternalistic, the IHS readily resorted to degrees of compulsion "for their own good," from body casts and straitjackets to the Indian Health Regulations, which essentially criminalized the ill. The promise of opportunities for medical training and employment in Indian hospitals likewise proved illusory. IHS mirrored broader social and economic inequities through rigid racialized and gendered medical hierarchies that left Aboriginal workers the least trained and worst paid. That Aboriginal employees (and patients) were often "graduates" of residential schools not only highlights the pervasive role of state institutions; it also exposes the state's hand in producing its own workforce. Nevertheless, as cultural brokers and interpreters, First Nations employees could mitigate the atmosphere of coercion and confinement that characterized the hospitals.

Blunt and unequivocal in his 1946 announcement, the minister of health rationalized the IHS and its hospitals as a humanitarian measure to protect the Canadian public. Aboriginal peoples' interests were subsumed in the medical bureaucracy's slippery understanding of humanitarianism. Constructed as objects of Ottawa's benevolence, Aboriginal people had little say in their own health care. Meanwhile, their bodies were readily exploited for research and teaching. As for postwar Canadians, Indian hospitals seemed to confirm that theirs was a vigilant yet compassionate state. As promises of a comprehensive welfare state quickly faded, Canadians could be assured that the most vulnerable were not forgotten. As the minister promised, the IHS established Indian hospitals in redundant military facilities and renovated residential schools. Meanwhile, the same bureaucracy's National Health Grants funded an unprecedented increase in hospital construction and expansion, adding thirty new institutions each year in the decade after 1948 and increasing the number of hospital beds by two-thirds. Indian hospitals had the added benefit of assuring Canadians that their new community hospitals would remain white, at least initially.

The logic of Indian hospitals for the 1940s combined enlightened self-interest, the rising social and political authority of medicine, and broad anxieties about the "Indian problem." But the 1960s saw profound transformations in national health. Massive investments in hospital infrastructure led to escalating operating costs, which yielded the national hospital insurance program and, with much political wrangling, health insurance in 1968. With the federal government sharing costs with the provinces, the seemingly redundant Indian hospitals could be "quietly closed." Responsibility for Aboriginal health care (and welfare) now shifted to the provinces. But the jurisdictional disputes that accompanied Medicare exposed Aboriginal people to the excesses of aggrieved provincial administrations and local hospital boards, which dismissed them as interlopers and less worthy of care. More ominous still was the understanding that Medicare would enable the federal government to fulfil its assimilationist goal and abandon its legal and treaty obligations.

Medicare's threat – or promise – to accomplish that aim was most clearly articulated in the protracted struggle over the North Battleford Indian Hospital. That bitter dispute exposed an obdurate and calculating bureaucracy that relentlessly undercut First Nations' efforts to address the links between ill health and the poverty that led to it. The effort to sever the legal and treaty relationship through the "equality" of Medicare continued for more than a decade after the White Paper's withdrawal, despite clear evidence that curative medical services had little impact on community health status. Medicare, not the medicine chest, would determine the state's role in health care.

To most Canadians, then as now, this was as it should be. The liberal democratic principles of individual political and legal equality imbued both the White Paper and Medicare. But Prime Minister Trudeau, who eventually admitted it was shortsighted, abandoned the White Paper within the year, saying, "we had perhaps the prejudices of small 'l' liberals and white men at that who thought that equality meant the same law for everybody."[1] Yet, shifting policies in the 1960s for hospital and health care insurance, and their implications for collective rights based on treaties and self-government, were not easily assailed. In the 1960s the court rejected First Nations attempts to assert a treaty right to health care, while the IHS bureaucracy directed them to discuss treaty issues with Indian Affairs. Nevertheless, dividing the authority between Indian Affairs, which was responsible for matters such as water quality, sanitation, and housing, and Health and Welfare, in charge of health services, did little to alleviate public health problems. Medicare threatened to exacerbate the problem by cutting the links between the roots of illness and health care services, not to mention the treaty relationship itself. Amid the socially and politically disruptive demands from Aboriginal people and Quebecers in the 1960s for collective rather than individual rights, the seemingly apolitical Medicare program bestowed a veneer of national unity that may account for its iconic status.[2] A cherished social program for a Canada that embraced liberal notions of social and political equality as the basis for good health, Medicare damaged the aspirations of many First Nations. Canadians remain eminently satisfied with Medicare, proudly proclaiming its values of equity, fairness, and solidarity as "intimately tied to their understanding of citizenship."[3] But Aboriginal citizenship was always incomplete and contingent. Denied the most basic right of the franchise before 1960, First Nations faced serial projects aimed at terminating their rights after. Medicare bestowed its benefits unevenly: "Aboriginal status" remains one of the key social determinants of health that includes other primary factors such as income, education, housing, and employment.[4]

The 1979 Indian Health Policy continues as the federal government's guiding statement on health care. Drafted in response to the determined resistance by First Nations to the state's continued attempts to shift responsibilities to the provinces, the policy pledged to preserve the federal government's "special relationship" with Aboriginal people. It employs the language of self-determination in its laudable goal "to achieve an increasing level of health in Indian communities, generated and maintained by the Indian communities themselves."[5] With a stronger federal commitment, the broken-down Indian hospitals, once powerful symbols in the long struggle for effective health care, were replaced by health clinics to provide primary care in communities. To address the problem of chronically understaffed hospitals in northern regions, IHS partnered with university medical schools to provide qualified personnel, who in turn benefited from the expanded opportunities for teaching and research. Nevertheless, significant disparities in health status persist between Aboriginal and non-Aboriginal Canadians. As T. Kue Young concluded in his study of the Anishinaabe of northwestern Ontario and the Sioux Lookout Indian Hospital, real change in health status required resources dedicated to community authority and control of health care, not highly specialized medical services.[6] In 1988, as Young's book went to press, five men from Sandy Lake First Nation went on a hunger strike at the Indian hospital to draw attention to years of worsening health care and deteriorating relations between First Nations communities and the Department of Health and Welfare.[7]

A decade after its inception, the broader promise of the 1979 Indian Health Policy, to address health care in communities, was abandoned for an exclusive focus on federal transfers to First Nations for some aspects of health care delivery. As minister of health Jake Epp told the Assembly of First Nations health transfer conference in 1987, "We, in Health and Welfare, and many others in the health field, are convinced that the future health of the Indian people rests in your hands, not in ours ... God bless you all." Author Dara Culhane Speck wondered if the minister's statement was a threat or a promise.[8] Critics suggested that the transfer policy merely offloaded the responsibility for health care to communities without actually sharing any power to develop or control programs. Was health transfer another "hidden agenda" of termination like the White Paper? The Assembly of First Nations argued that until First Nations had actual control over resources and economic development, communities would simply be "administering their own misery."[9] The policy's "non-enrichment" clause froze funding at levels in place at the time of transfer, with no provision for on-reserve population increases or shifting community needs. Other critics noted that the transfer program failed to address the wider social, economic, and environmental sources of ill health, while reinforcing a medical model of health that maintained colonial relations of power over Aboriginal people.[10] Tellingly, non-insured health benefits were excluded from the transfer program, which led to suspicions that the benefits might be withdrawn, and they would certainly be administered by government criteria.[11] A recent study concluded that the transfer policy was less concerned with self-determination than with cutting costs; it does little more than meet the Indian Act's original commitment to health – to control the spread of disease and provide sanitary conditions.[12]

In its brief to the Royal Commission on Aboriginal Peoples roundtable on health issues in 1993, the Federation of Saskatchewan Indian Nations (FSIN) asked how the transfer policy would affect the treaty right to health care. If First Nations assumed the government's authority for health care, did that mean that treaty groups had absolved the state of its treaty responsibility? The FSIN brief, presented by Alma Favel-King in her capacity as the Executive Director of Health and Social Development portfolio, reflected the concerns of all treaty communities to define and protect the right to health care. But Favel-King had also been involved in the bitter twenty-year-long struggle over closing the North Battleford Indian Hospital two decades earlier. Better than most, she understood how health care policy was beholden to political caprice and bureaucratic interference. Echoing Chief Swimmer, the activist community had then argued the government's eyes "needed to be opened" to the clear link between ill health and IHS's arbitrary management of care. Although the Constitution Act (1982) reaffirmed existing treaty and Aboriginal rights, the interpretation of the treaty right to health care continues to be contested. As Favel-King told the Royal Commission, with the Aboriginal right to self-government and treaty rights clearly defined, together with adequate resources, First Nations could plan housing, sanitation, training, and community development to deal with ill health, family violence, and addictions, "in fact, all issues with a direct impact on the health status of First Nations people."[13] Until health policy was built on those acknowledged rights, she argued, health care remained vulnerable to the shifting political winds.[14]

It is only in the new century that "separate beds" has come to connote community management and control of some health care programs. With a fairly clear understanding of the health transfer's limitations, communities have embraced the opportunity for self-empowerment by managing nursing services, community health and addictions programs, prenatal nutrition, and mental health care.[15] In 2004, as part of the transfer process, the Touchwood and File Hills Qu'Appelle Tribal Councils took control of the sixty-eight-year-old Fort Qu'Appelle Indian Hospital and replaced it with the All Nations Healing Hospital, across the railroad tracks on Treaty Four reserve lands. The facility provides acute health care, community health programs, Indigenous ceremonies, and clinical counselling services in a holistic approach to health care to the whole community. The 1988 hunger strike at the Sioux Lookout Indian Hospital ended after the federal government agreed to permit the community to determine their own health needs and assert some control of the health delivery system.[16] After years of planning, the four parties – First Nations, federal, provincial, and municipal governments – agreed to amalgamate the resources of the Indian and provincial hospitals. In 2010 the sixty-bed Sioux Lookout Meno Ya Win Health Centre opened for First Nations and non-Aboriginal residents, offering acute and long-term care, mental health and addiction services, as well as community-based and Indigenous healing services.[17] Unlike earlier attempts, this "integration" has been accomplished, at least to some extent, on First Nations' terms. The inclusion of Indigenous healing with biomedical services reminds us of fundamentally different, though not incompatible, definitions of health and healing.

The history of Indian hospitals and health care policy since the 1920s reveals the limits of Canada's liberal democracy. Colonized in the interests of nineteenth-century state formation, Aboriginal people were marginalized in the construction of the welfare state. Lines of segregation and isolation, tended by the power of the state, and rationalized in the language of medical humanitarianism, did not negate Canada's liberal democratic values. In fact they were integral to the formation of national health as normal white citizenship. More than a half-century of contradictory and arbitrary policies that served the interests of the non-Aboriginal population left a destructive legacy in Aboriginal communities and beyond. Health disparities – constructed not found – have come to be seen as normal or inevitable. It is a measure of the strength and resolve of Aboriginal communities that the federal government finally was compelled to acknowledge its commitments to health care. It is with similar resolve that communities embark on, or more properly return to, the management of their health care. Whether the health transfer truly represents a new departure that will translate into better health or if the rhetoric of self-government masks yet another attempt to offload responsibility for health care remains an open question.

Notes

Introduction

1 *Edmonton Journal*, 27 August 1946.
2 The hospital began admitting patients in January 1946, before the official opening.
3 "Indian hospital" will be used throughout to reflect historical usage and the specific character of the institutions. In reference to communities, I use the national names preferred by contemporary First Nations, and where that is neither intended nor possible, I use First Nations or Aboriginal (Inuit and First Nations, or "status Indians" recognized by the state as coming under the authority of the Indian Act). The Metis are now defined as Aboriginal by the Constitution Act (1982), but in the period under study the federal government did not recognize any responsibility for their health care. Metis people's encounters with provincial hospitals would likely have been marked by the same community prejudices encountered by First Nations people, and they received no IHS support. That history remains to be written and is not treated here.
4 Mary-Ellen Kelm, *Colonizing Bodies: Aboriginal Health and Healing in British Columbia, 1900–1950* (Vancouver: University of British Columbia Press, 1998); Maureen Lux, *Medicine That Walks: Disease, Medicine and Canadian Plains Native People, 1880–1940* (Toronto: University of Toronto Press, 2001).
5 Amna Khalid and Ryan Johnson, "Introduction," in *Public Health in the British Empire: Intermediaries, Subordinates, and the Practice of Public Health, 1850–1960*, ed. Ryan Johnson and Amna Khalid (New York: Routledge, 2012), 20.
6 Waltraud Ernst, "Beyond East and West: From the History of Colonial Medicine to a Social History of Medicine(s) in South Asia," *Social History of Medicine* 20 (December 2007): 509–10, 513.

7 James Waldram, D. Ann Herring, and T. Kue Young, *Aboriginal Health in Canada: Historical, Cultural, and Epidemiological Perspectives*, 2nd ed. (Toronto: University of Toronto Press, 2006), 142.
8 For an overview of Aboriginal medical traditions see ibid., chapter 5; for the prairies, Lux, *Medicine That Walks*, chapter 2.
9 The responsibility for health care is not clearly defined in the Constitution Act (1982), where "Indians and Lands reserved for Indians" are the exclusive legislative authority of the federal government, while health and social services are provincial responsibilities. The Indian Act (1876) grants the Governor-in-Council the authority to make regulations to prevent, mitigate, and control the spread of diseases; to provide medical treatment and health services for Indians; to provide compulsory hospitalization and treatment for infectious diseases among Indians. Indian Act (R.S., c I-6, s 73).
10 Minister Brooke Claxton, Special Joint Committee of the Senate and the House of Commons Appointed to Examine and Consider the Indian Act, *Minutes of Proceedings and Evidence* No. 3 (6 June 1946), 65.
11 John L. Tobias, "Protection, Civilization, Assimilation: An Outline History of Canada's Indian Policy," *Western Canadian Journal of Anthropology* 6, no. 2 (1976): 13–30.
12 Ian McKay, "The Liberal Order Framework: A Prospectus for a Reconnaissance of Canadian History," *Canadian Historical Review* 81, no. 4 (December 2000): 625.
13 Uday S. Mehta, "Liberal Strategies of Exclusion," in *Tensions of Empire: Colonial Cultures in a Bourgeois World*, ed. Frederick Cooper and Ann Laura Stoler (Berkeley: University of California Press, 1997), 61.
14 Ian McKay, "Canada as a Long Liberal Revolution," in *Debating the Canadian Liberal Revolution*, ed. Jean-Francois Constant and Michel Ducharme (Toronto: University of Toronto Press, 2009), 351.
15 Quoted in Carolyn Strange and Alison Bashford, eds, *Isolation: Places and Practices of Exclusion* (London: Routledge, 2003), 5.
16 Adele Perry, "Women, Racialized People, and the Making of the Liberal Order in Northern North America," in *Debating the Canadian Liberal Revolution*, ed. Jean-Francois Constant and Michel Ducharme (Toronto: University of Toronto Press, 2009), 285.
17 Ian McKay, "Canada as a Long Liberal Revolution," 397.
18 McKay, "The Liberal Order Framework," 637.
19 See especially P.H. Bryce, *The Story of a National Crime: Being an Appeal for Justice to the Indians of Canada* (Ottawa: James Hope and Sons, 1922); John Milloy, *A National Crime: The Canadian Government and the Residential*

School System, 1879–1986 (Winnipeg: University of Manitoba Press, 1999); J.R. Miller, *Shingwauk's Vision* (Toronto: University of Toronto Press, 1996).

20 P.H. Bryce, *Report on the Indian Schools of Manitoba and the North-West Territories* (Ottawa: Government Printing Bureau, 1907), 18, RG10 (Records of the Department of Indian Affairs), v 4037, file 317,021, Library and Archives Canada (LAC); Bryce found that of the 1,537 school children, 35 per cent were either sick or dead, while 69 per cent of the children who had attended File Hills school in Saskatchewan were dead.

21 Bryce to Pedley, 5 Nov 1909, RG10 v 3957, file 140,754–1, LAC.

22 Brian Titley, *A Narrow Vision: Duncan Campbell Scott and the Administration of Indian Affairs in Canada* (Vancouver: University of British Columbia Press, 1986), 88.

23 Alison Bashford and Carolyn Strange, "Isolation and Exclusion in the Modern World," in Strange and Bashford, *Isolation*; Renisa Mawani, "Legal Geographies of Aboriginal Segregation in British Columbia," in Strange and Bashford, *Isolation*; Norbert Finzsch and Robert Jütte, eds, *Institutions of Confinement: Hospitals, Asylums, and Prisons in Western Europe and North America, 1500–1950* (Cambridge: Cambridge University Press, 1996); Michel Foucault, *Discipline and Punish: The Birth of the Prison*, trans. A. Sheridan, 2nd ed. (New York: Vintage, 1995); *Madness and Civilization: A History of Insanity in the Age of Reason* (New York: Vintage, 1984).

24 Colin Jones and Roy Porter, eds, "Introduction" to *Reassessing Foucault: Power, Medicine and the Body* (London: Routledge, 1994), 1–2.

25 David Arnold, "Medicine and Colonialism," in *Companion Encyclopedia of the History of Medicine*, ed. W.F. Bynum and Roy Porter (London: Routledge, 1993), 2:1411; see also David Arnold, ed., *Imperial Medicine and Indigenous Societies* (Manchester: Manchester University Press, 1988); Roy MacLeod and Milton Lewis, eds, *Disease, Medicine, and Empire* (London: Routledge, 1988); Randall M. Packard, *White Plague, Black Labor: Tuberculosis and the Political Economy of Health and Disease in South Africa* (Berkeley: University of California Press, 1989); Megan Vaughan, *Curing Their Ills: Colonial Power and African Illness* (Palo Alto, CA: Stanford University Press, 1991).

26 Strange and Bashford, *Isolation*, 3.

27 Robert Menzies and Ted Palys, "Turbulent Spirits: Aboriginal Patients in the British Columbia Psychiatric System, 1879–1950," in *Mental Health and Canadian Society: Historical Perspectives*, ed. James E. Moran and David Wright (Montreal and Kingston: McGill-Queen's University Press, 2006), 166.

28 Tuberculosis today is understood as an infectious disease caused by *Mycobacterium tuberculosis*. Spread through droplet infection, it most

commonly affects the lungs but can involve almost any organ of the body. Symptoms include fatigue, lethargy, and weight loss, progressing to coughing of sputum and blood and shortness of breath. It has a variable incubation period, and factors such as the quality of nutrition and crowding determine whether the disease develops. William D. Johnston, "Tuberculosis," in Kenneth Kiple, ed., *The Cambridge World History of Human Diseases* (Cambridge: Cambridge University Press, 1993), 1059–68.

29 Mary-Ellen Kelm, "Diagnosing the Discursive Indian: Medicine, Gender, and the 'Dying Race,'" *Ethnohistory* 52, no. 2 (2005): 373, 378.

30 Stewart to Premier Bracken, 14 November 1934, RG29 (Department of National Health and Welfare), v 1225, file 311-T7-16, LAC; quoted in "House of Commons Discusses Estimates for Indian Affairs Branch," *Bulletin of the Canadian Tuberculosis Association* 15, no. 4 (June 1937): 4; D.A. Stewart, *The Social Ramifications of Tuberculosis* (Winnipeg: Veterans Press, n.d.), 6, RG10–30-A-1, box 10, Archives of Ontario.

31 Warwick Anderson, *The Cultivation of Whiteness: Science, Health and Racial Destiny in Australia* (New York: Basic Books, 2003), 97.

32 The causes for tuberculosis decline in the Western world are not clear, but improvements in personal hygiene, increased prosperity, and improved sanitation, housing, and workplaces all had an impact; for Britain see Linda Bryder, *Below the Magic Mountain* (Oxford: Clarendon Press, 1988), 2; F.B. Smith, *The Retreat of Tuberculosis, 1850–1950* (London: Croom Helm, 1988), 1; Thomas McKeown, *The Modern Rise of Population* (London: Edward Arnold, 1976), 92; for the United States see Rene and Jean Dubos, *The White Plague: Tuberculosis, Man and Society* (Boston: Little, Brown, 1952), 185. G.J. Wherrett, the executive secretary of the CTA, wrote the CTA's celebratory history, *The Miracle of the Empty Beds: A History of Tuberculosis in Canada* (Toronto: University of Toronto Press, 1977).

33 Foucault, *Discipline and Punish*, 82.

34 Strange and Bashford, *Isolation*, 2; Strange and Bashford, "Cultures of Confinement," in Strange and Bashford, *Isolation*, 135.

35 G.D. Stanley, "Early Days at the Muskoka San," *Calgary Historical Bulletin* 18 (May 1953): 18–19.

36 *Katherine Ott, Fevered Lives: Tuberculosis in American Culture since 1870* (Cambridge: Harvard University Press, 1996), 1.

37 Quoted in C. Stuart Houston, *R.G. Ferguson: Crusader against Tuberculosis* (Toronto: Dundurn Press, 1991), 51.

38 Kelm, *Colonizing Bodies*, 122; Lux, *Medicine That Walks*, 197, 215; Houston, *R.G. Ferguson*, 92.

39 Bryder, *Below the Magic Mountain*; Smith, *Retreat of Tuberculosis*; Sheila Rothman, *Living in the Shadow of Death: Tuberculosis and the Social Experience of Illness in American History* (New York: Basic Books, 1994); Barbara Bates, *Bargaining for Life: A Social History of Tuberculosis, 1876–1938* (Philadelphia: University of Pennsylvania Press, 1992); Georgina Feldberg, *Disease and Class: Tuberculosis and the Shaping of Modern North American Society* (New Brunswick, NJ: Rutgers University Press, 1995); Katherine McCuaig, *The Weariness, the Fever, and the Fret: The Campaign against Tuberculosis in Canada, 1900–1950* (Montreal and Kingston: McGill-Queen's University Press, 1999); Amy Fairchild and Gerald Oppenheimer, "Public Health Nihilism vs Pragmatism: History, Politics and the Control of Tuberculosis," *American Journal of Public Health* 88, no. 7 (1998): 1105–17.

40 Smith, *Retreat of Tuberculosis*, 244–5.

41 Strange and Bashford, "Cultures of Confinement," in Strange and Bashford, *Isolation*, 135.

42 A.L. Paine and Earl Hershfield, "Tuberculosis: Past, Present and Future," *Canadian Family Physician* 25 (1979): 55–9.

43 Wherrett, *Miracle of the Empty Beds*, 41.

44 Dr Wherrett, "Back to Work after a Bout of Tuberculosis," *Canada at Work* (broadcast N-537, 5 December 1954), 3, MG28, I75, Canadian Tuberculosis Association, v 21, file 10, LAC.

45 Ibid., 4.

46 Jordan Goodman, Anthony McElligott, and Lara Marks, eds, *Useful Bodies: Humans in the Service of Medical Science in the Twentieth Century* (Baltimore: Johns Hopkins University Press, 2003), 12.

47 Donna Dryden, Elva Taylor, Rona Beer, Ron Bergman, and Margaret Cogill, *The Camsell Mosaic: The Charles Camsell Hospital, 1945–1985* (Edmonton: Charles Camsell History Committee, 1985), 7, 98–100.

48 On these transformations in Canada see, for example, David Gagan and Rosemary Gagan, *For Patients of Moderate Means: A Social History of the Voluntary Public General Hospital in Canada, 1890–1950* (Montreal and Kingston: McGill-Queen's University Press, 2002); for the United States, see Charles Rosenberg, *The Care of Strangers: The Rise of America's Hospital System* (New York: Basic Books, 1987); David Rosner, *A Once Charitable Enterprise: Hospitals and Health Care in Brooklyn and New York, 1885–1915* (New York: Cambridge University Press, 1982).

49 James Wishart, "Class Difference and the Reformation of Ontario Public Hospitals, 1900–1935," *Labour/Le Travail* 48 (2001): 27–61; Mark Cortiula, "Social Class and Health Care in a Community Institution: The Case of Hamilton City Hospital," *Canadian Bulletin of Medical History* 6 (1989):

133–45; Gagan and Gagan, *For Patients of Moderate Means*, 39–40; for an American example see Vanessa Northington Gamble, *Making a Place for Ourselves: The Black Hospital Movement, 1920–1945* (New York: Oxford University Press, 1995).

50 The impact of this investment is at times elided by histories of postwar health policy that tend to focus on the failures of the federal Liberal government to make good on its wartime promises of health insurance and a comprehensive program of social security. Alvin Finkel, "Paradise Postponed: A Re-examination of the Green Book Proposals of 1945," *Journal of the Canadian Historical Association* 4 (1993): 120–42; Alvin Finkel, *Our Lives: Canada after 1945* (Toronto: James Lorimer, 1997), 18–20; P.E. Bryden, "The Liberal Party and the Achievement of National Medicare," *Canadian Bulletin of Medical History* 26, no. 2 (2009): 315–32.

51 Malcolm Taylor, "The Canadian Health Care System: After Medicare," in *Health and Canadian Society: Sociological Perspectives*, 2nd ed., ed. David Coburn, Carl D'Arcy, George Torrance, and Peter New (Toronto: Fitzhenry and Whiteside, 1987), 74.

52 "Fort Alexander Reserve," 1 July 1957, RG29, v 2913, file 851-A501 pt. 3, LAC.

53 B.L. Van Der Berg, MD, to Wood, 9 August 1958; "Investigation Drinking Water Supplies, Fort Alexander Reserve," July 1958, RG29, v 2931, file 851-X200, pt. 3, LAC.

54 W.J. Wood, IHS, to M.R. Elliot, Public Health, Winnipeg, 19 September 1958, RG29, v 2931, file 851-X200, pt. 3, LAC.

55 M.V. Peever, Field Nurse, to Moore, 10 October 1958, RG29, v 2931, file 851-X200, pt. 3, LAC.

56 "Investigation Drinking Water Supplies, Fort Alexander Reserve," July 1958, RG29, v 2931, file 851-X200, pt. 3, LAC.

57 "Fort Alexander Reserve," 1 July 1957, RG29, v 2913, file 851-A501 pt. 3, LAC.

58 Ibid.

59 While one monthly adult ration provided 2,500 calories, Indian Affairs used a diminishing scale so that four adult rations provided only slightly more than twice as much food as a single ration. Rations consisted of flour, rolled oats, baking powder, sugar, lard, beans, rice or potatoes, cheese, meat or fish, salt, and matches. "Fort Alexander Reserve," 1 July 1957, RG29, v 2913, file 851-A501 pt. 3, LAC.

60 Ian Mosby, "Administering Colonial Science: Nutrition Research and Human Biomedical Experimentation in Aboriginal Communities and Residential Schools, 1942–1952," *Histoire Sociale/Social History* 46, no. 91 (May 2013): 152.

61 "Fort Alexander Reserve," 1 July 1957, RG29, v 2913, file 851-A501 pt. 3, LAC.

62 "Fort Alexander Indian Hospital," n.d. (visited 25 February 1960) RG29, v 2931, file 851–1-X200, pt. 4, LAC.

63 See for instance Natalia Ilyniak, "Mercury Poisoning in Grassy Narrows: Environmental Injustice, Colonialism, and Capitalist Expansion in Canada," *McGill Sociological Review* 4 (February 2014): 43–66.

64 For the sake of consistency I will use Indian Health Service (IHS) to refer to the bureaucracy responsible for health care. Known as Indian Health Service when it was housed in the Department of Indian Affairs, it retained the name when health services were transferred to National Health and Welfare in 1945. Reflecting an increasing interest in the north, the name was changed to the Indian and Northern Health Service (INHS) in 1955. In 1962 another government reorganization saw the elimination of INHS and the creation of the Medical Services Branch (MSB), an amalgamation of seven former independent services – Civil Aviation, Civil Service Health, Northern Health, Quarantine, Immigration, Sick Mariners, and the largest, Indian Health Service; in 2000 it was renamed the First Nations and Inuit Health Branch (FNIHB).

65 For a time in the 1950s, Inuit patients were kept at the federal government's Parc Savard Immigration Hospital in Quebec City.

66 P.E. Moore, "No Longer Captain: A History of Tuberculosis and Its Control amongst Canadian Indians," *Canadian Medical Association Journal* 84 (May 1961): 1012–16; Wherrett, *Miracle of the Empty Beds*; former staff at the largest hospital collected reminiscences from patients and staff (Dryden et al., *Camsell Mosaic*). It was a premature celebration. Recent scholarship judges the history of tuberculosis as "a story of medical failure." Alimuddin Zumla and Matthew Gundy, "Epilogue: Politics, Science, and the 'New' Tuberculosis," in *The Return of the White Plague: Global Poverty and the "New" Tuberculosis*, ed. Matthew Gundy and Alimuddin Zumla (London: Verso, 2003), 237.

67 Myra Rutherdale, "Nursing in the North and Writing for the South: The Work and Travels of Amy Wilson," and Laurie Meijer Drees, "Training Aboriginal Nurses: The Indian Health Services in Northwestern Canada," in *Caregiving on the Periphery: Historical Perspectives on Nursing and Midwifery in Canada*, ed. Myra Rutherdale (Montreal and Kingston: McGill-Queen's University Press, 2010); Kathryn McPherson, "Nursing and Colonization: The Work of Indian Health Service Nurses in Manitoba, 1945–1970," in *Women, Health, and Nation: Canada and the United States since 1945*, ed. Georgina Feldberg, Molly Ladd Taylor, Alison Li, and Kathryn McPherson (Montreal and Kingston: McGill-Queen's University Press, 2003); by 1960 IHS operated thirty clinics, thirty-seven nursing stations, and eighty-three health centres.

68 T. Kue Young, *Health Care and Cultural Change: The Indian Experience in the Central Subarctic* (Toronto: University of Toronto Press, 1988).

69 Pat Sandiford Grygier, *A Long Way from Home: The Tuberculosis Epidemic among the Inuit* (Montreal and Kingston: McGill-Queen's University Press, 1994); Laurie Meijer Drees, "The Nanaimo and Charles Camsell Indian Hospitals: First Nations' Narratives of Health Care, 1945 to 1965," *Histoire Sociale/Social History* 43, no. 85 (2010): 165–91; these narratives are reprinted in Meijer Drees's *Healing Histories: Stories from Canada's Indian Hospitals* (Edmonton: University of Alberta Press, 2013).

70 Adele Perry develops the notion in relation to nineteenth-century state formation that treats the project of marginalizing Aboriginal people and the building of a white settler society as separate and discrete processes; the fiction's power rests on the assumption that settler domination was inevitable. *On the Edge of Empire: Gender, Race and the Making of British Columbia, 1849–1871* (Toronto: University of Toronto Press, 2001), 19.

Chapter One

1 See especially P.H. Bryce, *The Story of a National Crime: Being an Appeal for Justice to the Indians of Canada* (Ottawa: James Hope and Sons, 1922); John Milloy, *A National Crime: The Canadian Government and the Residential School System, 1879–1986* (Winnipeg: University of Manitoba Press, 1999); J.R. Miller, *Shingwauk's Vision* (Toronto: University of Toronto Press, 1996).

2 D.C. Scott, "Notes on Dr. Bryce's Report with Suggestions for Further Action," 7 March 1910, RG10 v 3957, file 140754-1, LAC.

3 In his *The Story of a National Crime: Being an Appeal for Justice to the Indians of Canada* Bryce blamed Scott for undermining his efforts to improve the schools, and for refusing to include responsibility for Aboriginal health in the newly created federal Department of Health in 1919. He reserved his most bitter attacks for the administration that failed to appoint him the health department's first deputy minister.

4 James Wishart, "Class Difference and the Reformation of Ontario Public Hospitals, 1900–1935," *Labour/Le Travail* 48 (2001): 27–61; Mark Cortiula, "Social Class and Health Care in a Community Institution: The Case of Hamilton City Hospital," *Canadian Bulletin of Medical History* 6 (1989): 133–45; for an American example see Vanessa Northington Gamble, *Making a Place for Ourselves: The Black Hospital Movement, 1920–1945* (New York: Oxford University Press, 1995); on hospital transformation see David Gagan and Rosemary Gagan, *For Patients of Moderate Means: A Social History of the Voluntary Public General Hospital in Canada, 1890–1950*

(Montreal and Kingston: McGill-Queen's University Press, 2002); for the United States see Charles Rosenberg, *The Care of Strangers: The Rise of America's Hospital System* (New York: Basic Books, 1987); David Rosner, *A Once Charitable Enterprise: Hospitals and Health Care in Brooklyn and New York, 1885–1915* (New York: Cambridge University Press, 1982).

5 See Constance Backhouse, *Colour-Coded: A Legal History of Racism in Canada, 1900–1950* (Toronto: University of Toronto Press, 1999). Scientist and broadcaster David Suzuki recalls in his autobiography that in Prince Rupert, British Columbia, in the 1940s Aboriginal people were not allowed to stay in most hotels, were refused service in restaurants, and were forced to sit in designated sections of movie theatres. *The Autobiography* (Vancouver: Greystone Books, 2006), 14. George Manuel, noted activist and chief of the National Indian Brotherhood by 1970, recalled the segregated movie theatres in the Kamloops of his youth in *The Fourth World* (New York: Free Press, 1974), 101. Violet Clark from Ahousaht First Nation recalled for historian Laurie Meijer Drees an incident in the 1950s when she and other Aboriginal hospital employees and a white doctor were refused service in a Duncan, British Columbia, restaurant until they sat in the back at a table separate from their white dining companion. *Healing Histories* (Edmonton: University of Alberta Press, 2013), 185.

6 Gagan and Gagan, *For Patients of Moderate Means*, 166–7.

7 Andrew Lam, Esther Fung, et al., Chinese Christian Youth Conference Committee, 5 April 1946, to W.H. Hatfield, Director Division of TB Control; JB Peters to Deputy Provincial Health Officer, 3 September 1946, GR 129, box 2, file 5, British Columbia Archives (hereafter BCA).

8 Memorandum, Forget, Accountant, 26 February 1917, RG29 v 2728, file 811-2 part 1 LAC; Mary-Ellen Kelm, *Colonizing Bodies: Aboriginal Health and Healing in British Columbia, 1900–1950* (Vancouver: University of British Columbia Press, 1998), 136–7; E. Martin, BC Minister of Health, to J.W. Monteith, Minister of National Health, 25 October 1961: "At one time it was a practice in some hospitals in BC to maintain Indian wards to which Indian patients were assigned exclusively." GR679, box 5, file 10, BCA.

9 W.H. Carter to Thomas Murphy, 4 February 1933, RG 29, v 2775, file 822-1-X200, part 1; ibid., H. McGill to Dr Bissett, 24 March 1938, part 2, LAC; J.D. Adamson to J. McEachern, 15 July 1939, RG 29, v 2590, file 800-1-D297, part 1, LAC.

10 Ken Coates, *Best Left as Indians; Native-White Relations in the Yukon Territory, 1840–1973* (Montreal and Kingston: McGill-Queen's University Press, 1991), 95.

11 Stanton to Chairman, 27 March 1950, RG 22, v 878, file 41-5-9, LAC. Unlike most administrators, Stanton was made to justify his policy in order to receive the newly established National Health Grants.
12 G.J. Wherrett, "Tuberculosis in Canada," Royal Commission on Health Services (Ottawa: Queen's Printer, 1965), 62.
13 J. Barnes to Dr H.A. Proctor, IHS, 30 September 1948; Barnes and J.D. Heaslip, MD, to chairman and members, Calgary Hospitals Board, 12 January 1949, RG 29, v 2936, file 851-1-X400, part 1, LAC. Alberta introduced hospital insurance in July 1950, but the municipally administered plan covered less than 75 per cent of the population by 1953; by 1954 only 38 per cent of all hospital income came from the provincial government. Malcolm Taylor, *Health Insurance and Canadian Public Policy*, 2nd ed. (Montreal and Kingston: McGill-Queen's University Press, 1987), 169–70.
14 Barnes and J.D. Heaslip, MD, to chairman and members, Calgary Hospitals Board, 12 January 1949, RG 29, v 2936, file 851-1-X400, part 1, LAC.
15 Ibid., Moore to Barnes, 1 April 1949.
16 Ibid., Stone to Director IHS, 5 January 1950
17 Lindsay Granshaw, "The Hospital," in *Companion Encyclopedia of the History of Medicine*, ed. W.F. Bynam and Roy Porter (London: Routledge, 1993), 2:1193.
18 Maureen Lux, *Medicine That Walks: Disease, Medicine and Canadian Plains Native People, 1880–1940* (Toronto: University of Toronto Press, 2001), 200–1.
19 F.A. Corbett to Graham, 7 December 1920, RG10, v 4092, file 546898, LAC.
20 Quoted in Elizabeth Churchill, "Tsuu T'ina: A History of a First Nations Community, 1890–1940" (PhD diss., University of Calgary, 2000), 396.
21 Ibid., 393–4.
22 Quoted in ibid., 413.
23 McGill Papers, M742, box 4, file 36, "Correspondence, 1928–41," Glenbow Archives Institute (GAI).
24 Baker Memorial Sanatorium, 1917–1937, file 73.315/37, box 2, Public Archives of Alberta (PAA); *Calgary the Denver of Canada* (Calgary: Calgary Herald Print, 1895), 5.
25 Sarah Carter, *Aboriginal People and Colonizers of Western Canada* (Toronto: University of Toronto Press, 1999), 76.
26 Diamond Jenness, *The Sarcee Indians of Alberta* Bulletin no. 90 (Canada: National Museum of Canada, 1938).
27 R.F. Battle, Regional Supervisor to Director, Indian Affairs Branch, 8 December 1955, RG 29, v 2936, file 851-1-X400, part 1, LAC.
28 In the 1920s small nursing stations, called "hospitals," were built on the Stoney (Iyarhe Nakoda) and Peigan (Piikani) reserves near Calgary; in

1928 the Catholic Blood Hospital managed by the Grey Nuns was rebuilt on the southern edge of the reserve at the nearby village of Cardston, across the street from the local municipal hospital. It is not clear if band funds or the DIA paid for these institutions.

29 Canada, House of Commons (CHC), Sessional Papers, 1911, 187; the fate of the Blackfoot Hospital is treated in chapter 5.

30 G.H. Gooderham, "Twenty-five Years as an Indian Agent to the Blackfoot Band," January 1972, M3947, GAI; "The Hospital," M4738, box 1, file 3, GAI.

31 Sally Mae Weaver, "Health, Culture and Dilemma: A Study of the Non-Conservative Iroquois, Six Nations Reserve, Ontario" (PhD diss., University of Toronto, 1967), 146–7.

32 S.L. Macdonald to Secretary DIA, 31 July 1923, RG 29, v 2795, file 831-1-D353 part 1, LAC.

33 Ibid., Joseph Guy, OMI to DC Scott, 1 December 1924; S.L. Macdonald to D.C. Scott, 15 April 1926.

34 Right Rev George Exton Lloyd, Bishop Diocese of Saskatchewan, to DC Scott, 30 July 1926, RG 29, v 2795, file 831-1-D353 part 1, LAC.

35 Author interview with Andrew and Rosabel (Ryder) Gordon, Pasqua First Nation, 14 July 2000; Gordon's father, Andrew Gordon Sr led the delegation that included First World War veterans Abel Watech and Harry Ball; Petition 30 October 1923, RG10, v 4093, file 600,023 LAC.

36 Scott to Graham, 1 December 1925; Graham to Scott, 1 February 1926, RG10, v 4084, file 495,800 LAC.

37 H.W. Hill, "The Epidemiology of Tuberculosis amongst British Columbia Interior Indians," 31, MG28, Canadian Tuberculosis Association, I75, II (a) file 33, "Indians – BC," LAC; "Conference on Tuberculosis among Indians in Canada, Ottawa, 1937," 37, MG28, I75, file II (a), LAC.

38 Canada, House of Commons, *Annual Report of the Department of Indian Affairs* 1928, 7–8.

39 Kelm, *Colonizing Bodies*, 120.

40 "Conference on Tuberculosis among Indians in Canada, Ottawa, 23 June 1937," 1.

41 J.G. Wherrett, *The Miracle of the Empty Beds* (Toronto: University of Toronto Press, 1977), 109; Wherrett puts the meeting in 1925.

42 Obituary, "Ervin Lockwood Stone," *Canadian Medical Association Journal* 98 (2 March 1968): 473.

43 T. Kue Young, *Health Care and Cultural Change: The Indian Experience in the Central Subarctic* (Toronto: University of Toronto Press, 1988), 86.

44 E.L. Stone, "Canadian Indian Medical Services," *Canadian Medical Association Journal* (July 1935): 82–5.

45 McGill to Indian agents, 14 January 1937, RG 29, v 1225, file 311-T7–16, LAC.
46 Norquay to Stone, 28 September 1937, RG 29 v 2915, file 851-1-A671 part 1(a), LAC.
47 F.R. Conroy, LLB, Barrister and Solicitor North Battleford, 20 September 1937, to DIA, Ottawa, and Department of Public Health, Regina; Director of Indian Affairs to S.L. Macdonald, Indian Agent, 23 October 1937, RG 29, v 2795, file 831-1-D353 part 1, LAC; "Appeals in Vain to Get Hospital Care for Child," *Saskatoon Star Phoenix*, 24 September 1937.
48 The Prince Albert Sanatorium, opened in 1930, admitted its first Aboriginal patient in 1935. Mary was admitted along with three other school children in 1937; the following year Prince Albert took in fifty-six Aboriginal patients, half of them schoolchildren. Increasing Aboriginal admissions reflected the declining need for sanatorium beds by the non-Aboriginal population. Saskatchewan Lung Association Files, A638, file IX.73a, Saskatchewan Archives Board (hereafter SAB).
49 D.A. Stewart, "The Red Man and the White Plague" (1936), 4, Lung Association, A638 file VII.27, SAB.
50 D.A. Stewart, Sanatorium Board of Manitoba, to R.A. Wardle, 22 January 1934, A638 file VII.27, SAB.
51 E.L.M. Thorpe, *The Social Histories of Smallpox and Tuberculosis in Canada: Culture, Evolution and Disease* (Winnipeg: University of Manitoba Anthropology Papers No. 30, 1989), 98, 106. Thorpe, a nurse by training, worked in hospitals in Britain and in British colonies in the Middle East and Far East during the Second World War. She established a psychiatric hospital in Jamaica in the 1950s, and eventually arrived in Manitoba as a consultant to the Sanatorium Board's efforts to decommission its sanatoria in the 1960s. At age sixty-five she undertook graduate studies in anthropology and used her many personal connections to Sanatorium Board personnel to critically assess the supposed racial explanations for disease in Aboriginal communities.
52 Wherrett, *Miracle of the Empty Beds*, 62.
53 Donna Dryden et al., *The Camsell Mosaic* (Edmonton: Charles Camsell History Committee, 1985), 133; Bruce Norton, "Northern Manitoba Treaty Party, 1949," *Manitoba History* 39 (Spring 2000): 15–24.
54 Thorpe, *Social Histories of Smallpox and Tuberculosis in Canada*, 106.
55 This refers to Bruce Curtis's observations of the historical practice of census making in Canada. He argues that the census was not taken, it was made. Bruce Curtis, *The Politics of Population: State Formation, Statistics, and the Census of Canada, 1840–1875* (Toronto: University of Toronto Press, 2001), 34.
56 Stewart, "The Red Man and the White Plague," 4.

57 John D. O'Neil, "Aboriginal Health Policy for the Next Century" in *The Path to Healing: Report of the National Round Table on Aboriginal Health and Social Issues* (Ottawa: Royal Commission on Aboriginal Peoples, 1993), 34.
58 R.G. Ferguson, *Tuberculosis among the Indians of the Great Canadian Plains* (Reprint, London: Adlard and Son, 1928); R.G. Ferguson and A.B. Simes, "BCG Vaccination of Indian Infants in Saskatchewan," *Tubercle* 30, no. 1 (1949): 5–11.
59 Simes to Stone, 20 March 1934; Privy Council Minute, 6 August 1934, RG29, v 2819, file 831-1-X328, LAC.
60 See M.K. Lux, "Perfect Subjects: Race, Tuberculosis and the Qu'Appelle BCG Vaccine Trial," *Canadian Bulletin of Medical History* 15 (1998): 277–96. Of the vaccinated group, 39 of 306 children died in the first year, and 38 of 303 controls died within the first year. Ferguson and Simes, "BCG Vaccination," 5.
61 McGill to deputy minister, Mines and Resources, 28 April 1938, RG22, v 1207, file 675/3 part 1, LAC.
62 Crerar, erstwhile leader of the failed Progressive Party and an articulate voice for western and Manitoba interests, returned to Parliament in 1935 as a Liberal in Mackenzie King's cabinet as minister of Indian Affairs until 1936. When the department became a branch of Mines and Resources, he assumed the new portfolio until his appointment to the Senate in 1945, where he served until his ninetieth birthday in 1966. RG29, v 3391, file 811-2-Crerar, LAC.
63 Minister to Governor General in Council, 1 December 1936, RG29, v 3391, file 811-2-Crerar, LAC.
64 MacInnes to Waite, 2 February 1937, RG29, v 3391, file 811–2-Crerar, LAC.
65 Wherrett, *Miracle of the Empty Beds*, 110, 112–13.
66 "House of Commons Discusses Estimates for Indian Affairs Branch," quoted in *Bulletin of the Canadian Tuberculosis Association* 15, no. 4 (1937): 3–4.
67 Stewart to Premier Bracken, 14 November 1934, RG 29, v 1225, file 311-T7-16, LAC.
68 "Conference on Tuberculosis among Indians in Canada, Ottawa, 23 June 1937," 11, MG28, I75, II (a), file 36, LAC.
69 Ibid., 13, 57–8, 73, 89.
70 Memorandum, E.L. Stone to Director, 29 June 1937, MG28, I75, II (a), file 36, LAC.
71 "Conference on Tuberculosis," 14; "preventoria" were intended to prevent, not treat illness, and to provide a middle-class home life for children of the tubercular indigent. Cynthia Connolly, *Saving Sickly Children: The Tuberculosis Preventorium in American Life, 1909–1970* (New Brunswick, NJ: Rutgers University Press, 2008), 2.

72 Memorandum, E.L. Stone to Director, 29 June 1937, MG28, I75, II (a), file 36, LAC.
73 "Outline of Tuberculosis Control for the Indian Population of Canada, 1937," MG28, I75, II (a), file 31 LAC.
74 E.L. Ross and A.L. Paine, "A Tuberculosis Survey of Manitoba Indians," *Canadian Medical Association Journal* 4 (Aug 1939): 180–4.
75 McGill, Director Indian Affairs to Deputy Minister, Mines and Resources, 28 April 1938, RG22, v 1207, file 675/3 part 1, LAC.
76 The Sanatorium Board of Manitoba subsequently agreed to manage tuberculosis treatment for Indian Health Service in return for per diem payments from the federal government. RG29, v 2590, file 800-1-D297, part 1, LAC.
77 "Hospitals Developed for Canadian Indians," *New York Times*, 7 January 1940.
78 Sinnott to Crerar, 2 May 1940, RG29, v 3391, file 811-2-Crerar, LAC.
79 J.D. Adamson to McEachern, 15 July 1939, RG 29, v 2590, file 800-1-D297, part 1, LAC. Sectarian voluntary hospitals were particularly vulnerable to financial distress during the Depression. Unlike municipal or city hospitals they could not turn to taxpayers for increased grants; neither could they increase rates charged to paying patients while other hospitals kept rates unchanged. In order to stave off financial ruin in the 1930s, Edmonton General Hospital, also owned by the Grey Nuns, converted its pediatric and maternity wards to tuberculosis wards to take advantage of provincial funds for tuberculosis treatment for the indigent. Pauline Paul, "A History of the Edmonton General Hospital: 1895–1970" (PhD diss., University of Alberta, 1994), 378–9.
80 McGill, "Memorandum for the Deputy Minister," 15 September 1939, RG 29, v 2590, file 800-1-D297, part 1, LAC.
81 Northwood to P.E. Moore, 3 April 1940, RG 29, v 2590, file 800-1-D297, part 1, LAC.
82 William D. Johnston, "Tuberculosis," in *The Cambridge World History of Human Diseases*, ed. Kenneth Kiple (Cambridge: Cambridge University Press, 1993), 1065. Other forms of collapse therapy included thoracoplasty (the surgical removal of several ribs to collapse the lung) and phrenic nerve crush (to paralyse the diaphragm).
83 "Report of the Resident Physician of Dynevor Indian Hospital," 31 December 1940, RG 29, v 2590, file 800-1-D297, part 1, LAC.
84 "Report of the Dynevor Indian Hospital for the Year 1945." Of the remaining patients, 27 per cent were deemed well enough to work, 22 per cent were "at school," and 9 per cent were "at home." RG 29, v 2591, file 800-1-D297, part 2, LAC.

85 Katherine McCuaig, *The Weariness, the Fever, and the Fret: The Campaign against Tuberculosis in Canada, 1900–1950* (Montreal and Kingston: McGill-Queen's University Press, 1999), 71–2; Darlene Zdunich, "Tuberculosis and World War One Veterans" (MA thesis, University of Calgary, 1984), 102.
86 Report, 31 December 1940, RG 29, v 2590, file 800-1-D297, part 1, LAC.
87 Report, 1945, RG 29, v 2591, file 800-1-D297, part 2, LAC.
88 "Meeting of the Indian Advisory Committee, March 10, 1938," MG28, I75, II (a), file 31, "Indians," LAC.
89 "Coqualeetza" is the Sto:lo word for place of cleansing or purification. "The Coqualeetza Story, 1886–1956," RG29, v 2596, file 800-1-D528, part 1 LAC.
90 Ibid., 8.
91 Moore to deputy minister, 7 June 1950, RG 29, v 2596, file 800-1-D528, part 1, LAC.
92 Charlotte Gray, "Profile: Percy Moore," *Canadian Medical Association Journal* 126 (15 February 1982): 416.
93 Wherrett produced comparable statistics for the previous ten years. Advisory Committee for the Control and Prevention of Tuberculosis among the Indians, "Proceedings of Meeting, 30 and 31 May 1945," 9 MG28, 175, II(a), file 36, LAC.
94 Ibid., 21.
95 Ibid., 31.
96 Ibid., 15, 28–9.
97 Ibid., 22.
98 Ibid., 24–5.
99 Ibid., 25.
100 Ibid., 129.
101 Ibid., 12.
102 Ibid., 118.
103 Ibid., 96.
104 Wherrett to Moore, 28 August 1946, MG28, 175, II(a), file 32, LAC.
105 "Proceedings of Meeting," 54.
106 Ibid., 62.
107 G.J. Wherrett, "Arctic Survey 1: Survey of Health Conditions and Medical and Hospital Services in the North West Territories," *Canadian Journal of Economics and Political Science* 11, no. 1 (1945): 48–60.
108 "Proceedings of Meeting," 86.
109 Ibid., 176.
110 Ibid., 162, 165.
111 Ibid., 206.

112 Department of Indian Affairs, "Regulations for the Medical Services, 1934," 22a, http://scaa.sk.ca/ourlegacy/solr?query=ID%3A32158&start=0&rows=10&mode=view&pos=0&page=1 (accessed February 2012).
113 "Proceedings of Meeting," 205.
114 Ibid., 210.
115 Moore to Curran, legal advisor, 14 May 1946, RG10 v 6811, file 470-2-3, part 11, LAC.

Chapter Two

1 Minister Brooke Claxton, Special Joint Committee of the Senate and the House of Commons Appointed to Examine and Consider the Indian Act, *Minutes of Proceedings and Evidence No. 3* (6 June 1946), 65.
2 G.J. Wherrett, *The Miracle of the Empty Beds: A History of Tuberculosis in Canada* (Toronto: University of Toronto Press, 1977).
3 John Tobias, "Protection, Civilization, Assimilation: An Outline History of Canada's Indian Policy," in *The Prairie West: Historical Readings*, 2nd ed., ed. R. Douglas Francis and Howard Palmer (Edmonton: University of Alberta Press, 1992), 219.
4 Sally Weaver, *Making Canadian Indian Policy: The Hidden Agenda, 1968–1970* (Toronto: University of Toronto Press, 1981), 46.
5 John Dent, "New Deal for Indians Is Planned by MP," *Saturday Night*, 30 March 1946.
6 See RG10, v 6811, file 470-3-6, part 1, LAC.
7 Hugh Shewell, *Enough to Keep Them Alive: Indian Welfare in Canada, 1873–1965* (Toronto: University of Toronto Press, 2004), 206.
8 Tobias, "Protection, Civilization, Assimilation," 220; Noel Dyck, *What Is the Indian "Problem": Tutelage and Resistance in Canadian Indian Administration* (St John's, NL: Institute of Social and Economic Research, 1991), 105.
9 Alvin Finkel, "Paradise Postponed: A Re-examination of the Green Book Proposals of 1945," *Journal of the Canadian Historical Association* 4, no. 1 (1993): 120–42.
10 Claxton, *Minutes of Proceedings*, 65.
11 K.S. Coates and W.R. Morrison, *The Alaska Highway in World War II: The U.S. Army of Occupation in Canada's Northwest* (Toronto: University of Toronto Press, 1992); Shelagh D. Grant, *Sovereignty or Security? Government Policy in the Canadian North, 1936–1950* (Vancouver: UBC Press, 1988), 123.
12 Donna Dryden, Elva Taylor, Rona Beer, Ron Bergman, and Margaret Cogill, *The Camsell Mosaic: The Charles Camsell Hospital, 1945–1985* (Edmonton: Charles Camsell History Committee, 1985), 8–9.

13 Mayor Fry to MacKenzie, 4 October 1945; Petition to Prime Minister, 13 October 1945, RG29, v 2592, file 800-1-D479, part 1, LAC.
14 H. Darling, RCMP 'K' Division, 26 November 1945, RG29, v 2592, file 800-1-D479, part 1, LAC.
15 J. Allison Glen to Mayor, 24 October 1945, RG29, v 2592, file 800-1-D479, part 1, LAC.
16 "Statement by the Hon Brooke Claxton" (n.d., likely November 1945) RG29, v 2592, file 800-1-D479, part 1, LAC.
17 Moore to deputy minister, 17 July 1946, RG 29, vol. 2592, file 800-1-D479, part 1, LAC.
18 Charles Camsell, *Son of the North* (Toronto: Ryerson, 1954).
19 Grant Dexter, *Dr. Charles Camsell* (Winnipeg: Winnipeg Free Press, 1958), 5.
20 Camsell, *Son of the North*, 44.
21 Dryden et al., *Camsell Mosaic*, xv.
22 Bill Waiser, "Camsell, Charles," in *Oxford Companion to Canadian History*, ed. Gerald Hallowell (Toronto: Oxford University Press, 2004), 99.
23 Mary Jane Logan McCallum, "Labour, Modernity and the Canadian State: A History of Aboriginal Women and Work in the Mid-Twentieth Century" (PhD diss., University of Manitoba, 2008), 85.
24 Grant, *Sovereignty or Security?* 317n10.
25 Dryden et al., *Camsell Mosaic*, xvi.
26 Stone to medical director, 12 June 1946, RG29, v 2592, file 800-1-D479, part 1, LAC.
27 Stone to Moore, 2 March 1946, RG29, v 2592, file 800-1-D479, part 1, LAC.
28 B.F. Wilson to H.E. Horne, business manager, 30 April 1954, RG29, v 2797, file 831-1-D479, part 4, LAC.
29 Moore to Falconer, 27 February 1950, RG29, v 2797, file 831-1-D479, part 2, LAC.
30 Moore, "Kitchen Floor CCIH," 23 January 1949; Moore to deputy minister, 6 February 1950, RG29, v 2797, file 831-1-D479, part 2, LAC.
31 Stone to Moore, 9 May 1946, RG29 v. 2796 file 831-1-D479, part 1; v 2797, file 831-1-D479, part 4, LAC.
32 Rutledge to McGivern, 11 April 1946, RG29, v 2769, file 822-1-D479, LAC.
33 Dryden et al., *Camsell Mosaic*, 15
34 Stone to Moore, 2 March 1946, RG29, v 2592, file 800-1-D479, part 1, LAC.
35 Dryden et al., *Camsell Mosaic*, 22; the forms and extent of patient discipline will be examined in a subsequent chapter.
36 See various letters, February and March 1946, RG29, v 2592, file 800-1-D479, part 1, LAC; administrative assistant Pat Blanchfield recalled that it was a "regular occurrence for him to write a blistering letter of

resignation" which she filed, rather than mailed, apparently much to Meltzer's relief. Dryden et al., *Camsell Mosaic,* 17.

37 Meltzer to Moore, 8 February 1947, RG29 v 2796 file 831-1-D479, part 1, LAC.
38 Meltzer to Moore, 28 March 1947, RG29 v 2796 file 831-1-D479, part 1, LAC.
39 Stone to Moore, 27 November 1946, RG29, v 2592, file 800-1-D479, part 1, LAC.
40 Moore to Meltzer, 3 October 1946, RG29, v 2592, file 800-1-D479, part 1, LAC.
41 Meltzer to Moore, 16 January 1947; Meltzer to Moore, 8 February 1947, RG29, v 2796 file 831-1-D479, part 1, LAC.
42 Deputy Minister National Health Cameron to the Minister, 4 February 1950, v 2769, file 822-1-D479, part 1, LAC.
43 H.A. Proctor to personnel division, 19 July 1949, RG29, v 3405, file 823-1-D579, LAC.
44 Indian Association of Alberta, Minutes of Annual Meeting, 24–5 June 1949, RG29, v 2959, file 851-3-Indian Association of Alberta, part 1, LAC.
45 Falconer to the Director, 10 March 1958, RG29, v 2959, file 851-3-Indian Association of Alberta, part 1, LAC.
46 Meltzer to Moore, 15 February 1954, RG29, v 2769, file 822-1-D479, part 2, LAC.
47 Charles Camsell Hospital records, Accession 73.315, box 2, file 33, Central Alberta (Baker) Sanatorium, Public Archives of Alberta (PAA).
48 Falconer to Director, 10 December 1957, RG29, v 2876 file 851-1-17, part 1, LAC.
49 "Admission Register, December 1956 to July 1958, Camsell Hospital." Despite the dates on the inside cover, the Admission Register recorded personal information and diagnoses only from January 1957 to February 1958; after that date no diagnoses are given and the recording of names is desultory, despite exhortations in the margins to "Please fill in this page!" The Register included diagnoses for 1,539 patients admitted in thirteen months, 204 for some form of tuberculosis and 1,335 for all other causes. Of the 951 children admitted, 92 were newborns, RG29, v 3635, LAC.
50 Falconer to Moore, 10 December 1957, RG29 v 2876, file 851-1-17, part 1, LAC.
51 Falconer to Moore, 18 December 1957, RG29 v 2876, file 851-1-17, part 1, LAC.
52 Matas to Falconer, 31 January 1958, RG29 v 2876, file 851-1-17, part 1, LAC.
53 Falconer to Moore, 18 December 1957, RG29 v 2876, file 851-1-17, part 1, LAC.
54 Quoted in Laurie Meijer Drees, "Indian Hospitals and Aboriginal Nurses: Canada and Alaska," *Canadian Bulletin of Medical History* 27, no. 1 (2010): 153.
55 Falconer to Moore, 28 January 1954; J.D. Blake to Moore, 5 May 1955, RG29 v 2926, file 851-1-D479, part 1, LAC.

56 Falconer to Moore, 18 December 1957, RG29 v 2876, file 851-1-17, part 1, LAC.
57 Moore to Regional Superintendent, Foothills, 15 July 1957; Moore to Regional Superintendent, Foothills, 20 January 1958, RG29 v 2876, file 851-1-17, part 1, LAC.
58 Moore to Regional Superintendent, Foothills, 29 November 1957, RG29 v 2876, file 851-1-17, part 1, LAC.
59 Moore to Regional Superintendent, Foothills, 20 January 1958, RG29 v 2876, file 851-1-17, part 1, LAC. For example, at this time Calgary hospitals agreed to charge IHS a per diem rate of $12.75, R.F. Battle, Regional Supervisor to Director, Indian Affairs Branch, 8 December 1955, RG 29, v 2936, file 851-1-X400, part 1, LAC.
60 Moore to Regional Superintendent, Foothills, 29 November 1957, RG29 v 2876, file 851-1-17, part 1, LAC.
61 Moore to Meltzer and Stone, 14 March 1946, RG29 v 2592, file 800-1-D479, part 1, LAC.
62 The extensive collection, consisting of hundreds of graphic and gruesome images, carefully cross-indexed by disease and patient name, was deposited at Library and Archives Canada only in 2003 by the hospital's historical society (RG29, R227-240-4-E, files 3726-32, LAC); the tuberculosis specimens were eventually destroyed (Dryden et al., *Camsell Mosaic*, 20).
63 Moore, "Memorandum to all Regional and Zone Superintendents," 11 July 1956, RG29, v 2620, file 800-2-1, LAC.
64 David Woods, "The Canadian Council on Hospital Accreditation in Canada," *Canadian Medical Association Journal* 110 (6 April 1974): 851.
65 Quoted in ibid., 852.
66 D.R. Campbell to Regional Superintendent, 5 October 1956, RG29, v 2620, file 800-2-1, LAC.
67 IHS labour problems are examined in detail in the next chapter.
68 Dr Blake to the Director, 7 November 1955, RG29, v 2620, file 800-2-1, LAC.
69 Six years later when little had changed, the Council deferred accreditation status for the hospital "pending further consideration of the hazard which exists in the physical plant." Canadian Council on Hospital Accreditation, 27 September 1963, RG29 v 2620, file 800-2-D479, part 1, LAC.
70 "List of Canadian Hospitals Approved for Advanced Graduate Training by the Royal College of Physicians and Surgeons," *Canadian Medical Association Journal* 78 (April 1958): 520.
71 Effective chemotherapy included the introduction of streptomycin in 1944, para-amino-salicylic acid (PAS) in 1946, and isoniazid (INH) in 1952. Katherine Ott, in *Fevered Lives: Tuberculosis in American Culture since 1870*

(Cambridge: Harvard University Press, 1996), states, "The surgical era of tuberculosis was brief. It began in the early 1900s … it ended in the 1940s with the slow rise to dominance of chemotherapy" (153); the Canadian experience was different.

72 Stone to Moore, 27 November 1946, RG29, v 2592, file 800-1-D479, part 1, LAC.

73 Dryden et al., *Camsell Mosaic*, 23.

74 Falconer to Moore, 28 January 1954, RG29 v 2926, file 851-1-D479, part 1, LAC.

75 Meltzer to Moore 15 February 1954, RG29 v 2769, file 822-1-D479, part 2, LAC.

76 Falconer to Moore, 28 November 1953, RG29, v 2797, file 831-1-D479, part 4, LAC.

77 Meltzer to Moore, 12 August 1954; Meltzer to Moore, 9 April 1957, RG29 v 2769, file 822-1-D479, part 2, LAC.

78 Indeed, Meltzer performed all chest surgeries and interpreted all chest X-rays (more than one thousand monthly) well into the 1960s; his surgical privileges were finally restricted in 1977 because he was seventy-one years old. B. Brett to L.M. Black, director general, 3 May 1977, RG29 v 2769, file 822-1-D479, part 4, LAC.

79 Meltzer to Moore, 15 February 1954, RG29 v 2769, file 822-1-D479, part 2, LAC; general and orthopaedic made up the remaining 32 per cent of surgeries.

80 Meltzer to Moore, 15 February 1954, RG29 v 2769, file 822-1-D479, part 2, LAC.

81 Dryden et al., *Camsell Mosaic*, 23.

82 H. Meltzer, "Results of Thoracoplasty," *Journal of Thoracic Surgery* (St Louis) 11, no. 1 (October 1941): 84–94.

83 Meltzer to Moore, 9 November 1954, RG29 v 2926, file 851-1-D479, part 1, LAC.

84 "Report on the Pembine Therapy Conference, Pembine, Wisconsin, 1953," Sanatorium Board of Manitoba, file G15, Archives of Manitoba (AM).

85 Author interview with Dave Melting Tallow, Siksika, Alberta, 9 August 2010.

86 Katherine McCuaig notes that the antibiotic era actually encouraged the surgical treatment of pulmonary tuberculosis. *The Weariness, the Fever, and the Fret: The Campaign against Tuberculosis in Canada, 1900–1950* (Montreal: McGill-Queen's University Press, 1999), 197.

87 Author interview with Roy Little Chief, Strathmore, Alberta, 8 August 2010.

88 IHS also managed its own hospitals in the province at Norway House, Fisher River, and Fort Alexander Indian Hospitals.

89 In 1955, for instance, the Sanatorium Board's income from IHS was $833,971.20; 93 per cent went for treatment in the segregated sanatoria, the remaining 7 per cent went to surveys and limited treatment in the provincial Manitoba Sanatorium (formerly Ninette). "Federal Funding of TB treatment and Control for Indians in Manitoba as Conducted by the Sanatorium Board of Manitoba," Sanatorium Board of Manitoba, file 29, T-5–7-15, Archives of Manitoba (AM).

90 Obituary, "Arthur Henry Povah," *Winnipeg Free Press*, 8 August 2001. Povah's career trajectory was not uncommon for physicians who contracted tuberculosis.

91 "Brandon Sanatorium Committee Minutes, 1947–1965," January 1953, Sanatorium Board of Manitoba, file P7102, AM.

92 "Brandon Sanatorium Committee Minutes, 1947–1965," March 1956: "We are now able to do four pulmonary resections per week." Sanatorium Board of Manitoba, file P7102, AM.

93 "Board Report Assiniboine Hospital, 3 February 1959," Sanatorium Board of Manitoba, file P7102, AM.

94 E.L. Ross, "Report on the Pembine Therapy Conference, Pembine, Wisconsin, 1952," 15, Sanatorium Board of Manitoba, file G15, AM.

95 E.L. Ross, "Report on the Pembine Therapy Conference, Pembine, Wisconsin, 1956," 16, Sanatorium Board of Manitoba, file G15, AM.

96 Dr P.E. Baldry, "Chest Diseases in Canada: A Report by the 1959 Scholar of the Chest and Heart Association" (typescript), Canadian Tuberculosis Association, MG28 I75, file 16, LAC.

97 Clarice Beaton, Prince Albert San, 1 January 1953, file A638 Lung Association, file VIII.66, "Lady Superintendent," Saskatchewan Archives Board (SAB).

98 Mountain Sanatorium, Weekly Report of Bed Compliment, 25 January 1957, RG29, v 2876, file 851-1-17, part 1, LAC; Pat Grygier, *A Long Way from Home: The Tuberculosis Epidemic among the Inuit* (Montreal and Kingston: McGill-Queen's University Press, 1994), xxi; "Dr. Karan's Report," 3 March 1958, CTA, MG28 I75, IIa, file 38, LAC.

99 "Annual Report Manitoba Sanatorium," March 1958, Sanatorium Board of Manitoba, file G13, AM.

100 David B. Stewart, *Holy Ground: The Story of the Manitoba Sanatorium at Ninette* (Killarney, MB: J.A. Victor David Museum, 1999), 111.

101 Wood to Dr Jeffrey, 5 October 1956, RG29, v 2876, file 851-1-17, part 1, LAC.

102 Rath to Orr, 30 November 1956, RG29, v 2934, file 851-1-X300, part 1, LAC.

103 Annual Report Medical Services, General Superintendent's Report 1965, Saskatchewan Lung Association files, A638, file IX.117, SAB.

104 A.L. Paine, "Supervision of Out-patient Tuberculosis Chemotherapy in Patients of Native Extraction" (typescript), February 1967, Sanatorium Board of Manitoba, file G15, AM.
105 Cameron to Minister Waldo Monteith, n.d. (likely March 1961), RG 29, vol. 2936, file 851-1-X400, part 1, LAC.
106 "Federal Funding of TB Treatment and Control for Indians in Manitoba as Conducted by the Sanatorium Board of Manitoba," Sanatorium Board of Manitoba, file 29, T-5-7-15, AM; 76 per cent of the sum went for treatment in the Manitoba Sanatorium. By 1975, when tuberculosis treatment became an insured service under Manitoba Health Services Commission, Sanatorium Board income from federal sources fell to $53,629.43 for "preventive services."
107 Paine, "Supervision of Out-patient Tuberculosis Chemotherapy in Patients of Native Extraction."
108 Stewart, *Holy Ground*, 116.
109 As cited in the previous chapter, Dr Stone noted: "It would be hard to prove that the Residential Schools, as a group, are not agencies for the spread of tuberculosis." Memorandum, Dr E.L. Stone to Director, 29 June 1937, MG28, I75, II (a), file 36, LAC.

Chapter Three

1 Minister Brooke Claxton, Special Joint Committee of the Senate and the House of Commons Appointed to Examine and Consider the Indian Act, *Minutes of Proceedings and Evidence No. 3*, 6 June 1946, 69.
2 Stone to medical director, 12 June 1946, RG29, v 2592, file 800-1-D479, part 1, LAC; emphasis in the original.
3 Aboriginal Nurses Association of Canada, *Twice as Good: A History of Aboriginal Nurses* (Ottawa: Aboriginal Nurses Association of Canada, 2007).
4 Mary Jane Logan McCallum, "Labour, Modernity and the Canadian State: A History of Aboriginal Women and Work in the Mid-Twentieth Century" (PhD diss., University of Manitoba, 2008), 244.
5 Laurie Meijer Drees, "Indian Hospitals and Aboriginal Nurses: Canada and Alaska," *Canadian Bulletin of Medical History* 27, no. 1 (2010): 156.
6 Aboriginal Nurses Association, *Twice as Good*.
7 Laurie Meijer Drees, "Training Aboriginal Nurses: The Indian Health Services in Northwestern Canada, 1939–75," in *Caregiving on the Periphery: Historical Perspectives on Nursing and Midwifery in Canada*, ed. Myra Rutherdale (Montreal and Kingston: McGill-Queen's University Press, 2010), 188.

8 Ryan Johnson and Amna Khalid, eds, *Public Health in the British Empire: Intermediaries, Subordinates and the Practice of Public Health, 1850–1960* (New York, London: Routledge, 2012).
9 McCallum "Labour, Modernity and the Canadian State," 246.
10 "Advisory Committee for the Control and Prevention of Tuberculosis among the Indians, Proceedings of Meeting, 30 and 31 May 1945," 162, 165, MG28, 175, IIa, file 36, LAC.
11 McCallum, "Labour, Modernity and the Canadian State," 255.
12 IHS Directorate report, 1960, as quoted in Meijer Drees, "Training Aboriginal Nurses," 197.
13 IHS policy was to pay some (male) patients $2.00 per day, in this case for translation for Inuit patients in the Clearwater Lake Indian Hospital in Manitoba. Moore to S.L. Carey, 15 March 1962, RG29, v 2590, file 800-1-D279, part 1, LAC.
14 Minnie Aodla Freeman, *Life among the Qallunaat* (Edmonton: Hurtig, 1978), 174.
15 Ibid., 176.
16 Ibid., 178.
17 Ibid., 189.
18 Ibid., 43.
19 Ibid., 56.
20 Maureen Lux, *Medicine That Walks: Disease, Medicine and Canadian Plains Native People, 1880–1940* (Toronto: University of Toronto Press, 2001), 218–20.
21 Author interview with Grace Anderson, Winnipeg, Manitoba, 20 February 2013
22 "Minutes of Committee Meeting, 23 October 1945," Clearwater Lake Hospital Committee minutes 1945–1965, P7101, Sanatorium Board of Manitoba Records, Archives of Manitoba.
23 Author interview with Grace Anderson, Winnipeg, Manitoba, 20 February 2013.
24 "A Review of the Historical Development, Objectives and Principles of the Indian and Northern Health Services," May 1967, accession PR1991.443, box 1, file 16, PAA.
25 The "invisibility" of Aboriginal women workers is treated in McCallum, "Labour, Modernity and the Canadian State"; Shula Marks also notes the invisibility of South African ward aides and attendants in *Divided Sisterhood: Race, Class and Gender in the South African Nursing Profession* (Johannesburg: University of Witwatersand University Press, 1994), 62.
26 Author interview with Frank Malloway Sr, Chilliwack, BC, 29 July 2010.
27 Author interview with Agnes Cyr, Echo Lodge, Fort Qu'Appelle, SK, 17 July 2009.

28 Manitoba Association of Registered Nurses, "Report – Labour Relations Committee," 1947, RG29, v 3405, file 823-1-X253, LAC.
29 Ken Coates, *Best Left as Indians: Native-White Relations in the Yukon Territory, 1840–1973* (Montreal and Kingston: McGill-Queen's University Press, 1991), 102.
30 "Resolution re Treatment of Tuberculosis and Venereal Disease in Natives in the Prince Rupert Health Unit," June 1944, RG29, v 2598, file 800-1-D579, part 1, LAC.
31 Crerar to Ralston, 5 September 1944, RG29, v 2598, file 800-1-D579, part 1, LAC.
32 "Formal Opening of Finely-Equipped Hospital at Miller Bay for TB Cases," Prince Rupert *Evening Empire*, 17 September 1946.
33 W.S. Barclay to Moore, 21 July 1944, RG29, v 2598, file 800-1-D579, part 1, LAC.
34 Ibid.
35 Campbell to Director, 17 January 1949, RG29, v 3405, file 823-1-D579, LAC.
36 Rutledge to Moore, 26 November 1946, RG29, v 3405 file 823-1-D353, part 1, LAC.
37 J.D. Galbraith to Moore, 27 February 1951, RG29, v 3405, file 823-1-D579, LAC.
38 Galbraith to Director, 13 March 1951; Galbraith to Director, 16 August 1951, RG29, v 3405, file 823-1-D579, LAC.
39 Galbraith to Rutledge, 9 October 1947, RG29, v 2598, file 800-1-D579, LAC.
40 Acting superintendent Burgess to Moore, 6 June 1950, RG29, v 2803, file 831-1-D579 part 5, LAC.
41 Martin to E.P. Applewaithe, MP, 22 September 1951, RG29, v 2803, file 831-1-D579 part 5, LAC.
42 Galbraith to Moore, 12 January 1953, RG29, v 3405, file 823-1-D579, LAC.
43 Quoted in Katherine Ott, *Fevered Lives: Tuberculosis in American Culture since 1870* (Cambridge: Harvard University Press, 1996), 150.
44 Alison Bashford and Carolyn Strange, "Cultures of Confinement," in *Isolation: Places and Practices of Exclusion*, ed. Bashford and Strange (London: Routledge, 2003), 133.
45 Kathryn McPherson, *Bedside Matters: The Transformation of Canadian Nursing, 1900–1990* (Toronto: Oxford University Press, 1996), 240.
46 Dr G.R. Howell, "Enquiry into Ward B Morale," 30 March 1954, RG29, v 2598, file 800-1-D579, part 1, LAC.
47 Marion Ballantine, RN, to Paul Martin, 14 November 1954, RG29, v 2598, file 800-1-D579, part 1, LAC; infectious hepatitis, or hepatitis A, is transmitted in food and water contaminated with infected fecal matter.
48 G.R. Howell, Grace Harris, RN, Sara Wyman, Social Worker, "A Study of Ward Morale in a Tuberculosis Hospital from the Miller Bay Indian Hospital," November 1954, RG29, v 2598, file 800-1-D579, part 1, LAC.

49 Marion Ballantine, RN, to Paul Martin, 14 November 1954, RG29, v 2598, file 800-1-D579, part 1, LAC.
50 Eric Preston, "Observations – Miller Bay Indian Hospital," 6 June 1956, RG29, v 2598, file 800-1-D579, part 1, LAC.
51 McPherson, *Bedside Matters*, 222
52 Rutledge to Moore, 26 November 1946, RG29, v 3405, file 823-1-D353, part 1, LAC.
53 Barclay to Zone superintendent, 7 February 1958, RG29, v 3405, file 823-1-D579, LAC.
54 Barclay to Director, 23 April 1958, RG29, v 3405, file 823-1-D579, LAC.
55 Barclay to Moore, 23 April 1958; Moore to Barclay, 5 May 1958, RG29, v 3405, file 823-1-D579, LAC.
56 "General Application for Authority," 22 April 1959, RG29, v 3405, file 823-1-D579, LAC.
57 "Director's Newsletter" (no date, likely Fall 1960), RG29 v 2598, file 800-1-D579, part 2, LAC.
58 Moore to Personnel Division, 25 May 1950, RG29, v 3405, file 823-1-X328, LAC.
59 Fyfe to Moore, 29 November 1952, RG29, v 3405, file 823-1-X328, LAC.
60 Moore to Personnel Division, 25 May 1950, RG29, v 3405, file 823-1-D353, part 1, LAC.
61 HA Proctor, "Nursing Establishment North Battleford," 10 August 1949, RG29, v 3405, file 823-1-D353, part 1, LAC.
62 Fyfe to Moore, 29 November 1952, RG29, v 3405, file 823-1-X328, LAC.
63 Moore to Falconer, 17 February, 1953, RG29, v 3405, file 823-1-X328, LAC.
64 David Gagan and Rosemary Gagan, *For Patients of Moderate Means* (Montreal and Kingston: McGill-Queen's University Press, 2002), 89; expenditures by Indian Health Services alone rose from about $2.5 million in the 1945–6 fiscal year to $10 million in 1950–1. Department of National Health and Welfare, *Annual Report*, 1945–6 and 1950–1.
65 Morton to Dr Head, 11 May 1955, RG29, v 3405, file 823-1-D353, part 1, LAC.
66 Head to Moore, 18 May 1955, RG29, v 3405, file 823-1-D353, part 1, LAC.
67 Dr Chou to Regional Superintendent, 17 October 1957, RG29, v 3405, file 823-1-D353, part 1, LAC.
68 Matron's Report, 14 November 1957, RG29, v 3405, file 823-1-D353, part 1, LAC.
69 Orford to Moore, 11 March 1958, RG29, v 3405, file 823-1-D353, part 1, LAC.
70 Moore to personnel officer, 29 April 1958, RG29, v 3405, file 823-1-D353, part 1, LAC.
71 Orford to Director, 2 June 1965, RG29, v 3405, file 823-1-D353, part 1, LAC.
72 Moore to Dr McCutcheon, 14 July 1941, RG29, v 3399, file 822-1-D173, LAC.

73 Stone to Moore, 29 July 1946, RG29, v 2769, file 822-1-D479, part 1, LAC.
74 Stone to Moore, 15 April 1946, RG29, v 2769, file 822-1-D479, part 1, LAC.
75 P.S. Tennant, acting regional superintendent, Vancouver to Moore, 6 January 1947, RG29, v 2769, file 822-1-D579, LAC.
76 T. Kue Young, *Health Care and Cultural Change: The Indian Experience in the Central Subarctic* (Toronto: University of Toronto Press, 1988), 103.
77 Meltzer to Moore, 30 September 1948, RG29, v 2769, file 822-1-D479, part 1, LAC.
78 Rutledge to deputy minister, 12 October 1948, RG29, v 2769, file 822–1-D479, part 1, LAC.
79 Cameron to Moore, 15 October 1948, RG29, v 2769, file 822-1-D479, part 1, LAC.
80 Rutledge to Moore, 29 Dec 1949, RG29, v 2769, file 822-1-D479, part 1, LAC.
81 Galbraith to Moore, 22 March 1951, RG29, v 2769, file 822-1-D579, LAC.
82 Galbraith to Moore, 14 January 1953, RG29, v 2769, file 822-1-D579, LAC.
83 Galbraith to Moore, 8 April 1953, RG29, v 2769, file 822-1-D579, LAC.
84 Moore to Barclay, 9 March 1955, RG29, v 2769, file 822-1-D579, LAC.
85 Falconer to Moore, 27 April 1953, RG29, v 2769, file 822-1-D479, part 2, LAC.
86 Meltzer to Matas, 20 July 1964, RG29, v 2769, file 822-1-D479, part 2, LAC.
87 Falconer to Moore, 16 May 1952, RG29, v 2769, file 822-1-D479, part 2, LAC.
88 Falconer to Moore, 30 May 1958, RG29, v 2769, file 822-1-D479 part 2, LAC.
89 Falconer to Moore, June 10 1960, RG29, v 2769, file 822-1-D479 part 2, LAC.
90 Sally Mae Weaver, "Health, Culture and Dilemma: A Study of the Non-Conservative Iroquois, Six Nations Reserve, Ontario" (PhD Diss., University of Toronto, 1967), 150.
91 Ibid., 153. Weaver conducted anthropological fieldwork on the reserve in 1964 and 1965, studying the "medical acculturation" of the three thousand "non-Conservative" Six Nations community (as opposed to the 1,500 Longhouse people, or the non-Christian "Conservative" members who retained their Iroquois social and cultural beliefs).
92 Ibid., 182.
93 Wiebe to Moore, 3 June 1953, RG29, v 3399, file 822-1-D173, LAC.
94 Wiebe to Moore, 31 December 1953, RG29, v 3399, file 822-1-D173, LAC.
95 Wiebe to Moore, 27 May 1954, RG29, v 3399, file 822-1-D173, LAC; emphasis added.
96 Wiebe to Moore, 27 May 1954, RG29, v 3399, file 822-1-D173, LAC.
97 Weaver, "Health, Culture and Dilemma," 182.
98 Wiebe to Moore, 16 February 1955, RG29, v 3399, file 822-1-D173, LAC.

99 Six Nations Council Resolution, 21 June 1960. While Moore knew that this individual wrote his qualifying examinations, it was not clear that he had passed, though neither Moore nor Wiebe considered that to be an obstacle to his employment. Moore to regional superintendent, 29 October 1959, RG29, v 3399, file 822-1-D173, LAC.

100 Wiebe to Director, 11 July 1960, RG29, v 3399, file 822-1-D173, LAC.

101 Weaver, "Health, Culture and Dilemma," 170.

102 Ibid., 327–9. The complaints were also raised in the House of Commons on 12 February 1962. Canada, House of Commons *Debates*, 761.

103 Wiebe to Moore, 12 February 1962, RG29, v 2904, file 851-1-A479, part 2, LAC.

104 Moore to minister Waldo Monteith, 9 March 1962, RG29, v 2904, file 851-1-A479, part 2, LAC.

105 Weaver, "Health, Culture and Dilemma," 330.

106 The Royal Commission on Government Organization was established in 1960 to enquire into the organization of federal departments and agencies. Despite the recommendation that the ageing Coqualeetza and Charles Camsell hospitals be neither rebuilt nor extended, the latter was rebuilt in 1967. The recommendations for changes to IHS took up a scant seven pages in the five-volume report, *Royal Commission on Government Organization, Report*, vol. 3, Report 15, "Health Services" (Ottawa: Queen's Printer, 1962) 197, 200–2.

107 Meijer Drees, "Indian Hospitals and Aboriginal Nurses."

108 Moore to Regional Superintendent, 21 May, 1962, RG29, v 2769, file 822-1-D479 part 2, LAC.

Chapter Four

1 Minnie Aodla Freeman, *Life among the Qallunaat* (Edmonton: Hurtig, 1978), 65.

2 Kathleen Steinhauer-Anderson, quoted in Donna Dryden, Elva Taylor, Rona Beer, Ron Bergman, and Margaret Cogill, *The Camsell Mosaic: The Charles Camsell Hospital, 1945–1985* (Edmonton: Charles Camsell History Committee, 1985), 101.

3 "Advisory Committee for the Control and Prevention of Tuberculosis among the Indians, Proceedings of Meeting, 30 and 31 May 1945," 206, MG28, 175, IIa, file 36, LAC.

4 Katherine McCuaig, *The Weariness, the Fever and the Fret: The Campaign against Tuberculosis in Canada, 1900–1950* (Montreal and Kingston: McGill-Queen's University Press, 1999), 98; F.B. Smith, *The Retreat of Tuberculosis, 1850–1950* (London: Croom Helm, 1988).

5 I.H. Mazer to Moore, 23 January 1946, RG29, v 2876, file 851-1-17, part 1, LAC.
6 McCuaig, *The Weariness, the Fever and the Fret*, 187.
7 Ibid., 188–9.
8 C. Stuart Houston, *R.G. Ferguson: Crusader against Tuberculosis* (Toronto: Dundurn Press, 1991), 104.
9 Stewart Murray, Metropolitan Health Committee (Vancouver) to Mr H.P.J. Gunn, Administrator Children's Hospital, 17 December 1957, GR-0129, Tuberculosis Control Division, box 39, file 1, BCA (emphasis in original); tuberculin, a solution containing substances extracted from the tubercle bacillus, became by the early twentieth century a simple skin test; a positive reaction indicated exposure to the disease, not the disease itself. The Mantoux test (purified protein derivative, or PPD) continues to be used to infer exposure to the disease. Katherine Ott, *Fevered Lives: Tuberculosis in American Culture since 1870* (Cambridge: Harvard University Press, 1996), 62–3.
10 Stefan Grzybowski and Zygmunt Dunaj, "Tuberculin Survey of the Population of Manitoulin Island," *Canadian Medical Association Journal* 81 (1 September 1959): 366–8.
11 McCuaig, *The Weariness, the Fever and the Fret*, 192.
12 W.J. Wood, regional superintendent, IHS, "Survey of BCG Vaccinated Indians in Manitoba," 13 June 1955, RG29 v 2868, file 851-1-4 part 2, LAC.
13 Armand Frappier, "Report on the opportuneness, possibility and practical means of applying routine preventive BCG vaccination," 11 January 1947, RG29 v 2868, file 851-1-4, part 1a, LAC.
14 WJ Wood, regional superintendent IHS, "Survey of BCG Vaccinated Indians in Manitoba," 13 June 1955, RG29 v 2868, file 851-1-4 part 2, LAC.
15 G.D.W. Cameron to Moore, 10 October 1952, RG29 v 2868, file 851-1-4, part 2, LAC.
16 BCG vaccination (not the skin test) is widely used throughout the developing world. The deaths between the 1990s and 2003 of six vaccinated Aboriginal infants with underlying immunodeficiency disorders led to the discontinuation of routine immunization in some Canadian provinces and territories. Routine BCG vaccination continues in Aboriginal communities in Alberta, Manitoba, Northwest Territories, northern Ontario, and Nunavut; its use in Aboriginal communities in Saskatchewan was discontinued in 2011, in Quebec in 2005, and other provinces in the 1990s. Canada, Public Health Agency of Canada, *Canadian Immunization Guide* http://www.phac-aspc.gc.ca/publicat/cig-gci/p04-bcg-eng.php#clae (accessed 22 March 2015); "BCG Vaccine use in Canada – Current and Historical," http://www.phac-aspc.gc.ca/tbpc-latb/bcgvac_1206-eng.php (accessed 16 April 2013).

17 Dr M. Matas, "Tuberculosis Programs of the Medical Services, Department of National Health and Welfare," in "Proceedings of the Third National Tuberculosis Conference," *Medical Services Journal Canada* 22 (1966): 881–2.

18 Ibid., 879.

19 Dryden et al., *Camsell Mosaic*, 134.

20 The debate over tuberculin testing and the efficacy of BCG continued in the 1980s. See Raj Narian, "Need for a BCG Trial in Canada's Native Populations," *Canadian Medical Association Journal* 127 (July 1982): 101–2; and reply by T. Kue Young, "A BCG Trial in Canada's Native Populations," *Canadian Medical Association Journal* (December 1982): 1166–7; McCuaig cites a 1995 study of the life-threatening hazards of BCG use among those most likely at risk for TB, the immunocompromised patients (*The Weariness, the Fever and the Fret*, 274).

21 Harold Lerat with Linda Ungar, *Treaty Promises Indian Reality: Life on a Reserve* (Saskatoon: Purich Publishing, 2005), 142; Dryden et al., *Camsell Mosaic*, 133; P.E. Baldry, "Chest Diseases in Canada, A Report by the 1959 Scholar of the Chest and Heart Association" (typescript), Canadian Tuberculosis Association, MG28 I 75, file 16, LAC.

22 E.L.M. Thorpe, *The Social Histories of Smallpox and Tuberculosis in Canada: Culture, Evolution and Disease* (Winnipeg: University of Manitoba Anthropology Papers No. 30, 1989), 106.

23 Bruce Noton, "Northern Manitoba Treaty Party, 1949," *Manitoba History* 39 (Spring/Summer 2000), http://www.mhs.mb.ca/docs/mb_history/39/treatyparty1949.shtml (accessed 12 April 2013).

24 Ibid.

25 "Indian Clinics," files T-6-2-2 to T-6-2-14, Sanatorium Board Manitoba, Archives of Manitoba.

26 Houston, *R.G. Ferguson*, 104, 105.

27 Baldry, "Chest Diseases in Canada."

28 Ott, *Fevered Lives*, 3.

29 Ann Meekitjuk Hanson, "Finding Hope and Healing in Memories of Our Past," *Above and Beyond: Canada's Arctic Journal* (March/April 2012), http://issuu.com/arctic_journal/docs/above_and_beyond_march_april_2012 (accessed 28 May 2013).

30 Ebba Olofsson et al., "Negotiating Identities: Inuit Tuberculosis Evacuees in the 1940s–1950s," *Études/Inuit/Studies* 32, no. 2 (2008): 131.

31 Megan Vaughan makes this point in reference to mass medical campaigns in colonial Africa in *Curing Their Ills: Colonial Power and African Illness* (Palo Alto, CA: Stanford University Press, 1991), 52.

32 Dryden et al., *Camsell Mosaic*, ix, 93–130.

33 George Manuel and Michael Posluns, *The Fourth World: An Indian Reality* (New York: Free Press, 1974), 65, 100.
34 Laurie Meijer Drees, *Healing Histories* (Edmonton: University of Alberta Press, 2013), 80–1.
35 Author interview with Dave Melting Tallow, 9 August 2010, Siksika, Alberta.
36 Quoted in "More Canadian Genocide: TB Sanitariums," *Windspeaker News*, September 1998, 44.
37 See chapter 3. "Formal Opening of Finely-Equipped Hospital at Miller Bay for TB Cases," *Prince Rupert Evening Empire*, 17 September 1946.
38 W.P.B. Pugh, Indian Agent, "Quarterly Report," 8 January 1947, RG29, v 2592, file 800-1-D479, part 1, LAC.
39 "Aged Chief Swimmer Pleads with Indians to Make Use of Hospital Facilities," *Saskatoon Star Phoenix*, 1 October 1953.
40 Interview with Gordon Albert by Alma Favel-King, North Battleford, September 2011.
41 Interview with Rose Atimoyoo by Alma Favel-King, North Battleford, September 2011.
42 Chief Cornelius Bignell, Councillors Tom Henderson, Donald Lathlin, and Matthew McGillivary to E. Law, Indian Agent, 4 July 1949, RG29, v 2590, file 800-1-D279, part 1, LAC.
43 E.L. Ross to Moore, 6 September 1949, RG29, v 2590, file 800-1-D279, part 1, LAC.
44 Freeman, *Life among the Qallunaat*, 174.
45 Ibid., 175–6.
46 G.R. Howell to Moore, 7 April 1954, RG29, v 2598, file 800-1-D579, part 1 LAC.
47 Dryden et al., *Camsell Mosaic*, 29–30.
48 *Lost Songs* (director Clint Tourangeau and Elaine Moyah, National Film Board, 1999).
49 Joanne Hader, "The Effect of Tuberculosis on the Indians of Saskatchewan, 1926–1965" (MA thesis, University of Saskatchewan, 1990), 162.
50 Miriam Wright, RN, in Dryden et al., *Camsell Mosaic*, 71.
51 Dryden et al., *Camsell Mosaic*, 95; author interview with Dave Melting Tallow, 9 August 2010, Siksika, Alberta.
52 M. Matas, Charles Camsell Hospital rules, 1 April 1959, RG29, v 2593, file 800-1-D479, part 2 LAC.
53 Hader, "The Effect of Tuberculosis on the Indians of Saskatchewan, 1926–1965," 160–1; Hader's informants, interviewed in the 1980s, remained anonymous.
54 Freeman, *Life among the Qallunaat*, 176.
55 Ibid., 45–6.

56 "Eskimo Correspondence," RG85, v 314, file 1012-8, part 3, LAC.
57 Annalisa Staples and Ruth McConnell, *Soapstone and Seed Beads: Arts and Craft at the Charles Camsell Hospital* (Edmonton: Jasper Printing, 1993).
58 G.R. Howell, "Enquiry into Ward B Morale," 30 March 1954, RG29 v. 2598, file 800-1-D579, part 1, LAC.
59 Dryden et al., *Camsell Mosaic*, 200–1.
60 G.R. Howell to Barclay, 24 August 1956, RG29 v. 2598, file 800-1-D579, part 1, LAC.
61 Petition to Rt Hon. John G Diefenbaker, 4 June 1962, RG29, v 2608, file 800-1-X328 part 1, LAC.
62 See chapter 3. Historian Mary Jane McCallum notes the state's role in the procurement of its own workforce. "Labour, Modernity and the Canadian State: A History of Aboriginal Women and Work in the Mid-Twentieth Century" (PhD diss., University of Manitoba, 2008), 67.
63 Author interview with Roy Little Chief, 8 August 2010, Strathmore, Alberta.
64 Dryden et al., *Camsell Mosaic*, 101.
65 Author interview with Dave Melting Tallow, 9 August 2010, Siksika, Alberta.
66 Author interview with Frank Malloway Sr, 29 July 2010, Chilliwack, BC.
67 The policy continued with the "Sixties Scoop," or the widespread practice by social welfare authorities of removing Aboriginal children from their families and placing them in non-Aboriginal homes. See Ernie Crey and Suzanne Fournier, *Stolen from Our Embrace. The Abduction of First Nations Children and the Restoration of Aboriginal Communities* (Vancouver: Douglas and McIntyre, 1998). The Truth and Reconciliation Commission bore witness to the legacy of the residential schools as a "sincere indication and acknowledgement of the injustices and harms experienced by Aboriginal people and the need for continued healing." http://www.trc.ca/websites/trcinstitution/index.php?p=3 (accessed 16 May 2013).
68 P.E. Moore, H.D. Kruse, F.F. Tisdall, and R.S.C. Corrigan, "Medical Survey of Nutrition among the Northern Manitoba Indians," *Canadian Medical Association Journal* 54 (March 1946): 233.
69 "New Deal for Indians," *Ottawa Citizen*, 3 February 1947; "Shifting Care of Indians," *Winnipeg Tribune*, 17 January 1947; "The Indian Still Waits," *Globe and Mail*, 14 May 1947.
70 Ian Mosby, "Administering Colonial Science: Nutrition Research and Human Biomedical Experimentation in Aboriginal Communities and Residential Schools, 1942–1952," *Histoire Sociale/Social History* 46 (May 2013): 148.
71 Meijer Drees, *Healing Histories*, 175.
72 Ibid., xxviii, 182, 202; author interviews with Dave Melting Tallow, 9 August 2010, and Frank Malloway Sr, 29 July 2010.

73 See Maureen Lux, *Medicine That Walks: Disease, Medicine and Canadian Plains Native People, 1880–1940* (Toronto: University of Toronto Press, 2001), 180.
74 Maureen Lux, "Perfect Subjects: Race, Tuberculosis, and the Qu'Appelle BCG Vaccine Trial," *Canadian Bulletin for Medical History* 15 (1998): 277–95; David S. Jones, *Rationalizing Epidemics: Meaning and Uses of American Indian Mortality since 1600* (Cambridge, MA: Harvard University Press, 2004), 195–220.
75 Barclay to Moore, 2 December 1947, RG29, v 2868, file 851-1-4 part 1a, LAC; Houston, *R.G. Ferguson*, 60.
76 Barnett to Stark, 20 May 1966, Saskatchewan Lung Association files, A638, VIII.157, SAB.
77 Barclay to the Director, 2 December 1947; Falconer to Barclay, 5 December 1947, RG29, v 2868, file 851-1-4 part 1a, LAC.
78 Freeman, *Life among the Qallunaat*, 175–6.
79 Dryden et al., *Camsell Mosaic*, 235.
80 Pat Sandiford Grygier, *A Long Way from Home* (Montreal and Kingston: McGill-Queen's University Press, 1994), 115.
81 Current definitions of informed consent are not applied here. Focus on the ethics of medical research and human experimentation, begun in the wake of the atrocities of the Second World War, continued in the mid-1960s, prompted by exposés of unethical medical research. H.K. Beecher, "Ethics and Clinical Research," *New England Journal of Medicine* 274 (1966): 1354–60.
82 See chapter 2. Moore to Meltzer and Stone, 14 March 1946, RG29, v 2592, file 800-1-D479, part 1, LAC.
83 "Submission to the Policy Review Committee on the Future of Charles Camsell Hospital," second draft, 15 May 1976, RG29 v 3379 file 800-1-D479, LAC.
84 John Robert Lymer and Arthur James Anderson, "An Evaluation of Several Orally Administered Para-aminosalicylic Acid Preparations," *Canadian Pharmaceutical Journal* (September 1957): 160–2.
85 A Cold War arm of the military established in 1947, the Defense Research Board operated its own facilities and also provided grants to universities and industry for research in areas of particular interest to Canada such as the Arctic. *The Canadian Encyclopedia*, http://www.thecanadianencyclopedia.ca/en/article/defence-research/#h3_jump_0 (accessed 19 May 2013).
86 Allan M. Edwards and Gordon C. Gray, "Observations on Juvenile Hypothyroidism in Native Races of Northern Canada," *Canadian Medical Association Journal* 84 (20 May 1961): 1116–24.
87 Edwards to Gray, 27 December 1962; Moore to Gray, 16 January 1963, RG29, v 2769, file 822-1-D479, part 2, LAC.

88 Informed consent became a national controversy in the 1970s when CBC Radio broadcast the stories of Aboriginal women who charged they were sexually sterilized in hospital without their knowledge or consent. Publicly, the minister of health defended the hospitals and claimed the public broadcaster was irresponsible; consent forms had been duly signed. Privately, however, it became clear to department officials that there were problems with the Inuktitut translations. Bureaucrats asked nine Inuk women "with above average education" to read the form consenting to sterilization; two thought it meant to have an abortion, five thought it meant to have an operation and have no more babies, and two could not discern what the message was about. It was clear to bureaucrats that "the form needs a bit of re-drafting to ensure that people are fully aware of what they are agreeing to." A.D. Hunt to M.L. Webb, 1 June 1973, RG29, v 2870, file 851-1-5 part 3b, LAC.

89 Laurie Meijer Drees, "The Nanaimo and Charles Camsell Indian Hospitals: First Nations' Narratives of Health Care, 1945 to 1965," *Histoire Sociale/ Social History* 43, no. 85 (2010): 165–91; reprinted in her *Healing Histories* (Edmonton: University of Alberta Press, 2013).

90 Robin Brownlie and Mary-Ellen Kelm, "Desperately Seeking Absolution: Native Agency as Colonialist Alibi?" *Canadian Historical Review* 75, no. 4 (1994): 543–56.

91 E. McPherson to Indian Affairs, 5 February 1946, RG29, v 2931, file 851-1-X200 part 1B, LAC ("George Hamilton" was not his real name).

92 See RG29, v 2931, file 851-1-X200 part 1B, LAC.

93 L.M. (Leo) Manning Report on Parc Savard visit, 22–5 February 1952, RG29, v 2947, file 851-2-2, part 1, LAC.

94 J.E. Labreque to H.D. Reid, 6 May 1955; Labreque to Director, 6 August 1956; contract with Maheu and Maheu Co. Pest Control, 14 March 1956; Labreque to WH Frost, 7 June 1957, RG29, v 2587, file 800-1-D117, part 3B, LAC.

95 P.E. Baldry, "Chest Diseases in Canada: A Report of the 1959 Scholar of the Chest and Heart Association," CTA, MG28 I 75, III, LAC.

96 G. Kinneard, MD, Director Regional Health Services Branch, to Dr F.B. Roth, Deputy Minister Health, 20 February 1953, R999 file I.70, SAB.

97 J.E. Hiltz, "Compulsory Treatment of Tuberculosis," *Canadian Medical Association Journal* 71 (December 1954): 569–71.

98 "Circular Letter to All Superintendents," Indian Health Regulations (sec. 72 Indian Act, Order in Council, P.C. 193-1129), 17 July 1953, RG29 v 2936, file 851-1-X400, part 2a, LAC. The Regulations targeted all infectious disease, but made special mention of tuberculosis and venereal disease.

99 Sharon Helen Venne, *Indian Acts and Amendments 1868–1975: An Indexed Collection* (Saskatoon: Native Law Centre University of Saskatchewan, 1981), 337.
100 Indian Health Regulations, 1.
101 Indian Health Regulations, sections 6, 18, 8.
102 Derek G. Smith, "The Emergence of 'Eskimo Status': An Examination of the Eskimo Disk List System and Its Social Consequences, 1925–1970," in *Anthropology, Public Policy, and Native Peoples in Canada*, ed. Noel Dyck and James Waldram (Montreal and Kingston: McGill-Queen's University Press, 1993), 50.
103 Author interview with Dave Melting Tallow, 9 August 2010, Siksika, Alberta.
104 Zone Superintendent, Nanaimo, to Regional Superintendent, 15 December 1959, RG29 v 2876, file 851-1-17 part 1, LAC; "Advisory Committee for the Control and Prevention of Tuberculosis among the Indians, Proceedings of Meeting, 30 and 31 May 1945," 210, MG28, 175, II(a), file 36, LAC.
105 Kathleen Steinhauer, quoted in Meijer Drees, *Healing Histories*, 174.
106 K.R. Brown, superintendent, Blood Indian Agency, to Regional Supervisor, 30 October 1958, RG29 v 2798, file 831-1-D479, part 6, LAC; M. Matas, Charles Camsell Hospital rules, 1 April 1959, RG29, v 2593, file 800-1-D479, part 2 LAC.
107 In a reversal of positions from the 1950s, when the Saskatchewan Anti-TB League's medical superintendent hoped to use the public health act to detain Metis patients in sanatorium in 1969, the provincial public health director opposed the notion: "I would not like to think that selected patients should be brought before a magistrate and sentenced to a stay in a sanatorium. This would have to be done for everybody and I am sure that you could not agree to this as a measure in the control of tuberculosis. As I have said before, we can legislate and organize for the generality of patients but there is the occasion when we have to admit defeat in some instances of extreme cases." Barnett to Walker, 7 February 1969; Walker to Barnett, 14 February 1969, Saskatchewan Lung Association files, A638 file VIII.25, SAB.
108 G.R. Howell to W.S. Barclay, 5 June 1956, "Report on Hospital Progress," RG29 v 2598 file 800-1-D579 part 1, LAC.
109 Falconer to Moore, 10 December 1957, RG29 v 2876, file 851-1-17 part 1, LAC.
110 See "Sanatorium Admissions and Discharges," Saskatchewan Lung Association files, A638, file IX.73a, SAB. In northern Saskatchewan, the Prince Albert Sanatorium with 276 beds admitted only 2 Aboriginal patients in 1935; during the 1940s it admitted an average of 44 Aboriginal patients per year, but an average of 120 Aboriginal patients from 1951 to 1955.

111 T.J. Orford, regional superintendent, to G.D. Barnett, 13 October 1961, Saskatchewan Lung Association files, A638, file VIII.48, SAB.
112 M. Matas, "Tuberculosis Programs of the Medical Services, Department of National Health and Welfare," in "Proceedings of the Third National Tuberculosis Conference" *Medical Services Journal Canada* 22 (1966): 882.
113 The 1996 Royal Commission on Aboriginal Peoples devotes a complete section to relocations, highlighting the experiences of thirteen different communities relocated to ease government's administrative needs, or to make way for resource development. http://www.collectionscanada.gc.ca/webarchives/20071115053257/http://www.ainc-inac.gc.ca/ch/rcap/sg/sgmm_e.html (accessed 24 May 2013).
114 Pat Sandiford Grygier, *A Long Way from Home* (Montreal: McGill-Queen's University Press, 1994).
115 J.M. Ridge to P.E. Moore, 28 October 1945, RG29, v 2590, file 800-1-D279, part 1, LAC.
116 *Lost Songs*, dir. Clint Tourangeau and Elaine Moyah, National Film Board, 1999.
117 Freeman, *Life among the Qallunaat*, 45.
118 Grygier, *A Long Way from Home*, 126.
119 Resident Physician's Report, February, June 1951, "Dynevor Indian Hospital Committee minutes, 1942–1957," Sanatorium Board of Manitoba files, P7096, Archives of Manitoba.
120 "It seems strange to hear people speaking of competition in the treatment field of tuberculosis when only a few years ago the hue and cry across Canada was for the federal government to provide more facilities for tuberculous Indians." P.E. Moore to G.D. Barnett, 2 April 1963, Saskatchewan Lung Association files, A638, file VIII.47, SAB.
121 "Saskatchewan Sanatoria Admissions and Discharges," Lung Association files, A638, file IX.73a, SAB.
122 C.B. Ross to Moore, 31 October 1955, RG29, v 2926, file 851-1-X100, part 1A, LAC.
123 J.S. Willis to medical superintendent, 21 March 1955, RG29, v 2926, file 851-1-X100, part 1A, LAC.
124 Report to the Board on Clearwater Lake Hospital, July 1962; Minutes of Medical Advisory Committee, 11 September 1962, RG29, v 2590, file 800-1-D279, part 1, LAC.
125 Clearwater Lake Hospital committee, minutes October 1962, Manitoba Sanatorium Board files, P7101, Archives of Manitoba.
126 Grygier recounts the experiences of Inuit patients delivered to the wrong communities, and others "lost" in the IHS system. *A Long Way from Home*,

121–8; see also Ebba Olofsson, "Negotiating Identities: Inuit Tuberculosis Evacuees in the 1940s to 1950s," *Études/Inuit/Studies* 32, no. 2 (2008): 127–49.

127 Memorandum, director DIA, 25 February 1947, RG29, v 2783, file 830-1-D479, part 1, LAC.

128 Northwood to Moore, 3 April 1940, RG 29, v 2590, file 800-1-D297, part 1, LAC.

129 E.L. Stone to director, 19 December 1946, RG29, v 2783, file 830-1-D479, part 1, LAC.

130 Falconer to Stone, 28 January 1947, RG29, v 2783, file 830-1-D479, part 1, LAC.

131 Hoey to Dr Moore, 25 February 1947, RG29, v 2783, file 830-1-D479, part 1, LAC.

132 Gooderham to Indian Affairs, 18 August 1947, RG29, v 2796, file 831-1-D479, part 1, LAC.

133 Dryden et al., *Camsell Mosaic*, 66. Former students at the Edmonton residential school, at a healing ceremony at the school site in 2004, recalled being paid to dig the graves and are still haunted by the experience of seeing the caskets being put in the ground without ceremony or markings. Carl Carter (Sweetgrass) "Journey Continues to Heal School Trauma," *Windspeaker* 11, no. 10 (2004).

134 J.G. McGilp, Regional Supervisor, to G.D. Barnett, 27 April, 1964, Saskatchewan Lung Association files, A638, file VIII.47, SAB.

135 T.J. Orford to G.D. Barnett, 13 April 1964, Saskatchewan Lung Association files, A638, file VIII.47, SAB.

136 In 1988 the government of the Northwest Territories initiated its Medical Patient Search Project to trace patients who went missing since the 1940s. *Summary: Final Report* (Department of Health Government of Northwest Territories, April 1991). A cairn in memory of ninety-eight Aboriginal people who died at the Camsell Hospital and were buried at the Edmonton Residential school, was designed and erected by former Camsell staff and dedicated in 1990. "St. Albert Cemeteries," file 991.03.01.06, St Albert Museum and Archives. In 2010 a cairn was erected memorializing the 300 Aboriginal patients who were buried in unmarked graves in the Belmont Hillside Cemetery near Manitoba's Ninette Sanatorium. *Winnipeg Free Press*, 3 August 2010.

137 Meltzer to Moore, 19 February 1946, RG29 v 2592, file 800-1-D479 part 1, LAC.

138 Minutes, Patients' Committee, 19 March 1956, RG29 v 2598, file 800-1-D579 part 1, LAC.

139 Dryden et al., *Camsell Mosaic*, 194–5.

140 Dryden et al., *Camsell Mosaic*, 66. Resident Physician's Report, February 1951, "Dynevor Indian Hospital Committee minutes, 1942–1957," Sanatorium Board of Manitoba files, P7096, AM.
141 *The Longer Trail*, dir. Fergus McDonell, produced by Julian Biggs, 30 min., National Film Board, 1956.
142 *No Longer Vanishing*, dir. Grant McLean, produced by Tom Daly, 27 min. 31 sec., National Film Board, 1955. In the training course for its Indian placement officers, Indian Affairs showed both films. Mary Jane Logan McCallum, "Labour, Modernity and the Canadian State: A History of Aboriginal Women and Work in the Mid-Twentieth Century" (PhD diss., University of Manitoba, 2008), 133.
143 Freeman, *Life among the Qallunaat*, 65.

Chapter Five

1 G.D.W. Cameron to Minister Waldo Monteith, 15 March 1961, RG 29, vol. 2936, file 851-1-X400, part 1, LAC (original emphasis).
2 J.R. Miller, *Skyscrapers Hide the Heavens: A History of Indian-White Relations in Canada*, rev. ed. (Toronto: University of Toronto Press, 1989), 222.
3 Cameron to Minister, 15 March 1961, RG 29, vol. 2936, file 851-1-X400, part 1, LAC.
4 The other was the Lady Willingdon Hospital at Six Nations in Ontario.
5 "The Hospital"; "Twenty-five Years as an Indian Agent to the Blackfoot Band," January 1972, 7, M4738, Gooderham fonds, box 1, file 3, Glenbow-Alberta Institute Archives (GAI).
6 For an overview of medical traditions in plains Aboriginal cultures see Lux, *Medicine That Walks* (Toronto: University of Toronto Press, 2001) chapter 2, and Waldram et al., *Aboriginal Health in Canada* (Toronto: University of Toronto Press, 2006) chapter 5.
7 John Milloy, *A National Crime: The Canadian Government and the Residential School System, 1879–1986* (Winnipeg: University of Manitoba Press, 1999), 77–107.
8 G.H. Gooderham, "The Blackfoot Hospital and Its Progress" 18 February 1926, RG29 v 2592, file 800-1-D443, part 1, LAC.
9 Carlotta Hacker, *The Indomitable Lady Doctors* (Toronto: Clarke, Irwin, 1974), 185–92. Windsor remained at the Blackfoot Hospital until her retirement in 1948.
10 Lux, *Medicine That Walks*, 176–7.
11 Kennedy to Graham, 7 April 1923, RG10, v 1542, LAC.

12 "Contestants in first baby show held on the Blackfoot (Siksika) reserve, 1926," PA-32-1, GAI.
13 G.H. Gooderham, "The Blackfoot Hospital and Its Progress," 18 February 1926, RG29 v 2592 file 800-1-D443, part 1, LAC.
14 Gooderham to the Secretary, 27 April 1935, RG29 v 2796, file 800-1-D443, LAC.
15 "White Attitudes towards Indians," 30 June 1938, Hanks Fonds, M8458–29, GAI.
16 Agent Monthly Report, November 1934, RG29 v 2796, file 800-1-D443, LAC. A new wing for staff quarters had freed space for beds while the building's verandas were closed in and heated with stoves, adding space for thirty more beds.
17 Gooderham to Dr E.L. Stone, 13 February 1935, RG29 v 2796, file 800-1-D443, LAC.
18 Riou to Baker, 29 November 1937, Baker Memorial Sanatorium, GR1973.0315, file 35, Provincial Archives of Alberta (PAA).
19 Dr Windsor to Gooderham, n.d. (1935), RG29 v 2796, file 800-1-D443, LAC.
20 Gooderham to H.W. McGill, 12 February 1935, RG29 v 2796, file 800-1-D443, LAC.
21 Gooderham to Dr E.L. Stone, 13 February 1935, RG29 v 2796, file 800-1-D443, LAC.
22 Hospital Accounts, Baker Memorial Sanatorium, GR1973.0315, file 25, PAA; G.J. Wherrett, *The Miracle of the Empty Beds: A History of Tuberculosis in Canada* (Toronto: University of Toronto Press, 1977), 183.
23 Gooderham to Dr E.L. Stone, 13 February 1935, RG29 v 2796, file 800-1-D443, LAC.
24 L. Hanks and J. Hanks, *Tribe under Trust: A Study of the Blackfoot Reserve of Alberta* (Toronto: University of Toronto Press, 1950), 49. To compare with the nearby Kainai reserve, using 1935 figures (the last year that detailed accounts were published), the Siksika numbered 783 and the DIA spent just $6,512, mostly for wages and maintenance for Gooderham and his clerk. All other costs were paid by the trust fund. At the Kainai reserve, with a population of 1,317, the DIA spent $51,117 ($33,653 for reserve operations, plus $17,463 for the Blood Hospital). *Sessional Papers* 1936, Canada, House of Commons, 15–16.
25 W.L. Falconer to Director, 27 May 1942, RG29 v. 2936 file 851-1-X400 part 1, LAC.
26 E.L. Stone to Superintendent, 19 June 1946, RG29 v 2592 file 800-1-D443, part 1, LAC.
27 Stone to Director, 11 February 1949, RG29 v 2796 file 831-1-D426, part 1, LAC.

28 W.P.B. Pugh, Agent, 12 February 1947, RG29 v 2592, file 800-1-D443, part 1, LAC.
29 Moore to Pugh, 20 March 1947, RG29 v 2592, file 800-1-D443, part 1, LAC.
30 Paul Martin to J. Allison Glen, 21 March 1947; Martin to Glen, 6 May 1947, RG29, v 2592 file 800-1-D443, part 1, LAC.
31 Director to Deputy Minister, 23 April, 1947, RG29, v 2592 file 800-1-D443, part 1, LAC.
32 Alvin Finkel, "Paradise Postponed: A Re-examination of the Green Book Proposals of 1945," *Journal of the Canadian Historical Association* 4 (1993): 120–42. Much opposition came from provincial premiers, who objected to the federal Liberals' centralizing tendencies such as national health insurance that required provinces to yield tax revenues and undercut provincial autonomy. P.E. Bryden, "The Liberal Party and the Achievement of National Medicare," *Canadian Bulletin of Medical History* 26, no. 2 (2009): 315–32.
33 As noted, between 1945 and 1954 hospital expenditures in Canada increased 275 per cent. D. Gagan and R. Gagan, *For Patients of Moderate Means* (Montreal and Kingston: McGill-Queen's University Press, 2002), 89.
34 Malcolm Taylor, *Health Insurance and Canadian Public Policy*, 2nd ed. (Montreal and Kingston: McGill-Queen's University Press, 1987), 163–4.
35 Pugh to Gooderham, Regional Supervisor, 15 January 1954, RG29 v 2592 file 800-1-D443, part 1, LAC.
36 Moore to Jones, 23 February 1954, RG29 v 2592 file 800-1-D443, part 1, LAC.
37 H.M. Jones to Moore, 1 February 1954, RG29 v 2592 file 800-1-D443, part 1, LAC.
38 Moore to Col. Jones, 12 July 1954, RG29 v 2592 file 800-1-D443, part 1, LAC.
39 Blackfoot Band Council Resolution, 21 September 1954, RG29 v 2592 file 800-1-D443, part 1, LAC.
40 Falconer to Moore, 28 October 1954; E.A. Gardner, Chief Architect, to Moore, 29 March 1955; G. Borthwick to Moore, 30 March 1955, RG29 v 2592 file 800-1-D443, part 1, LAC.
41 J.R. Wild to R.F. Battle, 21 June 1956, RG29 v 2592 file 800-1-D443, part 1, LAC.
42 Moore to Wild, 6 September 1956; Moore to Falconer, 8 February 1957; Battle to Falconer, 14 March 1957; Falconer to Moore, 19 March 1957; Moore to Jones, 8 August 1957, RG29 v 2592 file 800-1-D443, part 1, LAC.
43 Jones to Moore, 6 May 1958, RG29 v 2592 file 800-1-D443, part 1, LAC.
44 Moore, "Memorandum of Meeting with Blackfoot Delegation," 22 May 1958; J.C.L. Bouchard to IHS, 16 October 1958, "Blackfoot Indian Hospital – Occupancy and Staff," December 1957, RG29 v 2592 file 800-1-D443, part 1, LAC.
45 Author interview with Roy Little Chief, 8 August 2010, Siksika, Alberta.

46 B. Griffiths, "Poverty Threatens Blackfoot Tribe," *Calgary Herald*, 5 December 1958, 1, 6.
47 A few examples: "Eskimo Boy Flown Here to Save Injured Eye" (1949); "Plane Carries Sick Woman 1,590 Miles" (1961); "Eskimo Flown 1,800 Miles to Hospital in Edmonton" (1960), quoted in Donna Dryden, Elva Taylor, Rona Beer, Ron Bergman, and Margaret Cogill, *The Camsell Mosaic: The Charles Camsell Hospital, 1945–1985* (Edmonton: Charles Camsell History Committee, 1985), 154–7.
48 As a training centre for medical bureaucrats, in the previous ten years the hospital had produced three regional superintendents, two assistant regional superintendents, seven zone-hospital superintendents, three assistant zone superintendents, three directors of nursing, and a senior administrative officer at head office. "Notes on the Proposed New Charles Camsell Hospital," 23 November 1961, RG29, v 2798, file 831-1-D479, part 8, LAC.
49 Dryden et al., *Camsell Mosaic*, 68. The camaraderie was maintained through staff reunions, and by 1985 former staff formed the Camsell Hospital History Committee and published their highly nostalgic and celebratory history, *The Camsell Mosaic*.
50 RG29 v 2620, file 800-2-D479 part 1, LAC.
51 The other members of "Project Group 12" that compiled the recommendations included four physicians and two laymen. McCreary to Glassco, 31 January 1962, RG29, v 2798, file 831-1-D479, part 8, LAC.
52 *Royal Commission on Government Organization, Report*, vol. 3, Report 15, "Health Services" (Ottawa: Queen's Printer, 1962), 196, 201–2.
53 "Notes on the Proposed New Charles Camsell Hospital," 23 November 1961, RG29, v 2798, file 831-1-D479, part 8, LAC.
54 Moore to Fortier, 15 December 1961, RG29, v 2798, file 831-1-D479, part 8, LAC.
55 "Notes on the Proposed New Charles Camsell Hospital," 23 November 1961, RG29, v 2798, file 831-1-D479, part 8, LAC.
56 Moore to Fortier, 15 December 1961, RG29, v 2798, file 831-1-D479, part 8, LAC.
57 Cabinet meeting, 27 December 1963, RG2, Privy Council Office, series A-5-a, v 6254, LAC.
58 Dryden et al., *Camsell Mosaic*, 49.
59 "Transcript CFRN News Report, 29 December 1977," RG29, v 2595, file 800-1-D479 part 8(c), LAC.
60 "Official Opening Ceremonies of the Charles Camsell Hospital, Edmonton, 10 October 1967," RG29, v 2593, file 800-1-D479, part 2, LAC. Though the minister did not attend, deputy minister Dr John Crawford read his remarks.

61 Not all hospitals were to close, however. In 1965 Cabinet decided to rebuild the Peguis reserve's Fisher River Indian Hospital, where Moore got his start in IHS. It would be rebuilt at Hodgson, Manitoba, on the southern edge of the reserve and intended to serve the non-Aboriginal community as well. In 1964 Moore had approached the chief and Council with the proposal; they agreed to provide the reserve lands and also agreed that it would be named the Percy E. Moore Hospital. It finally opened in 1973. Benita E. Cohen, "The Development of Health Services in Peguis First Nation: A Descriptive Case Study" (MSc thesis, University of Manitoba, 1994), 89, 95.

62 J. Donovan Ross to R.G. Armstrong, Bassano Municipal Hospital, 16 June 1961; Ross to Mr Caldwell, Cardston Municipal Hospital, 17 July 1961, RG 29, v 2936, file 851-1-X400, part 1, LAC.

63 "Memorandum," 27 September 1961, RG 29, v 2936, file 851-1-X400, part 1, LAC. (original emphasis).

64 Aleck Ostry, "The Foundations of National Public Hospital Insurance," in *Making Medicare: New Perspectives on the History of Medicare in Canada*, ed. Gregory Marchildon (Toronto: University of Toronto Press, 2012), 34.

65 J.D. Wallace to P.E. Moore, 8 June 1961, RG 29, v 2936, file 851-1-x400, part 1, LAC.

66 The four communities – Samson Cree Nation, Ermineskin Cree Nation, Louis Bull First Nation, and Montana First Nation – comprise what was once known as the Hobbema Indian Agency. A crossroads more than a community in the 1950s, Hobbema is located approximately 90 kilometres south of Edmonton.

67 "Memorandum," 27 September 1961, RG 29, v 2936, file 851-1-X400, part 1, LAC.

68 Press release, Wetaskiwin General Hospital, 19 December 1961, RG 29 v 3378, file 800-1-D426, LAC.

69 Stone to Director, 20 April 1950, NA RG29 v 2796, file 831-1-D426, part 1, LAC.

70 Stone to Director, 11 February 1949, NA RG29 v 2796, file 831-1-D426, part 1, LAC.

71 E.L. Stone to Superintendent, Hobbema Indian Agency, 14 February 1951. Stone retired from IHS later that year and bureaucrats pushed to have the hospital named for him, but he declined the honour. Stone to Director, 30 July 1951, RG 29 v 3378, file 800-1-D426, LAC.

72 Alberta's hospital insurance, established in 1950, was a municipally administered and financed plan with provincial subsidies that provided less than 40 per cent of hospital income; Indian reserves were not considered municipalities. Taylor, *Health Insurance and Canadian Public Policy*, 170.

73 T.J. Orford, Zone Superintendent, Alberta, to W.L. Falconer, 3 July 1956; Orford to Kirkby, 6 July 1956, RG 29 v 3378, file 800-1-D426, LAC.
74 Orford to Regional Superintendent, 18 September 1956, RG 29 v 3378, file 800-1-D426, LAC.
75 Davies to Regional Superintendent, 22 January 1962; Davies to Regional Superintendent, 27 April 1962, RG 29 v 3378, file 800-1-D426, LAC.
76 Clippings from *Wetaskiwin Times* and Ponoka's *Western Weekly Supplement*, Falconer to J.D. Campbell, Hospitals Division, Edmonton, 22 August 1962, RG 29 v 3378, file 800-1-D426, LAC.
77 J.W. Monteith, Minister, to Harry Moore, 28 August 1962, RG 29 v 3378, file 800-1-D426, LAC.
78 Matas to Regional Superintendent, 11 March 1963; meeting held in the Office of the Provincial Minister of Health, 1 April 1963, RG 29 v 3378, file 800-1-D426, LAC.
79 Meeting held in the Office of the Provincial Minister of Health, 1 April 1963, RG 29 v 3378, file 800-1-D426, LAC.
80 "General Information 1 January 1963 to 30 June 1963," RG 29 v 3378, file 800-1-D426, LAC.
81 Moore to Deputy Minister, 22 March 1963, Charles Camsell Hospital records, 1991.0443, box 13, Provincial Archives of Alberta (PAA).
82 Quoted in Taylor, *Health Insurance and Canadian Public Policy*, 339.
83 Ibid., 340.
84 Saskatchewan's medical care insurance plan was funded through premiums and through increases in income tax, corporate tax, and retail sales tax. Taylor, *Health Insurance and Canadian Public Policy*, 288.
85 Moore to Deputy Minister, 22 March 1963, Charles Camsell Hospital records, 1991.0443, box 13, PAA.
86 Byron King Plant, "The Politics of Indian Administration: A Revisionist History of Intrastate Relations in Mid-Century British Columbia" (PhD diss., University of Saskatchewan, 2009), 83–4, 90.
87 George Manuel and Michael Posluns, *The Fourth World: An Indian Reality* (New York: Free Press, 1974), 106.
88 "Health Services to Indians," *Alberta Medical Bulletin* 33, no. 3 (August 1968): 107.
89 The popular term "medicare," originally a shortened form for The Medical Care Act (1966), since became conflated with The Hospital Insurance and Diagnostic Services Act (1957) to become "Medicare," though the two were not fused until the Canada Health Act (1984). Gregory Marchildon, "Canadian Medicare: Why History Matters," in Marchildon, *Making Medicare*, 5.

90 The Medical Care Act (1966) was implemented in July 1968 with British Columbia and Saskatchewan immediately qualifying; five more provinces including Alberta joined in 1969, and all other provinces enrolled by 1971.
91 Cam Traynor, "Manning against Medicare," *Alberta History* 43 (Winter 1995): 10, 11.
92 Taylor, *Health Insurance and Canadian Public Policy*, 376.
93 Rhoda Vold, secretary Asker ALCW to DIA, 8 October 1966, RG29 v 3378, file 800-1-D426, LAC.
94 Branch Policy Development Group, Minutes of Meeting, 21 August 1969, RG29, v 2936, file 851-1-X400 part 3 (a), LAC.
95 The province's payment per patient per day (per diem rate) was $40, but the Hospital Commission paid the principle and interest on capital debt (for the hospital's expansion) and then deducted those charges from the per diem rate, reducing it to just $17, RG29, v 2936, file 851-1-X400 part 3(a), LAC.
96 J.D. Henderson, Minister of Health, to R.B. Wardle, Wetaskiwin Hospital, 5 February 1970, RG29, v 2936, file 851-1-X400 part 3(a), LAC.
97 John Munro to Chief Threefingers, 14 May 1971, RG29, v 2936, file 851-1-X400 part 3(a), LAC.
98 O.J. Rath to Director, 16 March 1961, RG29 v 2936, file 851-1X400 part 1; HA Proctor, Gleichen Hospital, 10 August 1965, RG29, v 2936, file 851-1-X400, part 2(b), LAC.
99 W.B. Brittain to Director, 17 February 1961, RG29 v 2936, file 851-1X400 part 1, LAC.
100 Sally Weaver, *Making Canadian Indian Policy: The Hidden Agenda, 1968–70* (Toronto: University of Toronto Press, 1981), 25.
101 For example, see Moore to Rath, 21 March 1956; Wiebe to Wong, 17 December 1969; Munro to Coueslan, 10 February 1971, RG 29, v 3390, file 811–2-Broadview Union Hospital.
102 O.J. Rath to Director, 16 March 1961, RG 29, v 2936, file 851-1-x400, part 1, LAC.
103 Regional Director, memorandum, "Amendments to the Medical Services Program," 26 February 1968, RG29, v 2936, file 851-1-X400, part 2(b), LAC.
104 Rath to Director General, 29 April 1968, RG29, v 2936, file 851-1-x400 part 2(b), LAC.
105 "Health Services for Indians," 26 April 1968, RG29, v 2936, file 851-1-x400 part 2(b), LAC.
106 As Weaver makes clear, Trudeau's ideological opposition to "special status" or collective rights was formulated in response to Quebec nationalism. *Making Indian Policy*, 54–5.

107 "Health Plans Rile Indians: Services Linked to Need," *Calgary Herald*, 27 April 1968, 1.
108 Ross to Hon. Allan MacEachen, 14 March 1968, RG29, v 2936, file 851-1-x400 part 2(b), LAC.
109 Munro to Robert Thompson, MP, 31 October 1968, RG29, v 2936, file 851-1-x400 part 2(b), LAC.
110 Harold Cardinal to All Chiefs and Band Councils, 13 June 1969, RG29, v 2936, file 851-1-X400, part 3(a), LAC.
111 Munro to Cardinal, 6 May 1969, RG29, v 2936, file 851-1-X400, part 3(a), LAC.
112 H.B. Hawthorn, *A Survey of the Contemporary Indians of Canada: Economic, Political, Educational Needs and Policies*, 2 vols. (Ottawa: Queen's Printer, 1966–7), as quoted in Weaver, *Making Canadian Indian Policy*, 21.
113 Indian Chiefs of Alberta, *Citizens Plus*, 195. http://ejournals.library.ualberta.ca/index.php/aps/article/view/11690 (accessed 6 October 2013). The treaty right to care will be examined in greater detail in the next chapter.
114 Other counter-proposals to the White Paper included Union of British Columbia Chiefs' *A Declaration of Indian Rights* (1970); Manitoba Indian Brotherhood's *Wahbung: Our Tomorrows* (1971); Association of Iroquois and Allied Indians' *Position Paper* (1971). Weaver, *Making Indian Policy*, 188–9.
115 Indian Association of Alberta, "To Whom It May Concern," 22 July 1969, RG29, v 2936, file 851-1-X400, part 3(a), LAC.
116 "Minutes of a meeting to discuss Federal/Provincial responsibility for Hospital Services to Treaty Indians," 13 December 1972, RG29, v 2936, file 851-1-X400, part 4, LAC.
117 General Meeting of the Blood Hospital Committee, 15 February 1973, RG29, v 2936, file 851-1-X400, part 4, LAC.
118 Webb, Assistant Deputy Minister, to Rath, Regional Director, 8 November 1972, RG29, v 2609, file 800-1-X431, LAC.
119 See various letters, RG29, v 2609, file 800-1-X431, LAC.
120 O.J. Rath, Regional Director, to Acting Assistant Deputy Minister, 10 November 1972, RG 29, v 2936, file 851-1-X400, part 3, LAC.
121 T. Brown to J. Thorpe, 9 May 1974, RG29, v 3378 file 800-1-D443, part 2, LAC; "Hospital Soon to Be Retired after 70 Years of Service," *Windspeaker*, 1 January 1999. The heritage designation states: "The building's only decorative details are a stylized pediment above the main façade and a decorative raised brick panel and date stone over the main entrance. The designation is confined to the footprint of the building." http://www.historicplaces.ca/en/rep-reg/place-lieu.aspx?id=9737 (accessed 8 October 2013).
122 Director to L.M. Black, 11 October 1978, RG29, v 2595, file 800-1-D429 part 10, LAC.

123 Memo, Rawson, Deputy Minister to the Minister, 14 September 1972, RG29, v 1604 – Charles Camsell Hospital Role Study, LAC.
124 "Report on the Future of Charles Camsell Hospital," 21 November 1975, RG29, v 3379, file 800-1-D479, LAC.
125 Memo, Rawson, Deputy Minister to the Minister, 14 September 1972, RG29, v 1604 – Charles Camsell Hospital Role Study; "Submission to the Policy Review Committee," 15 May 1976. In the fiscal year 1975–6 the operating expenses were $8.4 million and revenue $4.4 million. RG29, v 3379, file 800-1-D479, LAC.
126 Rawson to Sam Raddi, Committee for the Original Peoples Entitlement; Eric Tagoona, Inuit Tapirisat; George Erasmus, Indian Brotherhood of NWT; Joe Dion, Indian Association Alberta, 7 November 1978, RG29, v 2595, file 800-1-D479, part 8(c), LAC; Miniely to Monique Bégin and Hugh Faulkner, 14 November 1978, RG29, v 2595, file 800-1-D479, part 10, LAC.
127 News release, "New Indian Health Program Unveiled," June 1980, RG29, v 3379, file 800-1-D479, LAC.
128 It had been used as a location for B-movies; reputed to be haunted, it attracts the occasional intrepid ghost hunter. "Derelict Hospital a Project Going Nowhere," *Edmonton Journal*, 29 May, 2010, 8 November 2012, http://blogs.edmontonjournal.com/tag/camsell-hospital/ (accessed 25 September 2013).
129 Roy Romanow, *Building on Values: The Future of Health Care in Canada* (Final Report on the Royal Commission on the Future of Health Care in Canada, 2002), xvi, http://publications.gc.ca/site/eng/237274/publication.html.
130 Hospital Committee Meeting, 14 February 1973, RG29, v 2936, file 851-1-X400, part 4, LAC.

Chapter Six

1 Arthur J. Ray, Jim Miller, and Frank Tough, *Bounty and Benevolence: A History of Saskatchewan Treaties* (Montreal: McGill-Queen's University Press, 2000), 214.
2 See ibid.
3 Peter Erasmus, *Buffalo Days and Nights* (Calgary: Fifth House, 1999), 253; Alexander Morris, *The Treaties of Canada with the Indians of Manitoba and the North-West Territories* (1880; reprint Saskatoon: Fifth House, 1991), 185, 214–15.
4 Morris, *Treaties of Canada*, 355.
5 James Waldram, D. Ann Herring, and T. Kue Young, *Aboriginal Health in Canada*, 2nd ed. (Toronto: University of Toronto Press, 2006), 176–7; Yvonne Boyer, *Aboriginal Health: A Constitutional Rights Analysis* (Ottawa: National Aboriginal Health Organization and Native Law Centre, University of Saskatchewan, 2003), 20.

6 *Dreaver v The King* (1935), 20, copy in RG22 v 844, file 6-29-1 (3), LAC.
7 North Battleford, established in 1905 by the Canadian Northern Railway, left Battleford, the former Territorial capital, isolated on the south side of the North Saskatchewan River; the two towns are referred to collectively as "The Battlefords."
8 P.W. Head, *Annual Report*, 22 January 1945, RG29 v 2591, file 800-1-D353, part 1, LAC; there were approximately 2,500 people in the Battleford Agency, 700 in the Onion Lake Agency, and 1,000 in the Carlton Agency.
9 There were twenty-nine patients in the sanatorium. Memorandum for the Deputy Minister, 15 February 1945, RG29, v 2591, file 800-1-D353, part 1, LAC. Opened in 1930, the provincial Prince Albert Sanatorium admitted fifty-six Aboriginal patients by 1939, half of them schoolchildren. Aboriginal admissions reflected the declining need for sanatorium beds by the white population. Saskatchewan Lung Association Files, A638, file IX.73a, Saskatchewan Archives Board (SAB).
10 O.J. Rath, Regional Superintendent to Zone Superintendent, 12 December 1956, RG29, v 2591, file 800-1-D353, part 1, LAC.
11 "Ailing Chief Swimmer Reflects on Changes His People Had Known," *Saskatoon Star Phoenix,* 28 April 1953.
12 Corrigan to Director, 23 February 1956, RG29, v 2591, file 800-1-D353 part 1, LAC.
13 Petition to Indian Health Service, 8 March 1962, RG29, v 2591, file 800-1-D353, part 1, LAC.
14 Orford to Director, 15 March 1962, RG29, v 2591, file 800-1-D353 part 1, LAC.
15 Orford to Director, 18 April 1962, RG29, v 2591, file 800-1-D353 part 1, LAC.
16 Moore to Orford, 4 May 1962, RG29, v 2591, file 800-1-D353 part 1, LAC.
17 A.H. Fry to Regional Superintendent, 17 April 1962, RG29, v 2591, file 800-1-D353 part 1, LAC.
18 Orford to Director, 16 July 1964, RG29, v 2916, file 851-1-A67 part 3(a), LAC.
19 Ed Melynchuk, "Observations while Acting Administrator North Battleford Indian Hospital, June to August 1965," RG29, v 2591, file 800-1-D353 part 1, LAC.
20 Proctor to Regional Supervisor, 12 May 1965, RG29, v 2591, file 800-1-D353 part 1, LAC; Orford was medical superintendent at the hospital in 1957 when an infant died through neglect and understaffing (see chapter 3).
21 Sidney Fineday to Proctor, 21 July 1965, RG29, v 2591, file 800-1-D353 part 1, LAC.
22 Orford to Director, 9 August 1965, RG29, v 2591, file 800-1-D353 part 1, LAC; within two years, only Aboriginal representatives sat on the Advisory Board.

23 Orford to Director, 24 August 1965, RG29, v 2591, file 800-1-D353 part 1, LAC.
24 "Board Charges Medical Bias against Indians," *Toronto Telegram*, 19 August 1965, RG 29, v 2591, file 800-1-D353, part 2, LAC.
25 Proctor, Director, to Orford, 18 October 1965, RG29, v 2591, file 800-1-D353, part 2, LAC; Percy Moore retired in 1965, replaced as director by his long-serving assistant Dr H.A. Proctor.
26 Proctor to Deputy Minister, 21 October 1965, RG29, v 2591, file 800-1-D353, part 2, LAC.
27 "Report of the Meeting of the Lay Advisory Board, 27 November 1966," RG29, v 2591, file 800-1-D353, part 2, LAC.
28 Webb to Zone Director, 17 February 1967, RG29, v 2591, file 800-1-D353, part 2, LAC.
29 In 1962 all the North Battleford Indian Hospital's Aboriginal employees were served with "Loss of Benefit" notices, a form letter informing them that they were considered to have sufficient private resources to pay insurance premiums and they would no longer receive medical care through IHS. RG29, v 2916, file 851-1-A67, part 3(a), LAC.
30 Director to J. Williams, 10 March 1965, RG29, v 2591, file 800-1-D353 part 1, LAC.
31 Favel to G.D.W. Cameron, 9 March 1965; Cameron to Favel, 18 March 1965, RG29, v 2916, file 851-1-A67, part 3(a), LAC.
32 *Regina v Walter Johnston*, J.M. Policha, JHC, 12 May 1965, copy in RG29, v 2916, file 851-1-A67, part 3(a), LAC.
33 Proctor to Orford, 14 May 1965, RG29, v 2916, file 851-1-A67, part 3(a), LAC.
34 Orford to Proctor, 14 May 1965, RG29, v 2916, file 851-1-A67, part 3(a), LAC.
35 Cameron to Minister, 18 May 1965, RG29, v 2916, file 851-1-A67, part 3(a), LAC.
36 La Marsh to Nicholson, 19 May 1965, RG29, v 2916, file 851-1-A67, part 3(a), LAC.
37 Battle to Deputy Minister, 21 May 1965, RG22, v 844, file 6–29–1 (3) LAC.
38 Orford to Director, 25 May 1965; Orford to Zone Superintendents, 17 May 1965, RG29, v 2916, file 851-1-A67, part 3(a), LAC.
39 Steuart to Nicholson, 25 May 1965, RG29, v 2916, file 851-1-A67, part 3(a), LAC.
40 R.E. Williams to Assistant Deputy Minister, Indian Affairs, 7 October 1965, RG22, v 844, file 6–29–1 (3), LAC.
41 R.F. Battle, Assistant Deputy Minister (Indian Affairs), to Deputy Minister, 21 May 1965, RG22, v 844, file 6–29–1 (3), LAC.
42 First elected in 1935 as the Liberal member for Gravelbourg in the Saskatchewan legislature and a failed contender for the party leadership in

1945, Culliton was appointed to the Court of Appeal in 1951 and became Chief Justice in 1962. "Culliton, Edward Milton," *Encyclopedia of Saskatchewan*, http://esask.uregina.ca/entry/culliton_edward_milton_1906-91.html (accessed 10 February 2012).

43 Alexander Morris, *The Treaties of Canada with the Indians of Manitoba and the North-West Territories* (1880; reprint Saskatoon: Fifth House, 1991).

44 Ibid., 184, 214–15.

45 Diamond Jenness, *The Indians of Canada*, 7th ed. (1932 reprint; Toronto: University of Toronto Press, 1977); the seventh edition has been reprinted nine times, most recently in 2003.

46 Ibid., 264.

47 Heidi Bohaker and Franca Iacovetta, "Making Aboriginal People 'Immigrants Too': A Comparison of Citizenship Programs for Newcomers and Indigenous Peoples in Postwar Canada, 1940s–1960s," *Canadian Historical Review* 90, no. 3 (September 2009): 427–61.

48 Peter Alan Barkwell, "The Medicine Chest Clause in Treaty No. 6," *Canadian Native Law Reporter* 4 (1981): 16–17.

49 "Memorandum for Prairie Region," 1 April 1969, RG29, v 2591, file 800-1-D353, part 2, LAC; actually called the Federation of Saskatchewan Indians, established in 1940s.

50 M.P.D. Waldron to Director, 20 May 1970, RG29, v 2591, file 800-1-D353, part 3, LAC.

51 Lay Advisory Board Meeting, 30 April 1970, RG29, v 2591, file 800-1-D353, part 3, LAC.

52 See Harold Cardinal, *The Unjust Society: The Tragedy of Canada's Indians* (Edmonton: Hurtig, 1969); J.R. Miller, *Skyscrapers Hide the Heavens: A History of Indian-White Relations in Canada*, rev. ed. (Toronto: University of Toronto Press, 1989), 231. A formal retraction of the White Paper did not come until March 1971. Sally Weaver, *Making Canadian Indian Policy: The Hidden Agenda, 1968–70* (Toronto: University of Toronto Press, 1981), 187.

53 Quoted in ibid., 185.

54 R.J. Mulligan, "Memorandum," 15 June 1970, RG29, v 2591, file 800-1-D353, part 3, LAC.

55 Special Joint Meeting, 5 January 1971, RG29, v 2591, file 800-1-D353, part 3, LAC.

56 F.H. Hicks, Memorandum, 16 June 1971, RG29, v 2591, file 800-1-D353, part 3, LAC.

57 Ibid.

58 C.A. Bentley to Ken Butler, 19 May 1977, RG29, v 2592, file 800-1-D353, part 5, LAC.

59 Minutes of the Lay Advisory Board Meeting, 30 July 1971, RG29, v 2591, file 800-1-D353, part 3, LAC.
60 *Saskatchewan Indian* 3, no. 3 (1972): 5.
61 Assistant Deputy Minister to Dr M. LeClair, Deputy Minister, National Health, n.d., (November 1971), RG29, v 2591, file 800-1-D353, part 3, LAC.
62 Transcript of tape recorded meeting, 22 November 1971, RG29, v 2591, file 800-1-D353, part 3, LAC.
63 Quoted in Peter Alan Barkwell, "The Medicine Chest Clause in Treaty No. 6," *Canadian Native Law Reporter* 4 (1981): 18.
64 Following the ruling in *Johnston*, the Manitoba Queen's Bench Court ruled in 1969 in *The Manitoba Hospital Commission v Klein and Spence* that Mrs Spence, a Treaty Indian from Peguis, could not claim a right to free hospital care under the "medicine chest" clause. W.M. Weekes, Director, Legal Services, to M.L. Webb, 13 March 1973, RG22, v 1207, file 851-1-X300, LAC.
65 "Chief David Ahenakew," in *Saskatchewan Indian*, August 1972; Director, Legal Services, to Webb, 13 March 1973, RG29, v 2934, file 851-1-X300, part 2, LAC.
66 Transcript of tape recorded meeting, 22 November 1971; "Background Information for the Meeting," 22 November 1971, RG29, v 2591, file 800-1-D353, part 3, LAC.
67 Advisory Board Meeting, 6 December 1971, RG29, v 2591, file 800-1-D353, part 3, LAC.
68 Advisory Board Meeting, 8 February 1972, RG29, v 2728, file 811-2, part 2, LAC.
69 Webb to Le Clair, 23 February 1972, RG29, v 2728, file 811-2, part 2, LAC.
70 W.M. Weekes to M.L. Webb, "Legal Interpretation of Medicine Chest Clause in Treaty 6," 13 March 1973, RG22, v 1207, file 851-1-X300, LAC.
71 Lalonde to Joseph Weenie, 31 July 1973, RG29 v 3378, file 800-1-D443, part 2, LAC.
72 Memorandum, Brian Brett, 24 November 1976, RG29, v 2592, file 800-1-D353, part 4, LAC.
73 The North Battleford District Chiefs, "Proposal for a Study Regarding the Closure of the Indian Hospital in North Battleford, Saskatchewan," RG29, v 2592, file 800-1-D353, part 4, LAC.
74 Rawson to Pooyak, 9 December 1976, RG29, v 2592, file 800-1-D353, part 4, LAC.
75 North Battleford District Chiefs, "Hospital Services for Indians in the North Battleford District," March 1977, RG29, v 2592, file 800-1-D353, part 5, LAC.
76 The nine reserves were Thunderchild, Little Pine, Onion Lake, Moosomin, Mosquito, Saulteaux, Red Pheasant, Poundmaker, and Sweetgrass.

77 North Battleford District Chiefs, "Hospital Services for Indians in the North Battleford District," March 1977, 11, RG29, v 2592, file 800-1-D353, part 5, LAC.
78 Lyle Black, Director to Dr K. Butler, 6 May 1977, RG29, v. 2592, file 800-1-D353, part 5, LAC.
79 "Report of the Task Force on the Provision of Health Services to Indians in North Battleford, 30 June 1977," p. 10, RG29, v 2592, file 800-1-D353, part 5, LAC.
80 "Report of the Task Force in the Provision of Health Services to Indians in North Battleford, 30 June 1977," p. 1, RG29, v. 2592, file 800-1-D353, part 5, LAC.
81 "Comparison Noting the Differences between the Original Task Force Report on North Battleford and the Report Presented to the Department by Dr Laroche," p. 3, RG29, v 2592, file 800-1-D353, part 6, LAC. Emphasis added.
82 Ibid.
83 "Comparison Noting the Differences between the Original Task Force Report on North Battleford and the Report Presented to the Department by Dr Laroche," p. 1, RG29, v 2592, file 800-1-D353, part 6, LAC.
84 Laroche, "Memorandum for Mr. Bruce Rawson," 30 June 1977, RG29, v 2592, file 800-1-D353, part 5, LAC.
85 Rawson to the minister, 19 July 1977, RG29, v 2592, file 800-1-D353, part 6, LAC.
86 Lalonde to Steuart, 17 August 1977; Laroche to Lalonde, 9 September 1977, RG29, v 2592, file 800-1-D353, part 6, LAC.
87 Lalonde to Ahenakew, 14 September 1977, RG29, v 2592, file 800-1-D353, part 6, LAC.
88 Rawson to Caron, 27 July 1977, RG29, v 2592, file 800-1-D353, part 6, LAC.
89 Lalonde to Steuart, 17 August 1977, RG29, v 2592, file 800-1-D353, part 6, LAC.
90 Clarkson to Lalonde, 6 August 1977, RG29, v 2592, file 800-1-D353, part 6, LAC.
91 Graham Clarkson, "A Functional Health Plan for the Indians in the North Battleford Area," December 1977, 1; Clarkson to Black, 8 October 1977, RG29, v 2592, file 800-1-D353, part 6, LAC.
92 Clarkson, "A Functional Health Plan," 39.
93 Ibid., 13.
94 Ibid., 16.
95 Ibid., 24.
96 Dr M.K. Sas to Bégin, 17 Mar 1978; E.H. Baergen to Bégin, 28 March 1978; Dr C.M. Furniss to Bégin, 4 April 1978, RG29, v 2917, file 851-1-A671, part 6, LAC.

97 Clarkson to Murphy, 10 April 1978, RG29, v 2917, file 851-1-A671, part 6, LAC.

98 Black, "Visit to North Battleford 1–3 February 1978," RG29, v 2917, file 851-1-A671, part 6, LAC.

99 "Openings for Physicians in North Battleford, Sask," *Canadian Medical Association Journal* 120 (3 February 1979): 270–1.

100 Battlefords Indian Health Centre Inc., *30 Years Later: July 1979–July 2009*, commemorative booklet.

101 Noel Starblanket, "The Dawn of a New Era," quoted in Hon. Thomas Berger, *Report of Advisory Commission on Indian and Inuit Health Consultation* (Ottawa, February 1980), Appendix 4.

102 T. Kue Young, *Health Care and Cultural Change: The Indian Experience in the Central Subarctic* (Toronto: University of Toronto Press, 1988), 93; Anne Gilmore, "Indian Health Care: What the Dispute Is All About," *Canadian Medical Association Journal* 121 (7 July 1979): 87–94.

103 Starblanket, "The Dawn of a New Era," quoted in Berger, *Report of Advisory Commission on Indian and Inuit Health Consultation.*

104 Battlefords Indian Health Centre Inc., *30 Years Later: July 1979–July 2009*, commemorative booklet (emphasis added).

105 Berger, *Report of Advisory Commission*, 17.

106 "Indian Health Care: A Treaty Right," Indian Association of Alberta, January 1979, 16, RG29 v 2959, file 851-3-Indian Association Alberta, part 2, LAC.

107 Health and Welfare Policy Paper, quoted in Berger, *Report of Advisory Commission*, 17.

108 "Indian Health Policy," quoted in Berger, *Report of Advisory Commission*, Appendix 2.

109 Edward T. Jackson, "A Working Inventory of Community-Based Initiatives in the Health Field Being Undertaken by the Indians and Inuit Peoples," in Berger, *Report of Advisory Commission*, Appendix 6.

110 Young, *Health Care and Cultural Change*, 125.

111 World Health Organization, *Alma Ata: Primary Health Care* (Geneva: World Health Organization, 1978), 16.

112 Rawson to the minister, 19 July 1977, RG29, v 2592, file 800-1-D353, part 6, LAC.

113 *Wuskwi Sipihk Cree Nation v Canada (Minister of National Health and Welfare), Canadian Native Law Reporter* 4 (1999): 293.

114 Constance MacIntosh, "Envisioning the Future of Aboriginal Health under the Health Transfer Process," *Health Law Journal* (Special Edition 2008): 86, http://papers.ssrn.com/sol3/papers.cfm?abstract_id=2101674 (accessed 10 February 2014).

Conclusion

1 Quoted in Sally Weaver, *Making Canadian Indian Policy: The Hidden Agenda, 1968–70* (Toronto: University of Toronto Press, 1981), 185.

2 This status might also be explained by the fact that though Medicare has its historians, we await its history. Gregory Marchildon suggests that the lack of a general history stems from the value-laden and policy-heavy nature of Medicare. Marchildon, *Making Medicare: New Perspectives on the History of Medicare in Canada* (Toronto: University of Toronto Press, 2012). Gerald W. Boychuk's comparative view argues that public health insurance in Canada fostered national unity and has come to be seen as a right of citizenship. Boychuk, *National Health Insurance in the United States and Canada: Race, Territory and the Roots of Difference* (Washington: Georgetown University Press, 2008), 142–3. Two studies stress a progressive view of Medicare as seemingly inevitable: Malcolm Taylor, *Health Insurance and Canadian Public Policy: The Seven Decisions That Created the Canadian Health Insurance System and Their Outcomes*, 2nd ed. (Montreal and Kingston: McGill-Queen's University Press, 1987), and C. Stuart Houston and Merle Massie, *36 Steps on the Road to Medicare: How Saskatchewan Led the Way* (Montreal and Kingston: McGill-Queen's University Press, 2013). In a larger work on the history of social policy Alvin Finkel devotes a chapter to the compromises that resulted in Medicare in *Social Policy and Practice in Canada: A History* (Waterloo, ON: Wilfrid Laurier University Press, 2006).

3 That national satisfaction swells not least in comparison with American health care, though the program only covers about 60 per cent of health care costs. Roy Romanow, *Building on Values: The Future of Health Care in Canada: Final Report on the Royal Commission on the Future of Health Care in Canada* (2002), xvi, 34, http://publications.gc.ca/site/eng/237274/publication.html.

4 Juha Mikkonen and Dennis Raphael, *The Social Determinants of Health: The Canadian Facts* (Toronto: York University School of Health Policy and Management, 2010), http://www.thecanadianfacts.org/The_Canadian_Facts.pdf (accessed 8 February 2014).

5 "Government of Canada Indian Health Policy," in Hon. Thomas Berger, *Report of Advisory Commission on Indian and Inuit Health Consultation* (Ottawa, February 1980), Appendix 2.

6 T. Kue Young, *Health Care and Cultural Change: The Indian Experience in the Central Subarctic* (Toronto: University of Toronto Press, 1988), 110, 134. The Sioux Lookout Indian Hospital, built by the federal government in 1949, sat alongside the Sioux Lookout General Hospital.

7 Scott-McKay-Bain Health Panel, *From Here to There: Steps along the Way: Achieving Health for All in the Sioux Lookout Zone* (June 1989), http://www.slmhc.on.ca/assets/files/From_Here_to_There_-_Steps_Along_the_Way.pdf (accessed 1 December 2013).
8 Quoted in Dana Culhane Speck, "The Indian Health Transfer Policy: A Step in the Right Direction, or Revenge of the Hidden Agenda?" *Native Studies Review* 5, no. 1 (1989): 189.
9 Ibid., 206.
10 John D. O'Neil, "Aboriginal Health Policy for the Next Century," *The Path to Healing: Report of the National Round Table on Aboriginal Health and Social Issues*, Royal Commission on Aboriginal Peoples (Ottawa: Canada Communications Group, 1993), 43.
11 Culhane Speck, "The Indian Health Transfer Policy," 200. A decade later some trial transfers of non-insured health benefits began.
12 Kristen M. Jacklin and Wayne Warry, "The Indian Health Transfer Policy in Canada: Toward Self-Determination or Cost Containment?" in Arachu Castro and Merrill Singer, eds, *Unhealthy Health Policy: A Critical Anthropological Examination* (Walnut Creek, CA: Alta Mira Press, 2004), 230.
13 Alma Favel-King, "The Treaty Right to Health," *The Path to Healing: Report of the National Round Table on Aboriginal Health and Social Issues*, Royal Commission on Aboriginal Peoples (Ottawa: Canada Communications Group, 1993), 123, 128.
14 The Battlefords Tribal Council (representing Mosquito, Little Pine, Sweetgrass, and Lucky Man First Nations) signed a transfer agreement in 1993. "Battlefords Tribal Council Signs Historic Health Service Agreement," *Saskatchewan Indian* 22, no. 6 (July 1993): 2.
15 By 2008 more than 80 per cent of 599 eligible First Nations communities had entered into some form of transfer agreement, though only three Alberta communities participated because of concerns that it would affect claimed treaty rights to health services. Constance MacIntosh, "Envisioning the Future of Aboriginal Health under the Health Transfer Process," *Health Law Journal* (Special Edition 2008): 73, http://papers.ssrn.com/sol3/papers.cfm?abstract_id=2101674 (accessed 10 February 2014).
16 Scott-McKay-Bain Health Panel, *From Here to There.*
17 "Meno Ya Win" is an Anishinaabe term that connotes health, wellness, well-being, and individual spiritual, mental, emotional, and physical wholeness (http://www.slmhc.on.ca/history) (accessed 3 December 2013).

Bibliography

PRIMARY SOURCES

Archival Collections

- Archives of Manitoba
  Records of the Sanatorium Board of Manitoba
- Archives of Ontario
  Public Health Nursing, Record Group 10–30
- British Columbia Archives
  Tuberculosis Control Division GR 129
- Glenbow Alberta Archives
  Gooderham Family Papers
  Dr H.W. McGill Papers
- Library and Archives Canada
  Department of Indian Affairs, Record Group 10
  Department of National Health and Welfare, Record Group 29
  Canadian Tuberculosis Association, MG28 I75
- Prince Rupert City and Regional Archives
  Wrathall Collection
- Public Archives of Alberta
  Charles Camsell Hospital
  Central Alberta (Baker) Sanatorium
- St Albert Museum and Archives
  St Albert Cemeteries
- Saskatchewan Archives Board
  Saskatchewan Lung Association Files, A638

Oral Interviews

- Gordon Albert, North Battleford, Saskatchewan
- Grace Anderson, Winnipeg, Manitoba
- Rose Atimoyoo, North Battleford, Saskatchewan
- Agnes Cyr, Echo Lodge, Fort Qu'Appelle, Saskatchewan
- Andrew and Rosabel (Ryder) Gordon, Pasqua First Nation
- Roy Little Chief, Strathmore, Alberta
- Frank Malloway Sr, Chilliwack, British Columbia
- Hazel McArthur (née Wolf), Stoughton, Saskatchewan
- Dave Melting Tallow, Siksika, Alberta

Newspapers

- Aboriginal Multi-Media Society *Windspeaker*
- *Calgary Herald*
- *Edmonton Journal*
- *Ottawa Citizen*
- *Prince Rupert Evening Empire*
- *Saskatchewan Indian*
- *Saskatoon Star Phoenix*
- *Toronto Globe and Mail*
- *Winnipeg Free Press*
- *Winnipeg Tribune*

Published Primary Documents

Baergen, E.H. "Openings for Physicians in North Battleford, Sask." *Canadian Medical Association Journal* 120 (3 February 1979): 270–1.

Battlefords Indian Health Centre Inc. *30 Years Later: July 1979–July 2009*. Commemorative booklet.

Beecher, H.K. "Ethics and Clinical Research." *New England Journal of Medicine* 274 (1966): 1354–60.

Berger, Hon. Thomas. *Report of Advisory Commission on Indian and Inuit Health Consultation*. Ottawa, February 1980.

Bryce, P.H. *Report on the Indian Schools of Manitoba and the North-West Territories*. Ottawa: Government Printing Bureau, 1907.

– *The Story of a National Crime: Being an Appeal for Justice to the Indians of Canada*. Ottawa: James Hope and Sons, 1922.

Calgary: The Denver of Canada. Calgary: Calgary Herald Print, 1895.

Canada. *Building on Values: The Future of Health Care in Canada: Final Report on the Royal Commission on the Future of Health Care in Canada* (2002).

– House of Commons. *Sessional Papers.*

– House of Commons. Special Joint Committee of the Senate and the House of Commons Appointed to Examine and Consider the Indian Act. *Minutes of Proceedings and Evidence No. 3.*

– Public Health Agency of Canada, "BCG Vaccine use in Canada – Current and Historical." http://www.phac-aspc.gc.ca/tbpc-latb/bcgvac_1206-eng.php. Accessed 16 April 2013.

– Royal Commission on Government Organization. *Report* vol. 3, Report 15 "Health Services." Ottawa: Queen's Printer, 1962.

– Royal Commission on Aboriginal Peoples 1996. http://www.collectionscanada.gc.ca/webarchives/20071115053257/http://www.ainc-inac.gc.ca/ch/rcap/sg/sgmm_e.html. Accessed 24 May 2013.

– Truth and Reconciliation Commission. http://www.trc.ca/websites/trcinstitution/index.php?p=3. Accessed 16 May 2013.

Camsell, Charles. *Son of the North.* Toronto: Ryerson, 1954.

Cardinal, Harold. *The Unjust Society: The Tragedy of Canada's Indians.* Edmonton: Hurtig, 1969.

Dent, John. "New Deal for Indians Is Planned by MP." *Saturday Night*, 30 March 1946.

Edwards, Allan M., and Gordon C. Gray. "Observations on Juvenile Hypothyroidism in Native Races of Northern Canada." *Canadian Medical Association Journal* 84 (20 May 1961): 1116–24.

Erasmus, Peter. *Buffalo Days and Nights.* Calgary: Fifth House, 1999.

"Ervin Lockwood Stone" *Canadian Medical Association Journal* 98 (2 March 1968): 473.

Ferguson, R.G. *Tuberculosis among the Indians of the Great Canadian Plains.* Reprint. London: Adlard and Son, 1928.

Ferguson, R.G., and A.B. Simes. "BCG Vaccination of Indian Infants in Saskatchewan" *Tubercle* 30, no. 1 (1949): 5–11.

Freeman, Minnie Aodla. *Life among the Qallunaat.* Edmonton: Hurtig, 1978.

Gilmore, Anne. "Indian Health Care: What the Dispute Is All About." *Canadian Medical Association Journal* 121 (7 July 1979): 87–94.

Government of Northwest Territories. Department of Health. *Medical Patient Search Project Summary: Final Report.* April 1991.

Grzybowski, Stefan, and Zygmunt Dunaj. "Tuberculin Survey of the Population of Manitoulin Island." *Canadian Medical Association Journal* 81 (1 September 1959): 366–8.

"Health Services to Indians." *Alberta Medical Bulletin* 33, no. 3 (August 1968): 107–8.

Hiltz, J.E. "Compulsory Treatment of Tuberculosis." *Canadian Medical Association Journal* 71 (December 1954): 569–71.

"Hospitals Developed for Canadian Indians." *New York Times*, 7 January 1940.

"House of Commons Discusses Estimates for Indian Affairs Branch." *Bulletin of the Canadian Tuberculosis Association* 15, no. 4 (1937): 3–4.

Indian Chiefs of Alberta, *Citizens Plus*. http://ejournals.library.ualberta.ca/index.php/aps/article/view/11690. Accessed 6 October 2013.

Jenness, Diamond. *The Indians of Canada*, 7th ed. 1932. Reprint. Toronto: University of Toronto Press, 1977.

– *The Sarcee Indians of Alberta*. Bulletin no. 90. Ottawa: National Museum of Canada, 1938.

"List of Canadian Hospitals Approved for Advanced Graduate Training by the Royal College of Physicians and Surgeons." *Canadian Medical Association Journal* 78 (April 1958): 520.

Lymer, John Robert, and Arthur James Anderson. "An Evaluation of Several Orally Administered Para-aminosalicylic Acid Preparations." *Canadian Pharmaceutical Journal* (September 1957): 160–2.

Matas, M. "Tuberculosis Programs of the Medical Services, Department of National Health and Welfare." In "Proceedings of the Third National Tuberculosis Conference," *Medical Services Journal Canada* 22 (1966): 878–83.

Meltzer, H. "Results of Thoracoplasty." *Journal of Thoracic Surgery* (St Louis) 11, no. 1 (October 1941): 84–94.

Moore, P.E. "No Longer Captain: A History of Tuberculosis and Its Control amongst Canadian Indians." *Canadian Medical Association Journal* 84 (May 1961): 1012–16.

Moore, P.E., H.D. Kruse, F.F. Tisdall, and R.S.C. Corrigan. "Medical Survey of Nutrition among the Northern Manitoba Indians." *Canadian Medical Association Journal* 54 (March 1946): 223–33.

Morris, Alexander. *The Treaties of Canada with the Indians of Manitoba and the North-West Territories*. 1880. Reprint. Saskatoon: Fifth House, 1991.

Ross, E.L., and A.L. Paine. "A Tuberculosis Survey of Manitoba Indians." *Canadian Medical Association Journal* 4 (August 1939): 180–4.

Scott-McKay-Bain Health Panel. *From Here to There: Steps along the Way: Achieving Health for All in the Sioux Lookout Zone* (June 1989). http://www.slmhc.on.ca/assets/files/From_Here_to_There_-_Steps_Along_the_Way.pdf. Accessed 1 December 2013.

Stanley, G.D. "Early Days at the Muskoka San." *Calgary Historical Bulletin* 18 (May 1953): 17–20.

Stone, E.L. "Canadian Indian Medical Services." *Canadian Medical Association Journal* (July 1935): 82–5.

Wherrett, G.J. "Arctic Survey 1: Survey of Health Conditions and Medical and Hospital Services in the North West Territories." *Canadian Journal of Economics and Political Science* 11, no. 1 (1945): 48–60.

– "Tuberculosis in Canada." *Royal Commission on Health Services*. Ottawa: Queen's Printer, 1965.

World Health Organization. *Alma Ata: Primary Health Care*. Geneva: World Health Organization, 1978.

Film

The Longer Trail. Directed by Fergus McDonell. 30 min. National Film Board, 1956.

Lost Songs. Directed by Clint Alberta. 24 min. 04 sec. National Film Board, 1999.

No Longer Vanishing. Directed by Grant McLean. 27 min. 31 sec. National Film Board, 1955.

SECONDARY SOURCES

Aboriginal Nurses Association of Canada. *Twice as Good: A History of Aboriginal Nurses*. Ottawa: Aboriginal Nurses Association of Canada, 2007.

Anderson, Warwick. *The Cultivation of Whiteness: Science, Health and Racial Destiny in Australia*. New York: Basic Books, 2003.

Arnold, David. "Medicine and Colonialism." In *Companion Encyclopedia of the History of Medicine*, vol. 2, edited by W.F. Bynum and Roy Porter, 1393–416. London: Routledge, 1993.

– ed. *Imperial Medicine and Indigenous Societies*. Manchester: Manchester University Press, 1988.

Backhouse, Constance. *Colour-Coded: A Legal History of Racism in Canada, 1900–1950*. Toronto: University of Toronto Press, 1999.

Barkwell, Peter Alan. "The Medicine Chest Clause in Treaty No. 6." *Canadian Native Law Reporter* 4 (1981): 1–23.

Bashford, Alison, and Carolyn Strange. "Cultures of Confinement." In *Isolation: Places and Practices of Exclusion*, edited by Carolyn Strange and Alison Bashford. London: Routledge, 2003.

– "Isolation and Exclusion in the Modern World." In *Isolation: Places and Practices of Exclusion*, edited by Carolyn Strange and Alison Bashford. London: Routledge, 2003.

Bates, Barbara. *Bargaining for Life: A Social History of Tuberculosis, 1876–1938*. Philadelphia: University of Pennsylvania Press, 1992.

Bohaker, Heidi, and Franca Iacovetta. "Making Aboriginal People 'Immigrants Too': A Comparison of Citizenship Programs for Newcomers and

Indigenous Peoples in Postwar Canada, 1940s–1960s." *Canadian Historical Review* 90, no. 3 (2009): 427–61.

Boychuk, Gerald W. *National Health Insurance in the United States and Canada: Race, Territory and the Roots of Difference*. Washington, DC: Georgetown University Press, 2008.

Boyer, Yvonne. *Aboriginal Health: A Constitutional Rights Analysis*. Ottawa: National Aboriginal Health Organization and Native Law Centre, University of Saskatchewan, 2003.

Brownlie, Robin, and Mary-Ellen Kelm. "Desperately Seeking Absolution: Native Agency as Colonialist Alibi?" *Canadian Historical Review* 75, no. 4 (1994): 543–56.

Bryden, P.E. "The Liberal Party and the Achievement of National Medicare." *Canadian Bulletin of Medical History* 26, no. 2 (2009): 315–32.

Bryder, Linda. *Below the Magic Mountain*. Oxford: Clarendon Press, 1988.

Carter, Sarah. *Aboriginal People and Colonizers of Western Canada*. Toronto: University of Toronto Press, 1999.

Coates, Ken. *Best Left as Indians: Native-White Relations in the Yukon Territory, 1840–1973*. Montreal and Kingston: McGill-Queen's University Press, 1991.

Coates, K.S., and W.R. Morrison. *The Alaska Highway in World War II: The U.S. Army of Occupation in Canada's Northwest*. Toronto: University of Toronto Press, 1992.

Connolly, Cynthia. *Saving Sickly Children: The Tuberculosis Preventorium in American Life, 1909–1970*. New Brunswick, NJ: Rutgers University Press, 2008.

Cortiula, Mark. "Social Class and Health Care in a Community Institution: The Case of Hamilton City Hospital." *Canadian Bulletin of Medical History* 6 (1989): 133–45.

Crey, Ernie, and Suzanne Fournier. *Stolen from Our Embrace. The Abduction of First Nations Children and the Restoration of Aboriginal Communities*. Vancouver: Douglas and McIntyre, 1998.

Culhane Speck, Dana. "The Indian Health Transfer Policy: A Step in the Right Direction, or Revenge of the Hidden Agenda?" *Native Studies Review* 5, no. 1 (1989): 187–213.

"Culliton, Edward Milton." *Encyclopedia of Saskatchewan*. http://esask.uregina.ca/entry/culliton_edward_milton_1906-91.html. Accessed 10 February 2012.

Curtis, Bruce. *The Politics of Population: State Formation, Statistics, and the Census of Canada, 1840–1875*. Toronto: University of Toronto Press, 2001.

Dexter, Grant. *Dr. Charles Camsell*. Winnipeg: Winnipeg Free Press, 1958.

Dryden, Donna, Elva Taylor, Rona Beer, Ron Bergman, Margaret Cogill. *The Camsell Mosaic: The Charles Camsell Hospital, 1945–1985*. Edmonton: Charles Camsell History Committee, 1985.

Dubos, Rene, and Jean Dubos. *The White Plague: Tuberculosis, Man and Society.* Boston: Little, Brown, 1952.

Dyck, Noel. *What Is the Indian "Problem": Tutelage and Resistance in Canadian Indian Administration.* St John's, NL: Institute of Social and Economic Research, 1991.

Ernst, Waltraud. "Beyond East and West. From the History of Colonial Medicine to a Social History of Medicine(s) in South Asia." *Social History of Medicine* 20 (December 2007): 505–24.

Fairchild, Amy, and Gerald Oppenheimer. "Public Health Nihilism vs Pragmatism: History, Politics and the Control of Tuberculosis." *American Journal of Public Health* 88, no. 7 (1998): 1105–17.

Favel-King, Alma. "The Treaty Right to Health." *The Path to Healing: Report of the National Round Table on Aboriginal Health and Social Issues.* Royal Commission on Aboriginal Peoples. Ottawa: Canada Communications Group, 1993.

Feldberg, Georgina. *Disease and Class: Tuberculosis and the Shaping of Modern North American Society.* New Brunswick, NJ: Rutgers University Press, 1995.

Finkel, Alvin. *Our Lives: Canada after 1945.* Toronto: James Lorimer, 1997.

– "Paradise Postponed: A Re-examination of the Green Book Proposals of 1945." *Journal of the Canadian Historical Association* 4, no. 1 (1993): 120–42.

– *Social Policy and Practice in Canada: A History.* Waterloo, ON: Wilfrid Laurier University Press, 2006.

Finzsch, Norbert, and Robert Jütte, eds. *Institutions of Confinement: Hospitals, Asylums, and Prisons in Western Europe and North America, 1500–1950.* Cambridge: Cambridge University Press, 1996.

Foucault, Michel. *Discipline and Punish: The Birth of the Prison.* Trans. A. Sheridan. 2nd ed. New York: Vintage, 1995.

– *Madness and Civilization: A History of Insanity in the Age of Reason.* New York: Vintage, 1984.

Gagan, David, and Rosemary Gagan. *For Patients of Moderate Means: A Social History of the Voluntary Public General Hospital in Canada, 1890–1950.* Montreal and Kingston: McGill-Queen's University Press, 2002.

Goodman, Jordan, Anthony McElligott, and Lara Marks, eds. *Useful Bodies: Humans in the Service of Medical Science in the Twentieth Century.* Baltimore: Johns Hopkins University Press, 2003.

Grant, Shelagh D. *Sovereignty or Security? Government Policy in the Canadian North, 1936–1950.* Vancouver: UBC Press, 1988.

Gray, Charlotte. "Profile: Percy Moore." *Canadian Medical Association Journal* 126 (15 February 1982): 416.

Granshaw, Lindsay. "The Hospital." In *Companion Encyclopaedia of the History of Medicine*, vol. 2, edited by W.F. Bynam and Roy Porter, 1180–203. London: Routledge, 1993.

Grygier, Pat Sandiford. *A Long Way from Home: The Tuberculosis Epidemic among the Inuit.* Montreal and Kingston: McGill-Queen's University Press, 1994.

Hacker, Carlotta. *The Indomitable Lady Doctors.* Toronto: Clarke, Irwin, 1974.

Hanks, Lucien, and Jane Richardson Hanks. *Tribe under Trust: A Study of the Blackfoot Reserve of Alberta.* Toronto: University of Toronto Press 1950.

Hanson, Ann Meekitjuk. "Finding Hope and Healing in Memories of Our Past." *Above and Beyond: Canada's Arctic Journal*, March/April 2012. http://issuu.com/arctic_journal/docs/above_and_beyond_march_april_2012. Accessed 28 May 2013.

Houston, C. Stuart. *R.G. Ferguson: Crusader against Tuberculosis.* Toronto: Dundurn Press, 1991.

Houston, C. Stuart, and Merle Massie. *36 Steps on the Road to Medicare: How Saskatchewan Led the Way.* Montreal and Kingston: McGill-Queen's University Press, 2013.

Ilyniak, Natalia. "Mercury Poisoning in Grassy Narrows: Environmental Injustice, Colonialism, and Capitalist Expansion in Canada." *McGill Sociological Review* 4 (February 2014): 43–66.

Jacklin, Kristen M., and Wayne Warry. "The Indian Health Transfer Policy in Canada: Toward Self-Determination or Cost Containment?" In *Unhealthy Health Policy: A Critical Anthropological Examination*, edited by Arachu Castro and Merrill Singer. Walnut Creek, CA: Alta Mira Press, 2004.

Johnson, Ryan, and Amna Khalid, eds. *Public Health in the British Empire: Intermediaries, Subordinates, and the Practice of Public Health, 1850–1960.* New York: Routledge, 2012.

Johnston, William D. "Tuberculosis." In *The Cambridge World History of Human Diseases*, edited by Kenneth Kiple, 1059–68. Cambridge: Cambridge University Press, 1993.

Jones, Colin, and Roy Porter, eds. *Reassessing Foucault: Power, Medicine and the Body.* London: Routledge, 1994.

Jones, David S. *Rationalizing Epidemics: Meaning and Uses of American Indian Mortality since 1600.* Cambridge: Harvard University Press, 2004.

Kelm, Mary-Ellen. *Colonizing Bodies: Aboriginal Health and Healing in British Columbia, 1900–1950.* Vancouver: University of British Columbia Press, 1998.

– "Diagnosing the Discursive Indian: Medicine, Gender, and the 'Dying Race.'" *Ethnohistory* 52, no. 2 (2005): 371–406.

Lerat, Harold, with Linda Ungar. *Treaty Promises Indian Reality: Life on a Reserve.* Saskatoon: Purich, 2005.

Lux, Maureen. *Medicine That Walks: Disease, Medicine and Canadian Plains Native People, 1880–1940.* Toronto: University of Toronto Press, 2001.

– "Perfect Subjects: Race, Tuberculosis and the Qu'Appelle BCG Vaccine Trial." *Canadian Bulletin of Medical History* 15 (1998): 277–96.

MacIntosh, Constance. "Envisioning the Future of Aboriginal Health under the Health Transfer Process." *Health Law Journal* (Special Edition 2008): 67–100. http://papers.ssrn.com/sol3/papers.cfm?abstract_id=2101674. Accessed 10 February 2014.

MacLeod, Roy, and Milton Lewis, eds. *Disease, Medicine, and Empire*. London: Routledge, 1988.

Manuel, George, and Michael Posluns. *The Fourth World: An Indian Reality*. New York: Free Press, 1974.

Marchildon, Gregory. "Canadian Medicare: Why History Matters." In *Making Medicare: New Perspectives on the History of Medicare in Canada*, edited by Gregory Marchildon. Toronto: University of Toronto Press, 2012.

Marks, Shula. *Divided Sisterhood: Race, Class and Gender in the South African Nursing Profession*. Johannesburg: University of Witwatersand University Press, 1994.

Mawani, Renisa. "Legal Geographies of Aboriginal Segregation in British Columbia." In *Isolation: Places and Practices of Exclusion*, edited by Carolyn Strange and Alison Bashford. London: Routledge, 2003.

McCuaig, Katherine. *The Weariness, the Fever, and the Fret: The Campaign against Tuberculosis in Canada, 1900–1950*. Montreal and Kingston: McGill-Queen's University Press, 1999.

McKay, Ian. "Canada as a Long Liberal Revolution." In *Debating the Canadian Liberal Revolution*, edited by Jean-François Constant and Michel Ducharme. Toronto: University of Toronto Press, 2009.

– "The Liberal Order Framework: A Prospectus for a Reconnaissance of Canadian History." *Canadian Historical Review* 81, no. 4 (December 2000): 625.

McKeown, Thomas. *The Modern Rise of Population*. London: Edward Arnold, 1976.

McPherson, Kathryn. *Bedside Matters: The Transformation of Canadian Nursing, 1900–1990*. Toronto: Oxford University Press, 1996.

– "Nursing and Colonization: The Work of Indian Health Service Nurses in Manitoba." In *Women, Health and Nation: Canada and the United States since 1945*, edited by Georgina Feldberg, Molly Ladd Taylor, Allison Li, and Kathryn McPherson. Montreal and Kingston: McGill-Queen's University Press, 2003.

Mehta, Uday S. "Liberal Strategies of Exclusion." In *Tensions of Empire: Colonial Cultures in a Bourgeois World*, edited by Frederick Cooper and Ann Laura Stoler. Berkeley: University of California Press, 1997.

Meijer Drees, Laurie. *Healing Histories: Stories from Canada's Indian Hospitals*. Edmonton: University of Alberta Press, 2013.

– "Indian Hospitals and Aboriginal Nurses: Canada and Alaska." *Canadian Bulletin of Medical History* 27, no. 1 (2010): 139–61.
– "The Nanaimo and Charles Camsell Indian Hospitals: First Nations' Narratives of Health Care, 1945 to 1965." *Histoire Sociale/Social History* 43, no. 85 (2010): 165–91.
– "Training Aboriginal Nurses: The Indian Health Services in Northwestern Canada, 1939–75." In *Caregiving on the Periphery: Historical Perspectives on Nursing and Midwifery in Canada*, edited by Myra Rutherdale. Montreal and Kingston: McGill-Queen's University Press, 2010.
Menzies, Robert, and Ted Palys. "Turbulent Spirits: Aboriginal Patients in the British Columbia Psychiatric System, 1879–1950." In *Mental Health and Canadian Society: Historical Perspectives*, edited by James E. Moran and David Wright. Montreal and Kingston: McGill-Queen's University Press, 2006.
Miller, J.R. *Shingwauk's Vision: A History of Native Residential Schools.* Toronto: University of Toronto Press, 1996.
– *Skyscrapers Hide the Heavens: A History of Indian-White Relations in Canada.* Rev ed. Toronto: University of Toronto Press, 1989.
Mikkonen, Juha, and Dennis Raphael. *The Social Determinants of Health: The Canadian Facts.* Toronto: York University School of Health Policy and Management, 2010. http://www.thecanadianfacts.org/The_Canadian_Facts.pdf. Accessed 8 February 2014.
Milloy, John. *A National Crime: The Canadian Government and the Residential School System, 1879–1986.* Winnipeg: University of Manitoba Press, 1999.
Mosby, Ian. "Administering Colonial Science: Nutrition Research and Human Biomedical Experimentation in Aboriginal Communities and Residential Schools, 1942–1952." *Histoire Sociale/Social History* 46, no. 91 (May 2013): 145–72.
Narian, Raj. "Need for a BCG Trial in Canada's Native Populations." *Canadian Medical Association Journal* 127 (15 July 1982): 101–2.
Northington Gamble, Vanessa. *Making a Place for Ourselves: The Black Hospital Movement, 1920–1945.* New York: Oxford University Press, 1995.
Noton, Bruce. "Northern Manitoba Treaty Party, 1949." *Manitoba History* 39 (Spring/Summer 2000). http://www.mhs.mb.ca/docs/mb_history/39/treatyparty1949.shtml. Accessed 12 April 2013.
Olofsson, Ebba, et al. "Negotiating Identities: Inuit Tuberculosis Evacuees in the 1940s–1950s." *Études/Inuit/ Studies* 32, no. 2 (2008): 127–49.
O'Neil, John D. "Aboriginal Health Policy for the Next Century." *The Path to Healing: Report of the National Round Table on Aboriginal Health and Social Issues.* Royal Commission on Aboriginal Peoples. Ottawa: Canada Communications Group, 1993.

Ostry, Aleck. "The Foundations of National Public Hospital Insurance." In *Making Medicare: New Perspectives on the History of Medicare in Canada*, edited by Gregory Marchildon. Toronto: University of Toronto Press, 2012.

Ott, Katherine. *Fevered Lives: Tuberculosis in American Culture since 1870*. Cambridge, MA: Harvard University Press, 1996.

Packard, Randall M. *White Plague, Black Labor: Tuberculosis and the Political Economy of Health and Disease in South Africa*. Berkeley: University of California Press, 1989.

Paine, A.L., and Earl Hershfield. "Tuberculosis: Past, Present and Future." *Canadian Family Physician* 25 (1979): 55–9.

Perry, Adele. *On the Edge of Empire: Gender, Race and the Making of British Columbia, 1849–1871*. Toronto: University of Toronto Press, 2001.

– "Women, Racialized People, and the Making of the Liberal Order in Northern North America." In *Debating the Canadian Liberal Revolution*, edited by Jean-François Constant and Michel Ducharme. Toronto: University of Toronto Press, 2009.

Ray, Arthur J., J.R. Miller, and Frank Tough. *Bounty and Benevolence: A History of Saskatchewan Treaties*. Montreal: McGill-Queen's University Press, 2000.

Rosenberg, Charles. *The Care of Strangers: The Rise of America's Hospital System*. New York: Basic Books, 1987.

Rosner, David. *A Once Charitable Enterprise: Hospitals and Health Care in Brooklyn and New York, 1885–1915*. New York: Cambridge University Press, 1982.

Rothman, Sheila. *Living in the Shadow of Death: Tuberculosis and the Social Experience of Illness in American History*. New York: Basic Books, 1994.

Rutherdale, Myra. "Nursing in the North and Writing for the South: The Work and Travels of Amy Wilson." In *Caregiving on the Periphery: Historical Perspectives on Nursing and Midwifery in Canada*, edited by Myra Rutherdale. Montreal and Kingston: McGill-Queen's University Press, 2010.

Shewell, Hugh. *Enough to Keep Them Alive: Indian Welfare in Canada, 1873–1965*. Toronto: University of Toronto Press, 2004.

Smith, Derek G. "The Emergence of 'Eskimo Status': An Examination of the Eskimo Disk List System and Its Social Consequences, 1925–1970." In *Anthropology, Public Policy, and Native Peoples in Canada*, edited by Noel Dyck and James Waldram. Montreal and Kingston: McGill-Queen's University Press, 1993.

Smith, F.B. *The Retreat of Tuberculosis, 1850–1950*. London: Croom Helm, 1988.

Staples, Annalisa, and Ruth McConnell. *Soapstone and Seed Beads: Arts and Craft at the Charles Camsell Hospital*. Edmonton: Jasper Printing, 1993.

Strange, Carolyn, and Alison Bashford. *Isolation: Places and Practices of Exclusion*. London: Routledge, 2003.

Stewart, David B. *Holy Ground: The Story of the Manitoba Sanatorium at Ninette.* Killarney, MB: J.A. Victor David Museum, 1999.

Suzuki, David. *The Autobiography.* Vancouver: Greystone Books, 2006.

Taylor, Malcolm. "The Canadian Health Care System: After Medicare." In *Health and Canadian Society: Sociological Perspectives*, edited by David Coburn, Carl D'Arcy, George Torrance, and Peter New. 2nd ed. Toronto: Fitzhenry and Whiteside, 1987.

– *Health Insurance and Canadian Public Policy: The Seven Decisions That Created the Canadian Health Insurance System and Their Outcomes*. 2nd ed. Kingston and Montreal: McGill-Queen's University Press, 1987.

Thorpe, E.L.M. *The Social Histories of Smallpox and Tuberculosis in Canada: Culture, Evolution and Disease.* Winnipeg: University of Manitoba Anthropology Papers No. 30, 1989.

Titley, Brian. *A Narrow Vision: Duncan Campbell Scott and the Administration of Indian Affairs in Canada.* Vancouver: University of British Columbia Press, 1986.

Tobias, John L. "Protection, Civilization, Assimilation: An Outline History of Canada's Indian Policy." *Western Canadian Journal of Anthropology* 6, no. 2 (1976): 13–30.

Traynor, Cam. "Manning against Medicare." *Alberta History* 43 (1995): 7–19.

Vaughan, Megan. *Curing Their Ills: Colonial Power and African Illness.* Palo Alto, CA: Stanford University Press, 1991.

Venne, Sharon Helen. *Indian Acts and Amendments 1868–1975: An Indexed Collection.* Saskatoon: Native Law Centre, University of Saskatchewan, 1981.

Waiser, W.A. "Camsell, Charles." In *Oxford Companion to Canadian History*, edited by Gerald Hallowell. Toronto: Oxford University Press, 2004.

Waldram, James, D. Ann Herring, and T. Kue Young. *Aboriginal Health in Canada: Historical, Cultural, and Epidemiological Perspectives.* 2nd ed. Toronto: University of Toronto Press, 2006.

Weaver, Sally. *Making Canadian Indian Policy: The Hidden Agenda, 1968–70.* Toronto: University of Toronto Press, 1981.

Wherrett, George Jasper. *The Miracle of the Empty Beds: A History of Tuberculosis in Canada.* Toronto: University of Toronto Press, 1977.

Wishart, James. "Class Difference and the Reformation of Ontario Public Hospitals, 1900–1935." *Labour/Le Travail* 48 (2001): 27–61.

Woods, David. "The Canadian Council on Hospital Accreditation in Canada." *Canadian Medical Association Journal* 110 (6 April 1974): 851–5.

Young, T. Kue. "A BCG Trial in Canada's Native Populations." *Canadian Medical Association Journal* 127 (December 1982): 1166–7.

– *Health Care and Cultural Change: The Indian Experience in the Central Subarctic.* Toronto: University of Toronto Press, 1988.

Zumla, Alimuddin, and Matthew Gundy. "Epilogue: Politics, Science, and the 'New' Tuberculosis." In *The Return of the White Plague: Global Poverty and the "New" Tuberculosis*, edited by Matthew Gundy and Alimuddin Zumla. London: Verso, 2003.

Theses and Dissertations

Churchill, Elizabeth. "Tsuu T'ina: A History of a First Nations Community, 1890-1940." PhD diss., University of Calgary, 2000.

Cohen, Benita E. "The Development of Health Services in Peguis First Nation: A Descriptive Case Study." MSc thesis, University of Manitoba, 1994.

Hader, Joanne. "The Effect of Tuberculosis on the Indians of Saskatchewan, 1926–1965." MA thesis, University of Saskatchewan, 1990.

McCallum, Mary Jane Logan. "Labour, Modernity and the Canadian State: A History of Aboriginal Women and Work in the Mid-Twentieth Century." PhD diss., University of Manitoba, 2008.

Paul, Pauline. "A History of the Edmonton General Hospital: 1895–1970." PhD diss., University of Alberta, 1994.

Plant, Byron King. "The Politics of Indian Administration: A Revisionist History of Intrastate Relations in Mid-Century British Columbia." PhD diss., University of Saskatchewan, 2009.

Weaver, Sally Mae. "Health, Culture and Dilemma: A Study of the Non-Conservative Iroquois, Six Nations Reserve, Ontario." PhD diss., University of Toronto, 1967.

Zdunich, Darlene. "Tuberculosis and World War One Veterans." MA thesis, University of Calgary, 1984.

Index